PHYSICAL ACTIVITY
AND MENTAL HEALTH

A PRACTICE-ORIENTED APPROACH

Michel Probst & **Attilio Carraro** (Eds)

Physical Activity
and
Mental Health

A Practice-Oriented Approach

edi·ermes

PHYSICAL ACTIVITY AND MENTAL HEALTH

A Practice-Oriented Approach

Edited by Michel Probst & Attilio Carraro

Copyright 2014 Edi.Ermes s.r.l., Milan (Italy)

ISBN 978-88-7051-386-8 - Paper edition

ISBN 978-88-7051-387-5 - Digital edition

A book is the final product of a very complex series of operations that requires numerous tests on texts and images. It is almost impossible to publish a book with no errors. We will be grateful to those who find them and notify us. For enquiries or suggestions about this volume, please use the following address:

External relations - Edi.Ermes srl - Viale Enrico Forlanini, 65 - 20134 Milan (Italy)
Voice +39.02.70.21.121 - Fax +39.02.70.21.12.83

The Publisher is available for intellectual property owners with whom it was not possible to communicate, as well as for any inadvertent omissions and inaccuracies in the quotation of sources or songs reproduced in this volume.

Individuals that appear in the photos in chapters 5, 6, 7, 8, 10, 11, 15 and 17 of this book were all students enrolled in courses at the Universities of Padua (Italy) and Leuven (Belgium).

Photos: Shutterstock© (cover, 115)

Paper edition printed in February 2014 by Prontostampa - Fara Gera d'Adda (BG)
for Edi.Ermes - viale Enrico Forlanini, 65 - 20134 Milan, Italy
http://www.ediermes.it - Tel. +39 02 7021121 - Fax +39 02 70211283

Preface

The phrase "a sound mind in a healthy body", or in the original Latin "*mens sana in corpore sano*", has been considered an ideal to strive for since antiquity, but often has not been adequately put into practice, particularly in the modern culture of the 21st century. When one Googles "physical exercise as therapy in mental health", one finds about 39 million hits. This outcome suggests that the public is well aware of the potential effect of exercise for improving mental health. In addition, if one checks the references on the U.S. National Library of Health (PubMed.gov) for the term "physical exercise in mental health", a major increase is clearly visible of between around 40 articles per year during the early 1990s to well beyond 300 in 2012. If one changes the term exercise into physical activity, a similar trend is observed.

This book uses a clear and coherent outline to summarize the development of physical activity and exercise as utilized within the management of persons with mental health disorders across different modalities, such as psychomotor, movement, and sport therapy. The book provides disorder-specific intervention guidelines, based on theoretical reasoning as well as research evidence and practical application.

As an organization interested in increasing the well-being and empowerment of persons with activity limitations and participation restrictions through the use of physical activity adaptations, we believe that this book opens a window to evidence-based practices that should be applied by Adapted Physical Activity professionals specializing in the psychiatric and mental health field. The International Federation of Adapted Physical Activity (IFAPA) would like to thank both the editors and the twenty-six contributing authors for their outstanding contribution to our field of study.

Yeshayahu "Shayke" Hutzler
Ph.D. Prof.
Wingate Institute, Israel
Zinman College for Physical Education and Sport Sciences
Past-President of IFAPA

Contributors

Contents

Section 2 - Physical activity and exercise in the approach of mental health problems

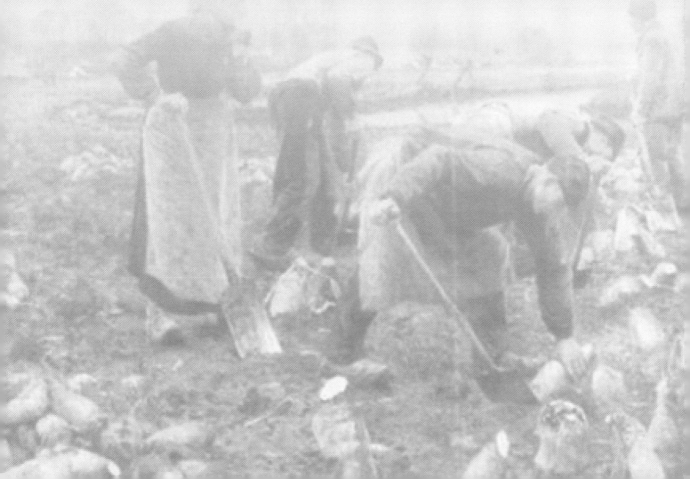

Section 1

The rationale
for **physical activity**
and **mental health**

Introduction: **why physical activity and mental health**

Michel Probst & Attilio Carraro

Modern scientific and non-scientific literature is paying a lot of attention to physical activity, exercise, movement, and sport-related activities for people with mental health problems.

Mental health is defined as a condition that permits the optimal psychological, intellectual, and emotional development of the individual (World Federation for Mental Health, WHO 1948); a mental health problem interferes with emotional and/or social abilities, but to a lesser extent than a mental illness. The care and cure for these persons is complex and requires specific competencies. The term "care" focuses on the present healthy possibilities of the subject to influence the psychological, social, and somatic functioning. The term "cure" is determined and systematic, addressing the dysfunctional part of the subject.

Exercise and body awareness within a psychosocial approach are important factors in rehabilitation programs in mental health.

A growing number of studies concern the obvious link beetween physical activity (in regard to mental health) and psychiatric rehabilitation (Faulkner & Biddle, 1999; Faulkner & Carless, 2006; Paluska & Schwenk, 2000; Penedo & Dann, 2005; Swarbrick, 2006). These efforts are being slowly integrated into clinical practice; however, many mental health professionals do not appear to view exercise as a worthwhile strategy. The discrepancy between theory and practice is an intriguing observation when faced with the knowledge that approximately one fourth of the population faces a mental dysfunction and seeing that physical exercises and the attention paid to the body are currently "hot topics" in our society.

Physical activity has been shown to enhance the effectiveness of psychological therapies and to have a role in improving the quality of life and symptom management for people with a wide range of mental health problems. Physical activity has a double benefit, since people with mental health problems are also at increased risk for a range of physical health problems, including cardiovascular disease, metabolic disorders, and obesity.

On one side, the use of physical activity as a health related or psycho-physiologic therapeutic approach is well described; on the other side, the use of physical activity in this manner is not known. The psychotherapeutic use of physical activity in psychiatric hospitals is well accepted in different countries under different names: "Psychomotor therapy" (Probst et al., 2011), "Bewegungstherapie" (Hölter, 2011), "Movement and dance therapy" (Vermeer, Bosscher, Broadhead, 1997), "Sport-therapie" (Deimel, 1983). These therapies are currently defined as methods of treatment that use physical activities as a lead in the approach and in which one tries – after having gone through an examination (observation or gruevaluation) in a

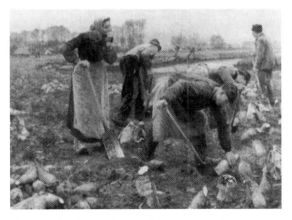

Figure 1.1 - Agriculture activity proposed in the psychiatric hospitals before of physical activity.

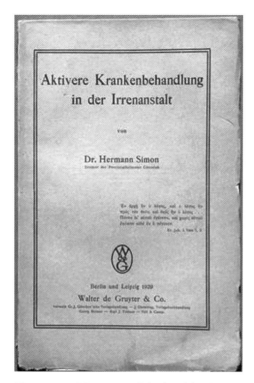

Figure 1.2 - The cover of the book by Simon.

methodical way and if possible in consultation with the patient – to realize clearly formulated goals that are relevant to the problems with which the patient needs help. All therapies integrates in their ap-

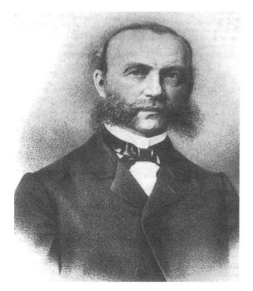

Figure 1.3 - A portrait of Wilhelm Griesinger (1817-1868).

proach and different extent some of psychotherapy elements. The physical activities considered act as complementary therapy or as a supplement to biomedical treatment and can be embedded in several psychotherapeutic approaches (behavior, cognitive, or psychodynamic therapy) for different diagnoses related to patient settings. It incorporates medical, psychological, pedagogic, kinesiological, and rehabilitative components.

Research in this field is progressing, and there is an increasing amount of clinical and scientific evidence. There are no real side effects and the rules of safety are transparent. The main idea behind this approach is the interaction between exercise and the mind. Through a wide variety of physical activities, everyday experiences and emotions are explored. Patients can discover that alternatives exist, which may trigger new emotions and experiences. The activities are not intrinsically therapeutic. The exercises are not goals in and of themselves, but are means by which to attain the desirable goals. The experiences during these activities and their subsequent responses function as dynamic powers of change. The sports hall functions as a laboratory for experimenting and learning how to deal with emotions. At the same time, the process of consciousness and verbalization can be stimulated.

1.1 A BRIEF HISTORY

Changes in the treatment of mentally ill persons occurred under the influence of Philippe Pinel (1745-1826), William Tuke (1745-1813), and Wilhelm Griesinger (1817-1868). The moral treatment approach, which included removing bondage and introducing daily rounds, was accepted and activities were propagated.

In Germany, the work of Griesinger influenced another German psychiatrist, Hermann Simon. With his book "Aktivere Krankenbehandlung in der Irrenanstalt" (Simon, 1929), he set a trend for a more active approache toward patients with mental illness. In contrast to the existing conception that patients with mental health illness should be locked up, these forms of therapy looked to address and activate the healthy part of the personality still present in each psychiatric patient.

In the USA, the American Journal of Insanity published in 1905 an article by S. I. Franz and G. V. Hamilton titled "The effects of exercise upon the retardation in conditions of depression."

Adolf Meyer also published a book where he underlined the positive effect of activities on health.

Thereafter, the application of movement activities for psychiatric patients has grown from the so-called active therapy (in some countries known as occupational therapy) in psychiatric hospitals. All kinds of activities have been recommended to fill daily schedules in the name of "active therapy."

The concepts laid forth by Simon were adopted by several Dutch, Belgian, and German psychiatrists, and after the Second World War, these ideas found growing traction in the psychiatric community. In the beginning, teachers in physical education developed a kind of movement therapy. The content existed in a therapeutic working method derived from physical education, dance, and sport for adults and later for children.

The institutions evolved to open psychiatric centers where more somatic treatment made room for an existential psychiatry. Philosophers such as Kierkegaard, Husserl, Heidegger, Merleau-Ponty, and Sartre had a notable influence on this new inversion. In psychiatry, the arsenal of therapies was adapted and movement therapists found acceptance in psychiatric institutions. Gradually the attention shifted from physical activity (mens sana in corpore sano) to how people move in relation to their environment and how they use physical activity in their tasks, activities, and responsibilities.

In summary, movement is devoted to addressing theoretical mediation and moderating factors ranging between cognitive, emotional, physical, social, and environmental influences on improving physical activity and health related complications.

1.2 THE ORGANIZATION OF THIS BOOK

This book collects the contributions of twenty-six authors, coming from thirteen Universities and clinic institutions in eight different countries. The book is formed by eighteen chapters, organized in three sections.

In the **first section**, titled *The rationale for physical activity and mental health*, Angela Favaro describes in chapter 2 the epidemiology and diagnostic criteria of psychiatric disorders as reported in the Diagnostic and Statistical Manual of Mental Disorders (DSM) and in the International

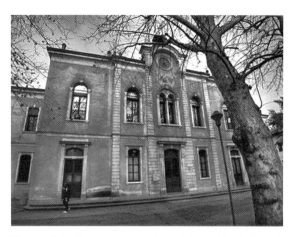

Figure 1.4 - The entrance of an old psychiatric hospital in Italy. Psychiatric hospital in the past were effectively "closed cities" within the community.

Classification of Diseases (ICD). In chapter 3 Simone Bolognesi, Arianna Goracci, and Andrea Fagiolini present the current state of research on the relationship between physical exercise and mental health, explaining the main psychological and neurobiological mechanisms involved in physical activity. In chapter 4 Antonio Fiorellini discusses the effects of psychopharmacological drugs on psychological, physical, and biological functions.

The **second section** is named *Physical activity and exercise in the approach of mental health problems*. This part of the book is comprised of twelve chapters focusing on several practice-oriented approaches to different mental health problems. In chapter 5 Markus Gerber and Uwe Pushe provide a comprehensive overview of the role of exercise in stress generation and regulation, underlining the protective role of exercise against the adverse health effects of stress. In chapter 6 Attilio Carraro suggests how to integrate exercise in alcohol dependence recovery. Davy Vancampfort, Jan Knapen, Ruud van Winkel, and Marc De Hert present in chapter 7 the rationale for physical activity in schizophrenia, in terms of physical and mental health benefits, and discuss the practical implications of physical activity interventions in this population group. In chapter 8 Katia E.L. Borges and Felipe A.S. Moura-Lima add to the theme of physical activity and schizophrenia, describing a movement-based community program oriented toward changing the lifestyles of schizophrenic people. Jan Knapen and Davy Vancampfort describe in

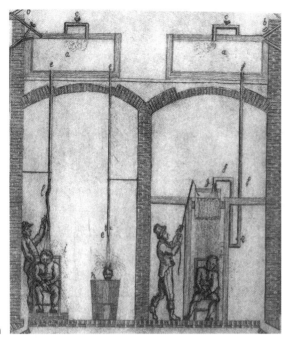

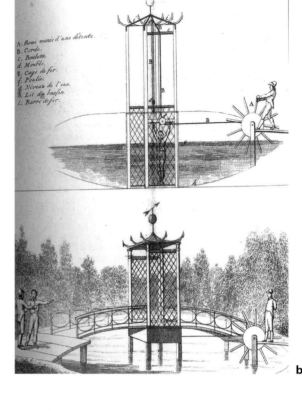

Figure 1.5 - Images of ancient invasive practices (like shocking methods), used to treat psychiatric disorders. **a**, warm or cold showers; **b**, walker falls unsuspecting in water.

chapter 9 an evidence-based approach for exercise in the treatment of depression and anxiety, offering recommendations for good clinical practice. In chapter 10 Michel Probst, Johana Monthuy-Blanc, and Milena Adamkova discuss the complex relationship between eating disorders and physical activity, and present a conceptual framework for body-oriented treatment of eating disorders. The discussion about eating disorders continues in chapter 11, where Johanna Monthuy-Blanc and Maud Bonanséa discuss the problem of eating disorders in athletes. Jannis Alexandridis in chapter 12 focuses on physical activity as a therapeutic treatment for obesity in clinical populations of obese adults. Two topics regarding children and adolescents are discussed; in chapter 13, where Marika Berchicci and Maurizio Bertollo point to the role of physical activity in the treatment of attention deficit hyperactivity disorder (ADHD), and in chapter 14 where Cristophe Maiano emphasizes the po-

tentialities of sport intervention for adolescents with conduct disorders. In chapter 15 Erica Gobbi, Ilaria Ferri, and Attilio Carraro review the literature on the role of physical activity for people with intellectual disabilities and describe several practical implementations for exercise-intervention in this population. In the last chapter of the second section Seppe Deckx discusses the place that psychomotor therapy and physical activity can have in the treatment of elderly with psychiatric disorders.

The **third section** of the book is devoted to the *Instruments*. In chapter 17 Attilio Carraro and Michel Probst present in a schematic way the reasons to adopt specific assessment tools in the field of physical activity and mental health and review several objective and subjective instruments. Finally, Ilaria Ferri and Amber DeHerdt report in chapter 18 on activities organized for people with mental disabilities by some Sport Federations and Organizations in Europe.

Epidemiology and **diagnostic criteria**
of psychiatric disorders

2

Angela Favaro

Mental disorders and psychiatric symptoms are highly prevalent in the general population. However, the definition of diagnosis and of the thresholds that delimit the presence of a psychiatric disorder is still a challenging issue. Classification is essential for research, but most importantly serves as a helpful guide to clinical practice and for faciliting communication among clinicians (APA, 1994). The revision process of DSM-5 is currently completed (American Psychiatric Association, 2013) and the change of many diagnostic criteria will follow the aim of reaching a deeper link between diagnosis and etiopathogenesis by one hand, and diagnosis and treatment planning/prognosis by the other.

In this chapter we will describe the DSM-IV diagnostic criteria of the main Axis I psychiatric disorders, report on the proposed revisions in DSM-5, and briefly illustrate data about the frequency of the disorder in the community. The DSM-5 revision of diagnostic criteria will follow some important guidelines in order to be more practical and clinically oriented. The multiaxial characteristic of DSM-IV (Axis I: Clinical Disorders; Axis II: Personality Disorders; Axis III: General Medical Conditions; Axis IV: Psychosocial and Environmental Problems; Axis V: Global Assessment of Functioning) will disappear to bring DSM-5 into greater harmony with the single-axis approach used by the World Health Organization's (WHO) International Classification of Diseases (ICD). In practice, the recommendation is to collapse the first three axes into one axis that contains all psychiatric and general medical diagnoses. In addition, particular attention will be given to the assessment of impairment and disability (Axis V) given by a specific mental illness (Kendler & First, 2010).

Experts working in the DSM-5 revision give a particular emphasis to the introduction of a cross-cutting *dimensional assessment*. Despite the predominance of a categorical approach, a dimensional approach is particularly interesting and fruitful in the study of, for example, personality characteristics (Kendler & First, 2010). A categorical approach is often recommended for a variety of reasons. In particular, it facilitates scientific communication and is more in tune with the medical tradition. However, the variation within diagnostic categories, the presence of symptoms that are characteristic of more than one category, and the influence of specific disorders on the clinical manifestations of other disorders are good reasons to consider the use of a dimensional approach in the study and clinical assessment of psychiatric disorders.

A spectrum approach appears to be a more suitable alternative for quantitative models that reflect the aetiology of multifactorial diseases such as psychiatric disturbances. Quantitative models more easily explain the effects of multiple genes and

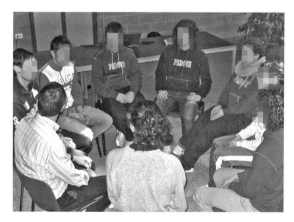

Figure 2.1 - Circle time discussion. Having the time to discuss feelings and emotions experienced during the activity is an essential component of psychomotor therapy.

multiple risk factors. However, spectrum models have important implications in the clinical field. They provide accurate diagnostic information to successfully individualize the treatment, as many psychiatric patients do not respond satisfactorily to standard treatments. To give an example, while the presence of specific traits, such as impulsive self-injurious behaviors in anorexia nervosa patients, does not necessarily indicate the presence of a full-syndrome personality disorder (Favaro et al., 2007), it often provides important information to the therapist to improve the patient's outcome and identify possible targets for treatment.

Finally, DSM-5 aims to give a specific interest to the assessment and definition of psychiatric disorders in children and adolescents.

2.1 SCHIZOPHRENIA AND OTHER PSYCHOTIC DISORDERS

Schizophrenia is the most studied and severe disorder in psychiatry. Usually, psychoses are considered those mental disorders in which impairment of mental function has developed to a degree that interferes grossly with insight, ability to meet ordinary demands of life, or to maintain adequate contact with reality. The symptoms that characterize psychoses are:
- delusions (a false belief that is held despite evidence to the contrary)
- hallucinations (a perception in the absence of a stimulus)
- disorganized speech and behavior (incoherence in thoughts, speech, or behavior)
- negative symptoms (apatia, alogia, avolition, affective flattening).

Symptoms of schizophrenia are not culture-bound and profiles of patients with schizophrenia look very similar in different cultures. Lifetime prevalence of schizophrenia is estimated around 1%, with some variations in incidence and prevalence in different populations. Onset of schizophrenia peaks in young adulthood with a difference between males and females (females peak about five years later, on average). There is large heterogeneity in onset, course and outcome of schizophrenia. Chronicity is very common (more than 60%) and a more benign course is associated with non-modern non-industrialised settings.

A poor prognosis is associated with extended prodromal symptoms or insidious onset, family history of schizophrenia, presence of neurological soft signs or cognitive impairment, and early onset.

The DSM-5 work group is recommending that schizophrenia subtypes not be included in DSM-5 and proposed the use of dimensions, instead.

Other types of psychotic disorders include: schizophreniform disorder (schizophrenia with less than 6 months of duration), schizoaffective disorder (schizophrenia with a coexistent mood disorder), delusional disorder (delusions involving situations that occur in real life, in the absence of schizophrenia and without impairment of functioning), brief psychotic disorder (acute psychotic symptoms present for less than one month) and attenuated psychotic symptoms syndrome (a new diagnosis proposed by DSM-5).

Textbox 2.1 shows the diagnostic criteria for schizophrenia (DSM-IV).

Schizophrenia: DSM-IV Diagnostic Criteria

Schizophrenia

A. *Characteristic symptoms*: Two (or more) of the following, each present for a significant portion of time during a 1-month period (or less if successfully treated):
 (1) delusions
 (2) hallucinations
 (3) disorganized speech (e.g. frequent derailment or incoherence)
 (4) grossly disorganized or catatonic behavior
 (5) negative symptoms, i.e. affective flattening, alogia, or avolition
B. *Social/occupational dysfunction*: For a significant portion of the time since the onset of the disturbance, one or more major areas of functioning such as work, interpersonal relations, or self-care are markedly below the level achieved prior to the onset (or when the onset is in childhood or adolescence, failure to achieve expected level of interpersonal, academic, or occupational achievement)
C. *Duration*: Continuous signs of the disturbance persist for at least 6 months

Schizophrenia Subtypes

The subtypes of Schizophrenia are defined by the predominant symptomatology at the time of evaluation.

Paranoid Type

A type of Schizophrenia in which preoccupation with one or more delusions or frequent auditory hallucinations are present.

Disorganized Type

A type of Schizophrenia in which disorganized speech, behavior, flat or inappropriate affect are predominant.

Catatonic Type

A type of Schizophrenia in which the clinical picture is dominated by motoric immobility as evidenced by catalepsy (including waxy flexibility), stupor, excessive motor activity (that is apparently purposeless and not influenced by external stimuli), extreme negativism or mutism, peculiarities of voluntary movement as evidenced by posturing (voluntary assumption of inappropriate or bizarre postures), stereotyped movements, prominent mannerisms, or prominent grimacing, echolalia or echopraxia.

Undifferentiated Type

A type of Schizophrenia in which symptoms that meet Criterion A are present, but the criteria are not met for the Paranoid, Disorganized, or Catatonic Type.

Residual Type

A type of Schizophrenia in which there is absence of prominent delusions, hallucinations, disorganized speech, and grossly disorganized or catatonic behavior and there is continuing evidence of the disturbance, as indicated by the presence of negative symptoms or two or more symptoms listed in Criterion A for Schizophrenia, present in an attenuated form.

Definitions of Mood episodes according to DSM-IV

1. Major Depressive Episode

A. Five (or more) of the following symptoms have been present during the same 2-week period and represent a change from previous functioning; at least one of the symptoms is either (1) depressed mood or (2) loss of interest or pleasure
  1. Depressed mood most of the day, nearly every day, as indicated by either subjective report (e.g. feels sad or empty) or observation made by others (e.g. appears tearful)
  2. Markedly diminished interest or pleasure in all, or almost all, activities most of the day, nearly every day (as indicated by either subjective account or observation made by others)
  3. Significant weight loss when not dieting or weight gain (e.g. a change of more than 5% of body weight in a month), or decrease or increase in appetite nearly every day
  4. Insomnia or hypersomnia nearly every day
  5. Psychomotor agitation or retardation nearly every day (observable by others, not merely subjective feelings of restlessness or being slowed down)
  6. Fatigue or loss of energy nearly every day
  7. Feelings of worthlessness or excessive or inappropriate guilt (which may be delusional) nearly every day (not merely self-reproach or guilt about being sick)
  8. Diminished ability to think or concentrate, or indecisiveness, nearly every day (either by subjective account or as observed by others)
  9. Recurrent thoughts of death (not just fear of dying), recurrent suicidal ideation without a specific plan, or a suicide attempt or a specific plan for committing suicide

2. Manic Episode

A. A distinct period of abnormally and persistently elevated, expansive, or irritable mood, lasting at least 1 week (or any duration if hospitalization is necessary)
B. During the period of mood disturbance, three (or more) of the following symptoms have persisted (four if the mood is only irritable) and have been present to a significant degree:
  1. Inflated self-esteem or grandiosity
  2. Decreased need for sleep (e.g. feels rested after only 3 hours of sleep)
  3. More talkative than usual or pressure to keep talking
  4. Flight of ideas or subjective experience that thoughts are racing
  5. Distractibility (i.e. attention too easily drawn to unimportant or irrelevant external stimuli)
  6. Increase in goal-directed activity (either socially, at work or school, or sexually) or psychomotor agitation
  7. Excessive involvement in pleasurable activities that have a high potential for painful consequences (e.g. engaging in unrestrained buying sprees, sexual indiscretions, or foolish business investments)

3. Mixed Episode

A. The criteria are met both for a Manic Episode and for a Major Depressive Episode (except for duration) nearly every day during at least a 1-week period
B. The mood disturbance is sufficiently severe to cause marked impairment in occupational functioning or in usual social activities or relationships with others, or to necessitate hospitalization to prevent harm to self or others, or there are psychotic features
C. The symptoms are not due to the direct physiological effects of a substance (e.g. recreational drug use, a medication, or other treatment) or a general medical condition (e.g. hyperthyroidism)

(continued)

4. Hypomanic Episode

A. A distinct period of persistently elevated, expansive, or irritable mood, lasting throughout at least 4 days, that is clearly different from the usual nondepressed mood

B. During the period of mood disturbance, three (or more) of the following symptoms have persisted (four if the mood is only irritable) and have been present to a significant degree:
   1. Inflated self-esteem or grandiosity
   2. Decreased need for sleep (e.g. feels rested after only 3 hours of sleep)
   3. More talkative than usual or pressure to keep talking
   4. Flight of ideas or subjective experience that thoughts are racing
   5. Distractibility (i.e. attention too easily drawn to unimportant or irrelevant external stimuli)
   6. Increase in goal-directed activity (either socially, at work or school, or sexually) or psychomotor agitation
   7. Excessive involvement in pleasurable activities that have a high potential for painful consequences (e.g. the person engages in unrestrained buying sprees, sexual indiscretions, or foolish business investments)

2.2 MOOD DISORDERS

The mood disorders are described using mood episodes and can be divided into two main groups: the Depressive Disorders (characterized by the presence of depressive episodes only) and the Bipolar Disorders (all types of mood episodes). There are four types of mood episodes: 1) major depressive episode; 2) manic episode; 3) mixed episode; 4) hypomanic episode (see Textbox 2.2 for diagnostic criteria of mood episodes). No substantial change is proposed in the revision of DSM-5 as regards the definitions of mood episodes, with the exception of mixed episode, which is slated to be replaced by "Mixed Features." In general, mood disorders are among the most common mental disorders around the world, accounting for a large amount of disability, and having high rates of recurrence.

Major depression disorder is a disorder characterized by the presence of one or more major depressive episodes. It is a relatively common disorder (10-25% in women, 5-12% in men) with a median onset in the young adulthood (25-30 years) and a high variability in rates around the world. Those who are female, younger, and unmarried are consistently at increased risk (Weissman et al., 1996). For diagnosis, it is important that depressive symptoms are not due to normal bereavement, physical illness, alcohol/substance use or drug side effects. Depressive disorders, however, are associated with the presence of several other medical conditions. In particular, they are associated with and influence the prognosis of cardiovascular diseases and cancer.

Bipolar I Disorder is characterized by the occurrence of one or more manic or mixed episodes. Usually individuals have also had at least one major depressive episode. The lifetime prevalence of this disorder is estimated between 0.4 and 1.6%, with no differences between sexes. Per definition, it is a recurrent disorder, with more than 90% of individuals going on to have future episodes. A family history of bipolar and depressive disorders is common. DSM-5 will introduce the concept of developmental onset, to give a more clear definition to childhood onset of this disorder.

Bipolar II Disorder is characterized by the occurrence of one or more hypomanic episodes and one or more major depressive episodes. This disorder seems to be more frequent in women than in men, and occurs at a lifetime prevalence of about 0.5% in the community. Other types of mood disorder include dysthymic disorder (a mild and chronic form of depression), cyclothymic disorder (a mild form of bipolar disorder), premenstrual dysphoric disorder (proposed as a new diagnosis in DSM-5), and mixed anxiety depression.

2.3 ANXIETY DISORDERS

A heterogeneous group of diseases are grouped as anxiety disorders in DSM-IV: panic disorder, specific and social phobias, obsessive compulsive disorder, generalized anxiety disorder, acute stress disorder, and posttraumatic stress disorder (APA, 1994). A new group labelled "Anxiety and obsessive-compulsive spectrum disorder" will be proposed in DSM-5 (APA, 2011). It will probably include obsessive-compulsive disorder, skin picking disorder (recurrent skin picking resulting in skin lesions), trichotillomania or hair pulling disorder (recurrent hair pulling resulting in hair loss), and body dysmorphic disorder (abnormal preoccupations with a perceived defect or flow in physical appearance that is not observable to others).

Obsessive-compulsive disorder is a severe and chronic disturbance present in the community with a lifetime prevalence of about 1%; obsessive-compulsive spectrum disorders as a whole are more frequent (5-8%). Onset typically occurs during adolescence or early adulthood, with no differences between sexes (Burijon, 2007). Textbox 2.3 shows the diagnostic criteria for obsessive-compulsive disorder.

The DSM-5 Task Force proposed a rewording of some criteria changing the word "impulses" to "urges," to avoid confusion with the impulsive-spectrum disorders. In addition, they propose to remove criteria 2 and 4 from the definition of obsessions and the B criterion.

TEXTBOX **2.3**

DSM-IV Diagnostic Criteria for Obsessive-Compulsive Disorder

Obsessive-Compulsive Disorder

A. Either obsessions or compulsions:

Obsessions as defined by (1), (2), (3), and (4):
1. Recurrent and persistent thoughts, impulses, or images that are experienced, at some time during the disturbance, as intrusive and inappropriate and that cause marked anxiety or distress
2. The thoughts, impulses, or images are not simply excessive worries about real-life problems
3. The person attempts to ignore or suppress such thoughts, impulses, or images, or to neutralize them with some other thought or action
4. The person recognizes that the obsessional thoughts, impulses, or images are a product of his or her own mind (not imposed from external sources as in thought insertion)

Compulsions as defined by (1) and (2):
1. Repetitive behaviors (e.g. hand washing, ordering, checking) or mental acts (e.g. praying, counting, repeating words silently) that the person feels driven to perform in response to an obsession, or according to rules that must be applied rigidly
2. The behaviors or mental acts are aimed at preventing or reducing distress or preventing some dreaded event or situation; however, these behaviors or mental acts either are not connected in a realistic way with what they are designed to neutralize or prevent, or are clearly excessive

B. At some point during the course of the disorder, the person has recognized that the obsessions or compulsions are excessive or unreasonable

C. The obsessions or compulsions cause marked distress, are time consuming (take more than 1 hour a day), or significantly interfere with the person's normal routine, occupational (or academic) functioning, or usual social activities or relationships

Specify if:

With Poor Insight: if, for most of the time during the current episode, the person does not recognize that the obsessions and compulsions are excessive

---

DSM-IV Diagnostic Criteria for Panic Disorder

Panic disorder
A. Both (1) and (2):
   1. Recurrent unexpected Panic Attacks
   2. At least one of the attacks has been followed by 1 month (or more) of one (or more) of the following:
      a. persistent concern about additional attacks
      b. worry about the implications of the attack or its consequences (e.g. losing control, having a heart attack, "going crazy")
      c. a significant change in behavior related to the attacks
B. Specify if: Presence (or absence) of Agoraphobia

Panic disorder is defined as the recurrence of panic attacks, i.e. an abrupt surge of intense fear or intense discomfort that reaches a peak within minutes. Panic attack includes both somatic and psychological symptoms, such as palpitations, sweating, trembling, shortness of breath, choking sensations, chest pain, nausea, dizziness, heat sensations or chills, paresthesias, derealisation or depersonalization, fear of losing control, fear of going crazy or dying. Defining the epidemiology of panic disorder is quite difficult, because of the high presence of untreated or unrecognized conditions in the community. It is estimated to be present in 2-3% of the population, with a typical onset in late adolescence or early adulthood. Women are at twice the risk of men and comorbidity with depression is quite common. Treatment reduces or prevents symptoms in 70-90% of patients. Textbox 2.4 shows the DSM-IV diagnostic criteria for panic disorder.

The DSM-5 proposed revisions suggest the elimination of the agoraphobia specification in panic disorder, proposing agoraphobia as a codable new disorder among the anxiety disorders.

Phobias are grouped in three categories: specific phobias, social phobias, and agoraphobia. They are quite common disorders with lifetime prevalences ranging around 10-11% in the community. Specific phobias include marked and disproportionate fear of animals (spiders), natural environment conditions (storms), blood, situations (flying), and others (fear of vomiting). Social phobias involve marked and disproportionate fear of one or more social situations, such as having a conver-

sation, eating or drinking, or performing in front of others. Agoraphobia is defined as a marked fear about at least two situations, such as being outside of the home alone, public transportation, open spaces, being in shops or cinemas, standing in line, or being in a crowd (Burijon, 2007).

Generalized anxiety disorder will be probably renamed as "Generalized Anxiety and Worry Disorder." It is characterized by the presence of excessive anxiety and worry (apprehensive expectation) about different types or domains of activity, such as family, health, work, or school. It is estimated to be present in 5% of the population in a lifetime, with a higher prevalence in females (about 2/3 of cases). It includes overanxious disorder in childhood (Burijon, 2007). Textbox 2.5 shows the DSM-IV diagnostic criteria for this disorder and the changes proposed by DSM-5.

Posttraumatic stress disorder is a complex disorder that follows exposure to a severe traumatic experience and is characterized by intrusive re-experience of the trauma, persistent avoidance of trauma-related stimuli, and symptoms of increased arousal. The prevalence of this disorder is difficult to estimate, because it largely depends on the definition of trauma. It is estimated to be 4-9% in the lifetime, and in similarly exposed people, it is more frequent in women than in men. There is no typical age of onset for this disorder and individuals seem to be more at risk when they are adolescent or in late adulthood. Comorbid psychiatric conditions, especially major depression, are very common. The DSM-5 Task Force proposed a dis-

DSM-IV and DSM-5 Diagnostic Criteria
for Generalized Anxiety Disorder

Generalized Anxiety Disorder (DSM-IV)
A. Excessive anxiety and worry (apprehensive expectation), occurring more days than not for at least 6 months, about a number of events or activities (such as work or school performance)
B. The person finds it difficult to control the worry
C. The anxiety and worry are associated with three (or more) of the following six symptoms (with at least some symptoms present for more days than not for the past 6 months)
    1. Restlessness or feeling keyed up or on edge
    2. Being easily fatigued
    3. Difficulty concentrating or mind going blank
    4. Irritability
    5. Muscle tension
    6. Sleep disturbance (difficulty falling or staying asleep, or restless unsatisfying sleep)
D. The anxiety, worry, or physical symptoms cause clinically significant distress or impairment in social, occupational, or other important areas of functioning

Generalized Anxiety and Worry Disorder (DSM-5)
A. Excessive anxiety and worry (apprehensive expectation) about two (or more) domains of activities or events (for example, domains like family, health, finances, and school/work difficulties)
B. The excessive anxiety and worry occur on more days than not for three months or more
C. The anxiety and worry are associated with one or more of the following symptoms:
    1. Restlessness or feeling keyed up or on edge
    2. Being easily fatigued
    3. Difficulty concentrating or mind going blank
    4. Irritability
    5. Muscle tension
    6. Sleep disturbance (difficulty falling or staying asleep, or restless unsatisfying sleep)
D. The anxiety and worry are associated with one or more of the following behaviors:
    a. Marked avoidance of situations in which a negative outcome could occur
    b. Marked time and effort preparing for situations in which a negative outcome could occur
    c. Marked procrastination in behavior or decision-making due to worries
    d. Repeatedly seeking reassurance due to worries
E. The anxiety, worry, or physical symptoms cause clinically significant distress or impairment in social, occupational, or other important areas of functioning *With Poor Insight*: if, for most of the time during the current episode, the person does not recognize that the obsessions and compulsions are excessive

tinction between conscious avoidance of trauma-related stimuli and less conscious mechanisms of numbing (APA, 2011). Textbox 2.6 shows the DSM-IV diagnostic criteria for this disorder and the changes proposed by DSM-5.

2.4 EATING DISORDERS

Eating disorders are severe and chronic psychiatric disorders characterized by an abnormal eating behavior and an excessive importance given to body weight and shape for self-esteem. They represent the psychiatric disorder with the highest female/male ratio (about 10-20/1) and their prevalence is high in the female general population (about 2% for anorexia nervosa and 4-5% for bulimia nervosa) (Favaro et al., 2003). The age with the highest incidence of both anorexia and bulimia nervosa is between 15 and 19 (about 200 new cases per 100,000 each year) (Favaro et al., 2009).

DSM-IV and DSM-5 Diagnostic Criteria
for Posttraumatic Stress Disorder

Posttraumatic Stress Disorder (DSM-IV)

A. The person has been exposed to a traumatic event in which both of the following were present:
   1. The person experienced, witnessed, or was confronted with an event or events that involved actual or threatened death or serious injury, or a threat to the physical integrity of self or others
   2. The person's response involved intense fear, helplessness, or horror
B. The traumatic event is persistently reexperienced in one (or more) of the following ways:
   1. Recurrent and intrusive distressing recollections of the event, including images, thoughts, or perceptions
   2. Recurrent distressing dreams of the event
   3. Acting or feeling as if the traumatic event were recurring (includes a sense of reliving the experience, illusions, hallucinations, and dissociative flashback episodes, including those that occur on awakening or when intoxicated)
   4. Intense psychological distress at exposure to internal or external cues that symbolize or resemble an aspect of the traumatic event
   5. Physiological reactivity on exposure to internal or external cues that symbolize or resemble an aspect of the traumatic event
C. Persistent avoidance of stimuli associated with the trauma and numbing of general responsiveness (not present before the trauma), as indicated by three (or more) of the following:
   1. Efforts to avoid thoughts, feelings, or conversations associated with the trauma
   2. Efforts to avoid activities, places, or people that arouse recollections of the trauma
   3. Inability to recall an important aspect of the trauma
   4. Markedly diminished interest or participation in significant activities
   5. Feeling of detachment or estrangement from others
   6. Restricted range of affect (e.g. unable to have loving feelings)
   7. Sense of a foreshortened future (e.g. does not expect to have a career, marriage, children, or a normal life span)
D. Persistent symptoms of increased arousal (not present before the trauma), as indicated by two (or more) of the following:
   1. Difficulty falling or staying asleep
   2. Irritability or outbursts of anger
   3. Difficulty concentrating
   4. Hypervigilance
   5. Exaggerated startle response
E. Duration of the disturbance (symptoms in Criteria B, C, and D) is more than 1 month.
F. The disturbance causes clinically significant distress or impairment in social, occupational, or other important areas of functioning

Posttraumatic Stress Disorder (DSM-5)

A. The person was exposed to one or more of the following event(s): death or threatened death, actual or threatened serious injury, or actual or threatened sexual violation, in one or more of the following ways:
   1. Experiencing the event(s) firsthand
   2. Witnessing, in person, the event(s) as they occurred to others
   3. Learning that the event(s) occurred to a close relative or close friend; in such cases, the actual or threatened death must have been violent or accidental

(*continued*)

4. Experiencing repeated or extreme exposure to aversive details of the event(s) (e.g. first responders collecting body parts; police officers repeatedly exposed to details of child abuse); this does not apply to exposure through electronic media, television, movies, or pictures, unless this exposure is work related

B. Intrusion symptoms that are associated with the traumatic event(s) (that began after the traumatic event[s]), as evidenced by 1 or more of the following:
   1. Spontaneous or cued recurrent, involuntary, and intrusive distressing memories of the traumatic event(s)
   2. Recurrent distressing dreams in which the content and/or affect of the dream is related to the event(s). Note: In children, there may be frightening dreams without recognizable content
   3. Dissociative reactions (e.g. flashbacks) in which the individual feels or acts as if the traumatic event(s) are recurring (Such reactions may occur on a continuum, with the most extreme expression being a complete loss of awareness of present surroundings)
   4. Intense or prolonged psychological distress at exposure to internal or external cues that symbolize or resemble an aspect of the traumatic event(s)
   5. Marked physiological reactions to reminders of the traumatic event(s)

C. Persistent avoidance of stimuli associated with the traumatic event(s) (that began after the traumatic event[s]), as evidenced by efforts to avoid 1 or more of the following:
   1. Avoids internal reminders (thoughts, feelings, or physical sensations) that arouse recollections of the traumatic event(s)
   2. Avoids external reminders (people, places, conversations, activities, objects, situations) that arouse recollections of the traumatic event(s)

D. Negative alterations in cognitions and mood that are associated with the traumatic event(s) (that began or worsened after the traumatic event[s]), as evidenced by 3 or more of the following:
   1. Inability to remember an important aspect of the traumatic event(s) (typically dissociative amnesia; not due to head injury, alcohol, or drugs)
   2. Persistent and exaggerated negative expectations about one's self, others, or the world (e.g. "I am bad," "no one can be trusted,")
   3. Persistent distorted blame of self or others surrounding the cause or consequences of the traumatic event(s)
   4. Pervasive negative emotional state -- for example: fear, horror, anger, guilt, or shame
   5. Markedly diminished interest or participation in significant activities
   6. Feeling of detachment or estrangement from others
   7. Persistent inability to experience positive emotions (e.g. unable to have loving feelings, psychic numbing)

E. Alterations in arousal and reactivity that are associated with the traumatic event(s) (that began or worsened after the traumatic event[s]), as evidenced by 3 or more of the following:
   1. Irritable or aggressive behavior
   2. Reckless or self-destructive behavior
   3. Hypervigilance
   4. Exaggerated startle response
   5. Problems with concentration
   6. Sleep disturbance – for example, difficulty falling or staying asleep, or restless sleep

F. Duration of the disturbance (symptoms in Criteria B, C, D and E) is more than one month

G. The disturbance causes clinically significant distress or impairment in social, occupational, or other important areas of functioning

Anorexia nervosa is characterized by a high risk of medical complications and it is considered the psychiatric disorder with the highest mortality rate. It is characterized by weight loss, low awareness of the illness and refusal of treatment, body image distortion, and an obsessive and in- flexible attention to eating and body weight. The diagnostic criteria for anorexia nervosa will be changed in order to reduce the prevalence of eat- ing disorders not otherwise specified (EDNOS) in patient samples (about 40-50% of all patients re- ferred to specialized units). Textbox 2.7 shows the

---

TEXTBOX **2.7**

DSM-IV and DSM-5
Diagnostic Criteria for Anorexia Nervosa

Anorexia nervosa (DSM-IV)
A. Refusal to maintain body weight at or above a minimally normal weight for age and height (e.g. weight loss leading to maintenance of body weight less than 85% of that expected; or failure to make expected weight gain during period of growth, leading to body weight less than 85% of that expected)
B. Intense fear of gaining weight or becoming fat, even though underweight
C. Disturbance in the way in which one's body weight or shape is experienced, undue influence of body weight or shape on self-evaluation, or denial of the seriousness of the current low body weight
D. In postmenarcheal females, amenorrhea, i.e. the absence of at least three consecutive menstrual cycles (A woman is considered to have amenorrhea if her periods occur only following hor- mone, e.g. estrogen, administration)

Specify type
Restricting Type: during the current episode of Anorexia Nervosa, the person has not regularly engaged in binge eating or purging behavior (i.e. self-induced vomiting or the misuse of laxatives, diuretics, or enemas).
Binge-Eating/Purging Type: during the current episode of Anorexia Nervosa, the person has regu- larly engaged in binge eating or purging behavior (i.e. self-induced vomiting or the misuse of laxa- tives, diuretics, or enemas).

Anorexia nervosa (DSM-5)
A. Restriction of energy intake relative to requirements leading to a significantly low body weight in the context of age, sex, developmental trajectory, and physical health. Significantly low weight is defined as a weight that is less than minimally normal, or, for children and adoles- cents, less than that minimally expected
B. Intense fear of gaining weight or becoming fat, or persistent behavior that interferes with weight gain, even though at a significantly low weight
C. Disturbance in the way in which one's body weight or shape is experienced, undue influence of body weight or shape on self-evaluation, or persistent lack of recognition of the seriousness of the current low body weight

Specify current type
Restricting Type: during the last three months, the person has not engaged in recurrent episodes of binge eating or purging behavior (i.e. self-induced vomiting or the misuse of laxatives, diuretics, or enemas).
Binge-Eating/Purging Type: during the last three months, the person has engaged in recurrent episodes of binge eating or purging behavior (i.e. self-induced vomiting or the misuse of laxatives, diuretics, or enemas.

DSM-IV Diagnostic Criteria for Bulimia Nervosa

Bulimia nervosa
A. Recurrent episodes of binge eating. An episode of binge eating is characterized by both of the following:
    (1) eating, in a discrete period of time (e.g. within any 2-hour period), an amount of food that is definitely larger than most people would eat during a similar period of time and under similar circumstances
    (2) a sense of lack of control over eating during the episode (e.g. a feeling that one cannot stop eating or control what or how much one is eating)
B. Recurrent inappropriate compensatory behavior in order to prevent weight gain, such as self-induced vomiting or misuse of laxatives, diuretics, enemas, or other medications; fasting, or excessive exercise
C. The binge eating and inappropriate compensatory behaviors both occur, on average, at least twice a week for 3 months
D. Self-evaluation is unduly influenced by body shape and weight
E. The disturbance does not occur exclusively during episodes of Anorexia Nervosa

Specify type
Purging Type: during the current episode of Bulimia Nervosa, the person has regularly engaged in self-induced vomiting or the misuse of laxatives, diuretics, or enemas.
Nonpurging Type: during the current episode of Bulimia Nervosa, the person has used other inappropriate compensatory behaviors, such as fasting or excessive exercise, but has not regularly engaged in self-induced vomiting or the misuse of laxatives, diuretics, or enemas.

DSM-IV criteria and the proposed changes introduced by the DSM-5 Task Force (APA, 2011). The main changes concern the amenorrhea criterion and a rewording of criteria A and B.

Bulimia nervosa is less severe than anorexia nervosa in terms of medical complications and mortality, but it tends to have a chronic course and high psychiatric comorbidity (especially major depressive disorder and borderline personality disorder). Like anorexia nervosa, subjects with bulimia are characterized by an excessive importance given to body weight and shape for self-esteem, the presence of episodes of objective loss of control over food (binge eating) and inappropriate use of compensatory behavior to control weight gain. A diagnosis of bulimia nervosa can be given only in the absence of anorexia nervosa and usually patients with bulimia nervosa are normal weight (Favaro & Santonastaso, 2008).

Textbox 2.8 shows the DSM-IV diagnostic criteria for this disorder. The DSM-5 Task Force proposed only a change in the threshold to define the frequency of binge eating and compensatory behavior (from twice a week to once a week) and the elimination of subtype distinction (APA, 2011).

The DSM-5 introduced a new eating disorder, named *Binge Eating Disorder*, characterized by recurrent binge eating in the absence of compensatory behavior to prevent weight loss. In addition, in DSM-5, eating and feeding disorders (pica, rumination) are part of the same category.

It is estimated that all these changes proposed by DSM-5 will reduce the EDNOS categories to 30% of cases or less.

Physical activity and **mental health,**
psychological and physiological mechanisms

3

Simone Bolognesi, Arianna Goracci, Andrea Fagiolini

This chapter will present the current state of research on the relationship between physical exercise and mental health, with focus on the relationships between exercise and mental disorders. We will also explain the main psychological and neurobiological mechanisms involved in physical activity and we will propose the importance of exercise in prevention and treatment of mental disorders. Finally, guidance for the operational translation of the theoretical indications treated will be provided.

3.1 MENTAL HEALTH AND PHYSICAL ACTIVITY

Physical activity is associated with a wide range of health benefits, and its absence may increase risk for cardiovascular diseases, diabetes, obesity, hypertension, and other high risk diseases. Sedentary lifestyle may also be associated with the development of mental illness. Indeed, a recent review evidences a "longitudinal relationship" between baseline depression and subsequent change in physical activity. Other studies found that depression was significantly related with a decline in the amount of physical activity, or with non-adherence to a prescribed exercise regimen, for example in the follow-up period after a coronary event (Moghaddam et al., 2009; Teychenne et al., 2008).

Despite overwhelming evidence demonstrating that leisure-time physical activity is associated with reduced mortality and extensive health benefits, the World Health Organization (WHO) notes that at least 60% of the world population fails to complete the recommended amount of physical activity required to achieve some health benefits. This is partly due to insufficient participation in physical activity during leisure time

and an increase in sedentary behavior during occupational and domestic activities. Furthermore, half of the people who initiate physical activity programs quit within the first 6 months, irrespective of the activity chosen (Yeung, 1996). The amount of physical activity is also correlated to the examined target population, being lower in women, older adults, people with disabilities, obese individuals, people of non-white races and people having less education or income (Wei et al., 1999).

Individuals with mental health disorders constitute an important population in which physical inactivity may contribute to increased morbidity and healthcare costs, as well as a higher risk of premature death than the general population. Ischemic heart disease is a common cause of excess mortality in this population (Lawrence et al., 2003). In addition, comorbid conditions (such as obesity) or the consumption of psychiatric drugs can contribute to a worse prognosis of psychiatric disorders, as they have a negative impact on general psychological and physical well-being and quality of life. Rates of co-occurring illnesses, such as hypertension, diabetes, respiratory disease, and cardiovascular disease, are as high as 60% among people with serious mental illnesses (Berren et al., 1994). For example, the high prevalence of the metabolic syndrome in patients with bipolar disorder (Fagiolini et al., 2005) suggests that the development and testing of specific interventions that target this epidemic are needed. A decrease in daily caloric intake and exercise should be recommended to any patient who has gained or is gaining weight. Even a limited weight loss (5%) can have positive effects. Counselling by a dietician and appropriate exercise should be encouraged, especially to maintain optimum weight (Fagiolini et al., 2007).

Depression and anxiety are significantly prevalent causes of physical illness, psychosocial impairment and mortality throughout the world (APA, 1994). Depressive and anxiety disorders are often recurrent, lifelong diseases that generate substantial individual and community costs (Glass, 1999). However, despite the existence of several effective therapeutic modalities, many patients with mental health disorders are being inadequately or inconsistently treated (Hirschfield et al., 1997). As such, physical activity may be an important, but underused, integration to currently accepted pharmacological and psychological therapies.

The psychological benefits of physical exercise have not, however, received much attention. Stable, adaptive-emotional, cognitive, and behavioral inclinations are imperative to the optimal functioning and wellbeing of an individual in society. Any factor that can enhance psychological wellbeing will therefore have a variety of potentially positive implications for the general wellbeing of an individual. The psychological effects of physical exercise need to be better understood, appreciated, and emphasized by both health professionals and their clients. Participation in regular physical activity has been associated with a variety of positive psychosocial effects ranging from a reduction in depressive symptoms (O'Neal et al., 2000) and anxiety (Petruzzello et al., 1991), to improvements in self-esteem (Fox, 2000), reduced age-related mental deterioration (Powell, 1974), enhanced alertness and faster reaction time (Kiesling, 1983), and a more positive perception of the self by others (Brody, 1981).

Even though the psychological benefits of regular exercise are well known, researchers have only recently begun to examine the impact of physical activity on the mental and physical health of individuals with serious mental illness. Strong relationships have been found both between physical activity and mental health and between physical activity and physical health within the general population (Biddle et al., 2000). People with serious mental illnesses often experience poor physical health along with significant psychiatric, social, and cognitive disabilities. Physical activity has the potential to improve the quality of life of people with serious mental illness through two routes: a) by improving physical health and b) by alleviating psychiatric and social disability.

3.1.1 Physical activity and depression

It has been known for many years that regular physical activity brings benefits to individuals with depressive symptoms (Dunn et al., 2005; Leppamaki et al., 2002). Patients with major depression have higher rates of health risk behaviors that can lead to a higher incidence of chronic diseases such as type II diabetes and cardiovascular disease (Goodman et al., 2002). In general, people with depression are less physically active and more deconditioned than non-depressed individuals (Martinsen, 1990). Clinical and epidemiological studies have shown a significant association between lack of physical activity and depressive symptoms (Rot et al., 2009).

In 2003, Goodwin published the results of the National Co-morbidity Survey, conducted over a sample of 8098 Americans (between 15 and 54 years), demonstrating that regular physical activity conducted in the workplace or leisure time was associated with a significantly reduced probability of experiencing a depressive disorder. Galper et al. (2006) described similar results, showing the inverse relationship between physical activity and amount of depressive symptoms, where inactive men and women were much more severely depressed than their active counterparts. In 2001 the British Medical Journal published a systematic review of the antidepressant effect of exercise, including 14 clinical trials, reporting that the effect of exercise is higher than not making any specific

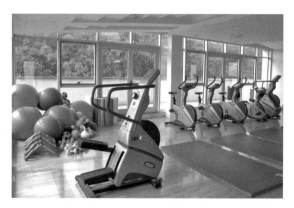

Figure 3.1 - Gymnasium. In this place people can exercise with different equipments and aerobic machines. The availability of balls, dumbbells, mats, cycle ergometers and others materials lets exercise specialists choose between single or group training.

treatment (Lawlor et al., 2001). In clinical practice this can be translated into a significant reduction of the scores in depression scales and presumably a reduction in the severity of depressive symptoms produced by exercise.

The relationship between improvement of mood and exercise, however, does not seem to be universal. Studies using cross-sectional data to demonstrate a negative association between physical activity and the prevalence or severity of depression are not suitable to demonstrate causality. Depression is considered to have a demotivating effect on exercise, and therefore depressed people may be less prone to perform physical activity. Likewise, people who exercise are considered less to develop major depression. In order to establish such causality in the "two-way binding-exercise depression" relationship, longitudinal studies are needed (Rot et al., 2009). Recent reviews have indeed investigated the evidence of the "longitudinal relationship" between baseline depression and subsequent changes in physical activity, and the relationship between baseline levels of physical activity and the subsequent risk of depression (Moghaddam et al., 2009; Teychenné et al., 2008). Many of the reviewed studies revealed that initial depression was significantly associated with a decline in the level of physical activity or loss of adherence to the prescribed regimen of physical exercises, for example subsequent to a coronary event. Moreover, the presence of baseline depression was significantly associated with the change of behavior from active to sedentary; in fact, depression after cardiovascular events was largely motivated by behavioral factors and especially by physical inactivity.

Studies have shown that individuals without psychiatric symptoms who exercise regularly experience better moods than those who do not (Sexton et al., 2001). Engels et al. (2002) demonstrated an association between mood improvement and medium- or long-term physical activity. Paluska et al. (2000) reported similar associations and improvement of various other aspects such as self-esteem, vitality, general wellbeing, and satisfaction with physical appearance. There is also evidence that regular physical activity may protect against the development of depression or that physical inactivity might be a risk factor for depression (Raglin, 1990), even if this putative protective effect has not been demonstrated experimentally.

Few studies have addressed the usefulness of physical activity in the treatment of depressive symptoms among *hospitalized or clinically depressed persons* (Craft et al., 1998). Investigators have noted beneficial effects within both groups across a variety of exercise modalities. Martinsen et al. (1985) and Sime (1987) investigated the effects of a vigorous and lasting (9-10 weeks) exercise program in subjects diagnosed with depression, noting a significant reduction in BDI depressive scores.

The effects of regular physical activity on mood have mainly been studied using aerobic exercise (Brosse et al., 2002). Dunn et al. (2005) have compared weekly aerobic exercise recommended by the American College of Sports Medicine to a lower intensity exercise in patients with moderate to major depression. After 12 weeks, aerobic exercise was more effective in reducing depressive symptoms, comparable to antidepressants than the lower intensity exercise.

Evidence indicates that anaerobic physical activity, such as bodybuilding or flexibility training, can also reduce depressive symptoms (Paluska et al., 2000). Singh et al. (2005) showed that anaerobic exercise, carried out according to the intensity recommended, not only reduced patients' depressive symptoms, but also improved the quality of their sleep and their perceived quality of life in general.

The benefit of exercise is known to be greater for longer programs and/or multiple sessions of physical activity, even though a single session proved to be more effective in reducing acute depressive symptoms (Hoffman et al., 2008), and the effects were reported to last for some hours or even up to one day (Hansen et al., 2001). At the moment it is not clear how long the antidepressant effect of exercise lasts after the end of a treatment program or a clinical trial. What is certain is that people who have started some sort of physical activity during a clinical trial or a specific project are more likely to continue and to improve physical activity after the end of the program.

Physical activity appears to be as effective as other therapeutic modalities for the treatment of mild or moderate depressive symptoms. Craft et al. (1998) reported a greater effect on moderately to severely depressed individuals than on those subjects who were initially classified as mildly to moderately depressed. Recent meta-analysis showed effects for exercise that were similar to those found in other psychotherapeutic interventions (Lawlor et al., 2001). Other reviews have also concluded that antidepressant effects of exercise may be comparable to that of psychotherapy and pharmacotherapy and that a combination of the two may be more effective than physical exercise alone (Martinsen, 1994, Trivedi et al., 2006). Even if this conclusion is not shared by all (Martinsen et al., 1989), the combined treatment of exercise with drug therapy may lead to a faster response and a faster improvement of depressive symptoms. This indication may be clinically relevant, considering that a significant result obtained only with antidepressant drug therapy may require several weeks. Exercise can be an appropriate enhancement strategy because it doesn't interfere with other treatments or therapies.

Results obtained from different series of studies on correlations between physical activity and mental health in subjects that were not previously diagnosed as being clinically depressed might be more relevant, as they are more representative of the general population (Brown, 1990). However, association between increased physical activity and improved mood in this "normal" population was less clear than from the community-based studies using nonclinical populations. In addition, the heterogeneity of study designs, research participants, psychological measures and duration of intervention limit the generalization of the studies' findings. King et al. (1989) found that regular exercise produced a significant change in perceived fitness and satisfaction with physical appearances, but did not generate any significant enhancement on depressed mood. In another study (Moses et al., 1989), subjects were randomly assigned to 1 of the following 4 categories: high intensity exercise, moderate intensity exercise, attention-placebo, or waiting list. Significant improvements in psychological responses were seen only in the group engaged in the moderate intensity exercise program, which probably improved patient satisfaction and exercise adherence (Glenister, 1996). Despite the mental health improvements noted among non-clinically depressed study populations, meta-analyses of the various studies have concluded that clinical and/or medically treated participants demonstrated the greatest decreases in depressive symptoms with exercise (North et al., 1990; Craft et al., 1998). Evidence supporting the preventive aspects of regular physical activity has been less conclusive than

studies focusing on the treatment of depression. Epidemiological surveys have noted cross-association between little or no leisure-time physical activity and increased risk for developing depression among previously healthy persons in a community sample (Farmer et al., 1988). However, no experimental data has definitively shown that either acute or chronic physical activity can prevent the onset of depression. Nevertheless, active individuals who develop mild depression may subsequently have a lower likelihood of severe depression (Raglin, 1990).

Overall, many of the currently available studies regarding depression and exercise have some important weaknesses: small sample sizes, short study durations and inadequate control groups limit their findings. Inconsistent definitions of depression with a variety of psychological measures also minimize generalization of the studies. Nonetheless, both aerobic and non-aerobic physical activities seem beneficial for the treatment of mild-to-moderate depressive symptoms. In addition, exercise seems to have similar efficacy to psychotherapy and provides no significant contraindication to the use of medications.

For more information about the role of exercise in the treatment of depression and anxiety see Chapter 9.

3.1.2 Physical activity and anxiety

Anxiety disorders constitute a large group of related mental health conditions that have a significantly lower worldwide prevalence than depressive disorders, but nonetheless affect the lives of millions of people (APA, 1994). Anxiety is characterized by feelings of uneasiness, apprehension, distress, and worry about the future, with or without identifiable cause. Cognitive and affective alterations are often accompanied by physiological arousal. In extreme form, anxiety can manifest itself as intense fear or dread and in worse cases it can lead to paralyzing panic.

The association between exercise and anxiety has received less attention than that between exercise and depression, and the majority of studies have examined only the transient psychological outcomes of single exercise sessions.

An extensive series of meta-analyses investigated the effects of acute and chronic physical activity on anxiety. The general finding is that exercise was associated with reduced anxiety symptom scores measured by standardized tests: state anxiety is significantly reduced following bouts of exercise, both for subjects with normal and elevated levels of anxiety. These reductions are statistically significant within 5-15 min after the cessation of exercise and remain decreased for the following 2-4 hours, before gradually returning to pre-exercise values. In contrast, the influence of long-term exercise programs on trait anxiety is less consistent (Raglin, 1990).

Physical activity has been associated with reduced symptoms of anxiety in both clinical (Martinsen et al., 1989) and nonclinical populations (Petruzzello et al., 1991). The exact association between physical exercise and reduction in anxiety is, however, yet to be firmly established: no results of the meta-analyses suggested a causal effect between physical activity and decreased anxiety. From a biochemical point of view, physical activity has been associated with alterations in serotonergic (Dishman, 1997), noradrenergic (Pagliari et al., 1995), cholinergic (Zhao et al., 1997), gamma-aminobutyric-acid (GABA) (Meeusen et al., 1997), and adenosine (Carey et al., 1994) neurotransmitter systems. Each of these neurotransmitter systems has been linked to the generation of anxiety. In its turn, physical activity might have an anxiety-reducing effect on a physiological level (O'Connor et al., 2000).

Considering the typology of exercise, aerobic exercise programs produced larger effect sizes than weight training/flexibility regimens, but studies using other methods of anxiety reduction (quiet rest, meditation, or relaxation) on control groups showed no significant difference between exercise and other treatments.

Martinsen et al. (1989) compared aerobic activity to strength/flexibility training in the treatment of anxiety disorders. The walking/jogging group and the strength/flexibility group achieved similar, significant reductions in their anxiety scores compared to their entrance levels. A weakness of the study was the lack of a non-exercise control group, so a causal relationship between exercise and anxiety symptoms could not be determined. In addition, the study population was drawn from hospitalized patients with heterogeneous anxiety disorders and co-morbidities who may not be representative of most community-dwelling individuals with elevated anxiety scores.

Bahrke et al. (1978) compared vigorous acute exercise activity, meditation activity and quiet reading, and found that after a single 20-minute study period all 3 groups had significant reductions in state anxiety. These findings were true for volunteers identified as having normal anxiety levels as well as those initially identified as having elevated state and/or trait anxiety. Since this study used only a single bout of acute exercise, it is not possible to make extrapolations regarding chronic anxiety.

Lobitz et al. (1983) investigated the impact of a 7-week aerobic physical exercise program compared with an anxiety management training program and with a no-treatment control group. Participants in the aerobic exercise and in the anxiety management groups achieved significant reductions in scores for state anxiety when compared to the control group. Importantly, only participants in the anxiety management group had reductions in trait anxiety scores.

Measures of trait anxiety were noted to improve following chronic physical activity but, interestingly, the program's length was found to be very important: programs needed to exceed 21 minutes of exercise per session for a minimum of 10 weeks in order to achieve significant reductions in trait anxiety (Petruzzello et al., 1991). Physical activity appeared to reach maximal benefit after 40 minutes per session, supporting findings that moderate duration exercise has the most beneficial effect on elevated anxiety measures (Osei-Tutu et al., 1998).

A specific anxiety disorder, *panic disorder*, has also been studied in relationship to physical activity. Since many people who have panic disorder fear that aerobic activity may trigger a panic attack, they often abstain from regular physical activity (Broocks et al., 1997). One study investigated the hypothesis that physical activity will increase anxiety symptoms among individuals with panic disorder and improve mood state among those with major depressive disorder (Rief et al., 1996). The authors assigned 3 groups of inpatients (diagnosed respectively with panic disorder, major depressive disorder, and healthy), to the same physical activity regimen. The authors noted that physical activity decreased depressive scores in all 3 groups, but increased anxiety scores among those with panic disorder. Since physical activity has appeared to increase anxiety ratings both objectively and subjectively in some patients with panic disorder, the possible contributions of exercise abstinence to the phobic avoidance behaviors noted in patients with panic disorder was studied. Subjects with panic disorder are generally concerned that physical activity could cause heart attack or other adverse cardiac event; this is why the majority of these individuals previously avoided intense physical activity. This subjective cardiac-related concern reflects findings that approximately 20% of patients seen with palpitations were subsequently diagnosed with panic disorder (Zimetbaum et al., 1998). Exercise avoidance may be an important component of panic disorder and potentially contribute to its pathophysiology.

A recent study compared the effects of a random assignment of regular aerobic exercise, clomipramine, or placebo pills among subjects with diagnoses of panic disorder and agoraphobia (Broocks et al., 1998). Participants in the exercise group and the clomipramine group had significantly decreased panic symptoms in comparison to the placebo group. The authors further concluded that clomipramine improved anxiety symptoms more effectively and earlier than exercise, but that both produced significant subjective improvements in individuals with panic disorder.

Orwin (1984) used exercise as a form of exposure in patients with agoraphobia, and reported positive results when patients exercised before approaching a fear-inducing situation. In a prospective study, patients with panic disorder and agoraphobia improved following an 8-week inpatient program, mainly consisting of daily aerobic exercise, but the majority relapsed by the 1-year follow-up (Martinsen et al., 1989).

Exercise intervention studies in other anxiety disorders are few. In a study without a control group, patients with generalized anxiety disorder improved during an 8-week inpatient program with daily aerobic exercise, and patients kept their gains at the 1-year follow-up. Patients with social phobia experienced no significant changes in anxiety. Exercise intervention studies with other anxiety disorders have not been published. Studies in children and adolescents are few, but there seems to be a small effect in favor of exercise in reducing anxiety scores in the general population of children and adolescents (Larun et al., 2006).

Overall, most studies have supported an association between acute exercise and state anxiety reduction, but have failed to demonstrate conclusively relationships among chronic exercise, phys-

ical fitness and improvements in trait anxiety (Biddle, 1995). For certain disorders, such as panic disorder, exercise may be helpful but is often falsely perceived as detrimental. Although consistent relationships between exercise and anxiety levels have been noted, most authors emphasised that no causal effect in alleviating anxiety symptoms has been substantiated by their research. It must be stressed that the adoption of a physically active lifestyle in an attempt to relieve or reduce anxiety is ultimately a more cost-effective mean of treating anxiety than the pharmacological and therapeutic alternatives offered by health professionals. In addition, exercise has been shown to be as effective as pharmacological treatments (such as clomipramine) in reducing symptoms of anxiety among patients diagnosed with a panic disorder (Broocks et al., 1998).

3.1.3 Physical activity and schizophrenia

Taylor et al. (1985) noted that only few case reports, anecdotes, and small group studies with heterogeneous populations suggest that physical activity and exercise can be beneficial for schizophrenic patients (for more information see Chapter 7).

Individuals with serious mental illnesses tend to be more sedentary than the general population and walking is the most common activity (Daumit et al., 2005). In one study of 140 individuals with schizophrenia, none of the responders reported any vigorous exercise during the previous week, and only 19% of men and 15% of women reported participating in at least one session of moderate-intensity physical activity (Brown et al., 1999). Very similar results were obtained by Davidson et al. (2001) wherein a cohort of 234 people with serious mental illness, 12% reported vigorous exercise during the previous two weeks, compared with 35% in the general population, and participation in light exercise was significantly decreased as well.

A review of exercise interventions for people with schizophrenia identified eight pre-experimental, three quasi-experimental, and only one experimental study (Faulkner et al., 1999). The authors concluded that exercise could alleviate secondary symptoms of schizophrenia, such as depression, low self-esteem, and social withdrawal. For some people, exercise can also be a useful coping strategy for the positive symptoms of schizophrenia, such as auditory hallucinations.

Physical activity may also play a role in reducing social isolation for people with serious mental illness. Still, Daumit et al. (2005) found that people with serious mental illness tend to report very little confidence in their ability to exercise when feeling sad or stressed and little, if any, social support for exercise is available. Lack of regular social contact appears to be a common correlate of inactivity in this population (McDevitt et al., 2006), and low self-efficacy is one of the strongest determinants of inactivity in general (Trost et al., 2002).

This aspect of physical activity remains an under-researched area, although case studies suggest that participation in physical activity can engage individuals in mental health services, promote a sense of normalization, and offer safe opportunities for social interaction (Carter-Morris et al., 2003).

This population values the support of health professionals. Physical activity interventions for persons with severe mental illness need to be tailored to individual preferences, e.g. toward the mode of exercise and for exercising alone versus with others. Education may be beneficial concerning opportunities for leisure-based and lifestyle activity on the basis of personal preferences as opposed to prescribed and structured exercise regimens (Richardson et al., 2005). In addition, mental health service users have a right to participate in recreational and leisure pursuits, such as physical activity, which are enjoyed by the community at large.

Another aspect to consider is that 40% to 80% of individuals on second-generation antipsychotic medications gain up to 20% of their ideal body weight. Clozapine and olanzapine are the worst offenders (Simpson et al., 2001). For people taking these medications, weight gain and its sequelae are major health concerns. Among people with schizophrenia, antipsychotic medications and poor lifestyle factors contribute to high rates of obesity, hyperlipidemia, hypertension and diabetes (Sernyak et al., 2003).

People with schizophrenia frequently experience motivation and energy problems, symptoms that reduce their capacity for healthy nutrition and regular physical activity (Allison et al., 1999). Also, the fear of weight gain may undermine medication compliance (Coldham et al., 2002),

which may lead to relapse. One approach to weight gain is regular exercise at a gym. Archie et al. (2003) tried to offer patients with schizophrenia a six-month membership to a YMCA fitness facility, but after 6 months high drop-out rate was found. The main reason given for poor attendance was lack of motivation. Motivating patients to participate in an exercise program poses a great challenge for clinicians. Archie et al. (2007) noted that many patients with psychotic disorders, after changing their eating and physical activity habits, saw increased intensity and frequency of physical activity, increased readiness to consider changing physical activity habits, and increased self-perceived satisfaction with body function and appearance.

More patients may be ready to consider lifestyle changes than clinicians realize. Mental health workers often overlook diet and exercise as viable interventions for people with mental illness (Callaghan, 2004).

3.1.4 The reverse of the medal: when exercise becomes a disorder itself

Exercise is, of course, the "good cure" for these situations. Because individuals not only enjoy the fitness and biochemical effects of exercise, but also have a "bond" with physical activity, which involves knowledge, motivations, and expected results, some may have a distorted and pathological view of physical activity. For example, in some individuals, physical activity becomes an obsession, resulting in an *exaggerated preoccupation with exercise and excessive training* even in the presence of medical counter indications, which can interfere with personal and occupational relationships. Studies on this subject have long characterized this condition as an analog of anorexia nervosa (Yates et al., 1982) or as an addiction (De Coverly Veale, 1987), and investigations have since been centered on a better definition of its characteristics. These studies point to differences between the characteristics of individuals that present excessive exercise associated with an eating disorder and individuals that present excessive exercise with no such association. Moreover, such reports stress that primary excessive exercise is rarely pathologic, since most exercise-dependent individuals show no signs of disease but rather present good mental health. However, case reports

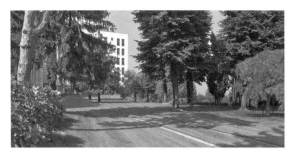

Figure 3.2 - The garden. Outdoor spaces such as this are comfortable and secure places to practice aerobic exercise or group games and sports.

(Spieker, 1996) leave no doubt regarding the possibilities of significant physical damage caused by excessive exercise.

Physical activity can also be associated with a condition of alterations in body image found among some weightlifters and bodybuilders: *muscle dysmorphia* whereby the individuals, although large and muscular, believe that they are weak and skinny. Pope et al. (1997) proposed the following criteria for the diagnosis of "muscle dysmorphia" based on the DSM-IV diagnostic criteria for body dysmorphic disorder: excessive preoccupation with the idea that their body is not sufficiently slim (in terms of a low fat content) and muscular. This preoccupation causes discomfort and significant impaired social functioning and cannot be explained by any other psychiatric disorder. In addition to its association with physical activity, evidence indicates a relationship between the presence of muscle dysmorphia and a history of mood, anxiety, and eating disorders (Olivardia et al., 2000). As muscle dysmorphia is often associated with *use of anabolic-androgenic steroids* (Pope et al., 1997) and anabolic-androgenic steroids are almost exclusively used by physically-active individuals, this is another situation likely to reflect an association between physical activity and impaired mental health. The effect of these substances is characterized by significant increases in irritability and aggressiveness and by the occurrence of manic-like and psychotic symptoms as well as of depressive symptoms during periods of abstinence (Peluso et al., 2000). In addition, it has been suggested that the continuous use of these substances can lead to a condition of dependence (Brower, 1993).

Physical activity is not associated only with improvement of mood. There are reports indicating *mood disturbances* compared to the state before exercise (Blanchard et al., 2001), which also seems to be the case after a few days of intense physical activity (O'Connor et al., 1991). On a medium- and long-term basis, worsened mood has been reported after high-intensity exercise lasting for 10 days to some weeks (Peluso, 2003). The studies that found these mood disturbances have mainly monitored elite athletes of sport modalities that require a high degree of aerobic fitness (the so-called endurance sports such as swimming, cycling, and long-distance running). For normal individuals, a constant and moderate physical activity, characterized by the so-called "sub-maximal endurance training," consisting of continuous and prolonged exercise in order to improve aerobic fitness which does not exceed the anaerobic threshold, is sufficient to achieve the physiological adaptations necessary to improve such aerobic fitness. The training season of high-level endurance athletes essentially consists of 3 different training periods: 1) an initial period at the beginning of the season with increasing numbers of mainly sub-maximal endurance training regimens; 2) a period during which sessions of a high quantity of submaximal endurance training are intercalated with sessions of high-intensity interval training (where the remaining time between training sessions doesn't allow complete recovery of the athlete due to "superadaptation" of the organism as a necessary event to support the large quantity and intensity of training); 3) a final period close to the competition during which training sessions are fewer and comprise lower intensity exercise which allow the athlete to rest so that they can reach their maximum potential at the time of the competition (Raglin, 1993). The monitoring of elite athletes during their training (Morgan et al., 1987; Steinacker et al., 2000) showed for most athletes a worsening of mood from the first to the second training period, followed by improvement from the second to the third period, i.e. mood improved just before competition when an increase in anxiety is expected. However, Peluso (2003) stated that mood changes associated with physical activity are much closer to the construct of depression than to the construct of anxiety.

Most athletes experience the mood deterioration observed without impairment in sport performance; in fact most of these athletes show improved performance at the end of the season. However, excessive training (or a lack of sufficient rest period) is not a rare event. In this case, the athlete starts to present more evident problems such as sleep disturbance, loss of weight and appetite, reduced libido, irritability, heavy and painful musculature, emotional lability, and even depression (Budgett, 1990). *Overtraining syndrome* was the first and continues to be the most widely used denomination. The diagnosis of overtraining syndrome should be considered when the athlete shows a decline in sport performance following or during a period of intense training that does not improve with short-term rest (1 or 2 weeks), accompanied by symptoms listed above. The similarity between the signs and symptoms of overtraining syndrome and depressive disorder, in addition to the importance of the presence of mood changes for diagnosis, led Eichner (1989) to suggest that overtraining syndrome is "a depression with a new face." In this respect, Armstrong et al. (2002) more recently proposed that both syndromes have the same aetiology and suggested the use of anti-depressive drugs for treatment.

3.2 PSYCHOLOGICAL AND PHYSIOLOGICAL MECHANISMS

Numerous psychological and physiological mechanisms have been suggested to explain the beneficial effects of exercise on mental health. Controversies surrounding the various psychological and physiological mechanisms have led several authors to conclude that an integrative psychobiological model that combines components of each hypothesis offers the most likely explanation (Petruzzello et al., 1991; North et al., 1990). In this section, a brief definition and description of the most studied psychological and physiological mechanisms will be presented. We will also describe the impact of the psychological mechanisms in different psychological domains, including cognitive performance, reaction to stressful events, and self-perception.

3.2.1 Psychological mechanism

There are many psychological mechanisms that are hypothesised to mediate in the relationship between physical activity and mental health, and well-being in general.

The *distraction hypothesis* suggests that diversion from unpleasant stimuli or painful somatic complaints leads to positive effect after an exercise session (Hill, 1987). Recent reviews (Yeung, 1996; North et al., 1990) have challenged the primary role of distraction in explaining changes in psychological well-being associated with chronic physical activity, but have suggested that distraction may account for some of the antidepressant effects of acute exercise.

Another popular psychological mechanism is the *self-efficacy theory* initially proposed by Bandura (1977). Proponents of this theory claim that confidence in the individual's ability to engage in a specific activity is strongly related to the individual's ability to perform the behavior. The importance of the self-efficacy theory, and the relationships between perceived self-efficacy and physical activity, will be examined in greater detail later in this text.

A third proposed psychological mechanism, the *mastery hypothesis*, suggests that command of a challenging pursuit such as exercise either promotes a sense of independence and success, or causes depression as result of a loss of control over one's body (Mellion, 1985). As participants become more confident and gain control over their physical skills, they may transpose this feeling of control and success into their everyday lives. By becoming their own supporter, it has been suggested, exercisers can use individual resources continue to improve their mental health (Griest et al., 1979).

Finally, the *social interaction hypothesis* postulates that the social relationships and mutual support that exercisers provide each other account for a substantial portion of the effects of exercise on mental health (Ransford, 1982). However, other studies comparing individual home programs and community group programs suggest that social interaction appears to be unnecessary for psychological benefits to occur (Glenister, 1996). This leads to the hypothesis that social interaction, although it cannot be considered the primary mediator of the antidepressant effects of physical activity, may have some importance at the beginning of an exercise program (North et al., 1990).

3.2.2 Exercise and cognitive performance

Many studies have investigated the relationship between exercise and cognitive functioning, seeking to shed light on how constant and proper physical activity can affect the mental performance of people. Thomas et al. (1994) present an early meta-analysis on the evaluation of the impact of exercise on cognitive functioning; among the variables taken into account in the reported studies we can find tests of mathematical ability, reaction time, standardized tests for cognitive performance, durability and intensity of the programs and characteristics of the subjects (in particular age and sex). The major effects of exercise on cognitive functioning have been found in pre-adolescent subjects or in women over 30 years old. In addition, it was noted that a constant training has more positive effects than single training sessions or short programs repeated after a period of time. These findings were confirmed by Etnier et al. (1997), which suggest that the influence of exercise on cognitive functioning is inversely correlated to short-term training programs, leading to limited changes in the physiology of the organism.

Thus, exercise would have an impact on cognitive functioning only if carried out regularly, and therefore positively impacting the global body's physiological functioning. It might be hypothesised that the value of these results are reduced due to the nature of most of the methodologies applied in the reviewed studies: they are non-experimental. However, Etnier (1997), considering only experimental studies, highlights that the described effect, though reduced, remains: in particular, it seems that it is not related to the duration in time of physical activity, or to its frequency. This result suggests a feature of the relationship among exercise and fitness and cognitive performance: they appear to act in parallel (and not as a consequence) with each other.

The impact of exercise on cognitive functioning has also been studied in relation to the process of cognitive impairment due to aging. Longitudinal studies conducted are few, and the results are unclear (Dustman et al., 1994). Most of the studies, all cross-cutting and non-experimental, show that physically active older people get higher scores in cognitive tests (Chodzko-Zajko et al., 1992; Emery et al., 1995). From the analysis of the literature it seems that for this population it is even more difficult to isolate the impact of important variables such as education level, level of residual cognitive functioning, and general state of health (Di Pietro et al., 1996). Furthermore, most studies examining the effects of exercise on the aging process have focused on physical and psychological effects, neglecting in part the importance of exercise for the maintenance and development of social relationships, while even World Health Organization guidelines (1997) deal with the effects of exercise on socio-cultural variables. In fact, aging involves a redefinition of social role, due to changes in job, health status, etc. Waning parental responsibilities or changes regarding employment require a redefinition of personal identity (McPherson, 1990), and physical activity may contribute to a smoother adjustment in this process, through a broadening of social networks, encouraging new relationships and new roles.

3.2.3 Exercise and reaction to stressful events

In recent years many studies have been published showing that exercise programs have beneficial effects on the ability to cope with perceived stress (Emery et al., 1988; Ossip-Klein et al., 1989). The term "stress" identifies responses that are generated by comparing features of the individual (skills, resources, etc.) and the stressful situation (stressor). A sense of discomfort occurs when the individual interprets events or situations experienced as "potentially threatening" or "potentially dangerous," or when resources are assessed as "insufficient to address and manage the situation." Regular exercise seems to help to counteract the harmful effects of stress on health: several studies have shown that the impact of negative life events on the perception of health status is lower among persons who perform regular exercise or who are characterized by high levels of aerobic fitness (Brown, 1991; Long et al., 1993). Regarding the impact of physical exercise as a contrast to stress, a distinction must be made between the benefit resulting from a change in the physiological response to stressful events and the subjectively perceived benefits: several experimental studies have evaluated the changes in *physiological responses* to stressful stimuli standardized before and after participation in training programs. Despite the significant increase in the level of aerobic fitness measured in all trials following the training program, the effects of training on stress reactivity (or recovery from stress) have been quite discouraging (De Geus et al., 1993). In general, changes in the levels of responsiveness to stressful stimuli after treatment in the group of aerobic exercise are not significantly greater than those observed in control subjects on the waiting list or in groups of patients undergoing alternative treatments, although in many studies, the average is in the expected direction (Blumenthal et al., 1990). Probably, the lack of significant effects is due to the short duration of training programs: enough to obtain a significant increase in fitness levels, but maybe not to create the necessary psychological and physiological basis for reduction in stress reactivity. To test this hypothesis, De Geus et al. (1993) provided subjects an eight month training program. The study considered a group of 55 male subjects, sedentary, aged between 26 and 40 years. To assess possible changes in response to a stressful stimulus, subjects were divided into two groups competing with each other in identifying a significant stimulus (a loud explosive noise) as quickly as possible to win a cash prize. Physiological parameters considered included heart rate, blood pressure and respiratory responses, and levels of catecholamines in the urine. The results show that even in this case the reaction to the stress was not different from that of the control group. Results seem to exclude the presence of significant effects of exercise in reducing reactivity to stressful stimuli. According to De Geus et al. (1993) these results do not exclude the possibility that exercise plays a role as mediator between stressors and health for many reasons. First, in research conducted a laboratory, the stressful stimuli for the subjects are generally new and unknown, while it is possible that exercise may act only on the individual's ability to cope with constant and known stressors. Claytor (1991), in fact, does not detect any difference between trained and sedentary subjects at the first administration of stressor, but after repeated presentation, subjects decreased their response to stressors (became familiar) to a greater extent than sedentary subjects. Second, exercise could act as a modulator on the effect of stressful events without causing any change in the physiological response to stress: a stressor, in order to have an affect on health, blood pressure or heart rate, must exceed a certain threshold value. Basically, individuals are generally far enough from this "danger zone," but are likely to cross the threshold in stressful situations. More fit individuals, having a better trained cardiovascular system, although responding to the stressors just like those who are more sedentary, may not reach (or

are less likely to reach) the danger area for their health, as they have the "threshold level" raised due to training.

With regard to the *subjective perception* of the negative effects of stressful events and the way this can be influenced by exercise, it is interesting to consider the model proposed by Long et al. (1993), based on the Lazarus and Folkman model of stress and coping (1984). According to this model, when there is a potentially stressful situation the individual assesses the significance (primary evaluation) and coping methods (secondary evaluation), and tries to identify the most appropriate responses in that situation (coping responses) and the resources actually available (coping resources). The *coping responses* are defined as "continuing efforts for cognitive and behavioral changes, carried out in order to manage specific internal and/or external needs" (Lazarus et al., 1984). These responses are actions for which the specific implementation, directly addressed to the problem (problem-centred coping) or dealing with their reaction to stressful stimuli (emotion-focused coping), will be decided when the stressful event occurs. *Coping resources* consist of the evaluations that individuals make of themselves and their own personal resources to cope with the stressful event (e.g. perceived social support, health status), and generally refer to the self-concept.

It is generally believed that exercise helps the individual to cope with the emotions that follow a stressful stimulus. Of course, exercise does not result in direct elimination or modification of the stressful event, but it can act both as an emotional regulator (Morgan, 1997), which helps to achieve a state of relaxation by reducing muscle tension (De Vries, 1976), or as a form of distraction (Howley et al., 1997). The stress-reduction function of exercise is now part of the lifestyle of many people: sport is not only an opportunity for one to improve fitness, but also a time to relax from the strain of everyday life. In this sense, if a work problem (stressor) creates a state of tension (stress), the person may decide to relieve it with an outdoor run (coping response focused on emotion). The effects of exercise are not limited to this. Physical activity also affects the constant knowledge that people develop about themselves, their value and level of personal effectiveness. For example, an athlete, conscious of having a good workout, is likely to develop a positive evaluation of himself, perhaps by thinking he is in good shape, and believing he will be able to successfully achieve his objectives. This would in turn generate an increase of coping resources and improved self-concept, with a positive impact on coping with difficulties in a different context (for example, the workplace), activating coping responses centred on the problem.

3.2.4 Exercise and self-concept: role of self-efficacy and self-esteem in physical activity

When choosing a sport, or a form of exercise in general, some psychological dimensions are crucial: concepts such as self-efficacy, self-esteem and physical self-concept have assumed great importance in the explanation of behavioral conduct linked to physical activity. Bandura (1977) defines *self-efficacy* as "beliefs about the ability to perform a task or, more specifically, to successfully adopt a certain behavior." These beliefs influence the choice of activity to perform, the amount of tolerated hard work, and the level of persistence in case of difficulty. Indeed, the runner mentioned above may have chosen running as physical activity because he feels suited to it, perceiving himself as able to achieve satisfactory results, and will train constantly, maybe even with bad weather. His level of self-efficacy could be derived from previous experiences, such as successful participation in sporting events (results are probably the most influential variable in determining the perception of our own physical ability), the comparison with other opponents or companions (vicarious experience), verbal persuasion by other people, some good perceptions coming from the body such as heart rate, muscle contractions, and so on.

Self-efficacy can be both an antecedent variable, which can affect the start and maintenance of exercise, and a variable resulting from physical exercise leading to success in the improving of the perception of personal abilities (McAuley, 1992). Individuals who have a high self-efficacy tend to perceive in any case the effort associated with physical activity as less demanding and stressful than those with low self-efficacy. The term *self-regulating efficacy*, coined by Bandura (1997), seems to better explain the beliefs that each of us have about the ability to perform in a way that will lead to the expected results. The self-regulating efficacy should not be confused with the expectations about outcomes, but refers to the feeling of

being able to "cope" successfully with the obstacles or challenges that may jeopardize the good outcome of the action. These beliefs have a proactive function: when the obstacles, whether real or perceived, are overcome successfully, the relationship between personal efficacy and exercise is strengthened.

The construct of self-efficacy, although relevant, cannot exhaust all the personal meanings in the relationship between exercise and well-being, since it mostly emphasizes the cognitive dimension. The evaluative dimension is rather seen as central to *self-esteem*, defined by Harter (1993) as the perception of self-worth and considered the most valid indicator of psychological well-being and social adaptation. The role of self-esteem in the relationship between exercise and health has been recognized by the International Society of Sport Psychology (1992), which identified the improvement of self-esteem as a key element, allowing the expression of psychological benefits resulting from participating to exercise programs, particularly in people with specific diseases such as hypertension, osteoporosis, type II diabetes and some psychiatric disorders.

Two hypotheses about the relationship between exercise and self-esteem have been developed. According to the *hypothesis of self-growth*, people, in order to maintain their sense of excellence (and therefore a high level of self-esteem), will try activities perceived as a challenge, in order to experience positive feelings or to demonstrate their skills (Fox, 1997; Biddle, 1997). On the other side, the *hypothesis of skills-development* states that exercise contributes to improved self-perception by improving general and motor skills. The relationship between physical activity and self-esteem seems to be circular: on one hand self-esteem increases the likelihood that the individual tries the exercise, on the other it is a factor that helps to improve the perception of themselves.

An interesting interpretation of the link between physical activity and perceived self-esteem is the use of the *multidimensional hierarchical model* of Shavelson et al. (1976), whereby self-concept is organized in hierarchical and structured components (e.g. academic self-concept, emotional, social, physical). Each component is itself composed of more elements and facets relating to more specific skills and context-dependent features. Within the concept of *physical self* the main elements are physical ability, including strength and coordination, and physical appearance, which is reflected by having smooth muscle or by taking care of aesthetics.

According to the theory of Shavelson, over the years the concept of Self becomes more differentiated and undergoes repeated changes, especially in the peripheral part of the hypothesized hierarchical structure. In this model, the concept of Self refers to descriptive and evaluative aspects, that include those judgments, positive or negative, that the person gives of themselves. These evaluations can be conducted on the basis of absolute ideals (e.g. to win a competition), personal standards (e.g. improving a previous performance), generalized expectations in relation to the expectations of significant others (e.g. parents or teachers) or vice versa, or are derived from a comparison with peers (Shavelson et al., 1976; Meleddu et al., 1998).

It should be noted, however, that the relationship between physical activity and the perception that people have of themselves is not easy to study, because it must consider many complex variables specific to the subject. To shed light on this complexity, Sonstroem (1997) proposes that the relationship between participation in physical activity and increased self-esteem would be mediated by the intervention of the perception of physical competence in relation to specific skills associated with exercise or with the athletic situation. This perception, in turn, would be able to increase the level of attraction of individuals with regard to physical activity. Perceived physical competence would therefore be a mediating variable between the physical aspects of motor activity and psychological level of self-esteem. A new model, known as EXSEM (Extension of the Self Esteem Model) incorporates the original Sonstroem's model, providing a better specification of the value that everybody applies to their physical self (physical self-worth): it considers the perceptions of effectiveness in relation to specific aspects of motor activity, already identified by Fox et al., (1989), such as the perception of physical competence, physical condition, and the force and attraction of the body, and relates them to concepts of self-efficacy and value associated with the body. This value is considered a key component of global self-esteem and a valid indicator of adaptation and psychological well-being. It was observed that the perceived self-efficacy correlates more strongly with some aspects, such as perceived physical competence, physical condi-

tion and strength, while the value associated with the figure correlates closely with the level of attractiveness of the body. The pattern of correlations proposed raises the risk that an individual's measure of their own attractiveness represents a potential source of confusion in the study of the relationship between physical self-concept, physical activity and health: the effect of an increase of self-efficacy on the value associated with the figure, obtained through the positive assessment of physical competence, physical fitness and strength, could be overshadowed by a negative assessment on the degree of attraction attributed to the body. Let's think about a person who seeks to lose weight through exercise: in case the individual does not succeed in this goal, thereby strengthening the negative assessment of the degree of attractiveness of the body, the results obtained in terms of fitness (related to the perception of physical competence, physical fitness, strength) may be underestimated or ignored, contributing to low self-esteem.

In summary, it is possible to highlight how the starting of physical activity poses challenges and requires a significant amount of effort and persistence. This is the reason why expectations about efficacy are important regulators of motivation, which can promote participation in physical activities not aimed at achieving results in competitions (Guicciardi et al., 1999). In the subsequent maintenance phase of physical activity, the crucial role of self-efficacy tends to be reduced, and more comprehensive assessments involving the various facets of physical self-concept become more important.

3.2.5 Physiological mechanism

Physiological changes that occur with physical activity have also received significant attention. Some different hypothesis have been developed, in order to explain the effect of physical activity on mental health, but at present there is no general accepted overall theory.

One well studied mechanism is the *monoamine hypothesis*, which proposes that exercise enhances brain aminergic synaptic transmission (Ransford, 1982). The primary monoamines in the brain, noradrenaline (norepinephrine), dopamine and serotonin, affect arousal and attention and also have been implicated in depressive and sleep disorders. A large body of studies and research describes the relationship between the pathophysiological theory of monamine for the development of depression, namely the lack of serotonin, norepinephrine and dopamine in the brain, and exercise. Results show that exercise increases the availability of serotonin and norepinephrine in the brain. Clinical evidence suggests that exercise stimulates the functions of serotonin in the brain. In animals, exercise increases the levels of tryptophan, the precursor of serotonin, in the blood and cerebrospinal fluid, promotes serotonergic transmission, and increases production of proteins involved in the functions of serotonin (Chaouloff, 1989; Meeusen et al., 1995). After exercise in men, increased concentration of the metabolite of serotonin, 5 idrossindolacetic acid, and reduced levels of branched-chain amino acids that compete with tryptophan for uptake into the brain were found in peripheral blood. Exercise in experimental animals induced an immediate increase in the number of brain cells producing norepinephrine. Moreover, continuous exercise increased levels of norepinephrine and its metabolites and the activation of tyrosine hydroxylase, an enzyme involved in the production of norepinephrine. This was consistent with the positive effects on mood. Recent reviews have supported the monoamine hypothesis as a tenable, although oversimplified, explanation of the antidepressant effects of exercise (Dunn et al., 1991). Actually, increased levels of dopamine could be detected in peripheral blood after exercise, even though they seem not to be statistically correlated to reduced depression (Bliss et al., 1991).

The observed effects of exercise on the *axis hypothalamus-pituitary-adrenal* (HPA) suggest that exercise can help reverse or reduce the potential failure of the HPA axis. Although acute exercise can increase levels of stress hormones such as cortisol and corticotropin (which can induce a state of mood activation), long-term exercise seems to blunt the body's response not only to stress due to exercise, but also to stress in general (Sutton et al., 1989; Stranahan et al., 2008). The effects of acute versus continuous exercise on the HPA axis are very interesting, parallel to those on norepinephrine, according to the interactions that exist between these two systems.

The monoamine hypothesis of depression is increasingly considered by newer theories that rotate around changes in neuronal plasticity, primarily in the hippocampus, at both the structural and the functional levels. The *neurotrophic hypothesis* of depression is based on the observation that stress hampers, while drug treatments help to improve, the ability to generate new brain cells and support existing ones. Both stress and antidepressants have been shown to affect levels of: brain-derived neurotrophic factor (BDNF), a factor that promotes the proliferation, survival and synaptogenesis of nerve cells; Insulin-Like Growth Factor 1 (ILGF-1), which promotes cell growth and inhibits programmed cell death; and Vascular Endothelial Growth Factor (VEGF), which promotes angiogenesis in nervous tissue. BDNF itself has antidepressant-like actions. One class of genes regulated by both BDNF and serotonin (5-HT) are neuropeptides such as VGF (non-acryonimic), which has a novel role in depression. Neuropeptides are important modulators of neuronal function, but their role in affective disorders is just emerging. Based on these results, it has been argued that factors governing the health of neurons subtend the pathophysiology of depression, rather than the neurotransmitters themselves. BDNF and other neurotrophins are also believed to play an important role in affective disorders: low levels of BDNF are found in patients with neurodegenerative diseases, including Alzheimer's disease and major depression. Moreover, it is well established that BDNF plays a role in the hypothalamic pathway that controls body weight and energy homeostasis. Exercise increases, in both humans and animals, neurotrophic factors in blood, and in particular BDNF (Van Praag, 2008). BDNF is likely to mediate some of the beneficial effects of exercise with regard to protection against neurodegenerative diseases. Gustafsson et al. (2009) investigated plasma-BDNF response during an incremental exercise test in patients suffering from moderate major depressive disorders, not treated with antidepressants or neuroleptics. The results shows no difference in basal BDNF levels between patients and controls. BDNF increased significantly during exercise with no significant differences between the groups. No correlation between BDNF and cortisol or Montgomery-Asberg Depression Rating Scale (MADRS) scores was found. Recent studies demonstrated that VGF is up-regulated by antidepressant drugs and voluntary exercise, and is reduced in animal models of depression. VGF enhances hippocampal synaptic plasticity as well as neurogenesis in the dentate gyrus but the mechanisms of antidepressant-like actions of VGF in behavioral paradigms are not known. Some experimental data underlie the emerging roles of BDNF, VGF and other neuropeptides in depression and how they may be acting through the generation of new neurons and altered synaptic activity (Thakker-Varia et al., 2008). Understanding the molecular and cellular changes that underlie the actions of neuropeptides and how these adaptations result in antidepressant-like effects will aid in developing drugs that target novel pathways for major depressive disorders.

The *endorphin hypothesis* is another popular hypothesis used to explain the effects of physical activity on mental health (Moore, 1982; Thoren et al., 1990). Endorphins, particularly ß-endorphin, are produced in several endogenous locations and have been shown to reduce pain and potentiate a euphoric state. Extended exercise significantly activates endorphin secretion, but it has not been clearly shown that this increase subsequently alters mood states.

This increase of endorphins can lead to the emergence of the phenomenon that the Anglo-Saxon authors call "runner's high," characterized by a sense of euphoria and insensitivity to pain experienced after strenuous physical activity. Clinical evidence shows an increased concentration of endorphins both in blood and cerebrospinal fluid after an intense exercise, and a reduction of the "runner's high" after administration of naloxone, an opioid antagonist (Morgan, 1985, Carr et al., 1981). It must be said that the "runner's high" does not occur in everyone and does not necessarily take place only after a race, and is perhaps due to dysregulation of the neuromodulator system. Therefore this phenomenon hardly explains the antidepressant effect of exercise.

Moreover, naloxone blocked the endorphin-generated pain threshold elevation but failed to decrease the mental health benefits seen following exercise. Some believe that endorphins primarily produce energy conservation during exercise. Therefore a psychological effect is subsequently facilitated rather than directly produced. Further research is needed to clarify the relationship between endorphins and mood states, and to identify the specific endorphins responsible.

Other less popular physiological hypotheses include the *thermogenic model*, suggesting that increase in body temperature is responsible for mood improvements following exercise, and the *visceral afferent-feedback hypothesis*, which impli-

cates the increase in afferent impulses arising from muscular and autonomic activity during exercise. Meta-analyses of these hypotheses have not supported clear relationships between these proposed mechanisms and mental health benefits, and other studies have refuted them (Yeung et al., 1996).

3.3 PHYSICAL ACTIVITY: HANDLE WITH CARE

While the clinical evidence supports a positive relationship between exercise and mood, exercise might present some problems and there is the necessity to be pragmatic in promoting physical activity in patients. The effectiveness of physical exercise as a tool for promoting and maintaining an individual's health principally relies on the willingness of the individual to adhere to a physically active lifestyle. Because exercise is a successful treatment, a large amount of energy, commitment, and motivation must be sought from patients. Optimizing long-term compliance is one of the most challenging objectives of all physical-activity interventions. Adherence to the program is a critical factor in the outcome of treatment; patients must engage in the exercise program for a period of time to experience the therapeutic benefits.

The drop out rate in the depressed population is around 20%, and this result is similar (in some cases better) to other therapies for depression (MacGillivray et al., 2003). Following regular physical activity according to the intensity and timing recommended for health benefits, at least initially, can be a challenge for depressed patients, especially for those who have always led a sedentary life or have a serious physical illness.

The *theory of decisional balance* (Janis et al., 1977) has been used in assessing, predicting, and enhancing behavioral changes among a variety of samples, including physically inactive individuals. Individuals who are physically active will perceive the benefits of exercise (e.g. weight loss, improved health, opportunity to meet people) and this will outweigh the barriers (e.g. bad weather, physical discomfort) of adopting a more physically active lifestyle (Prochaska et al., 1994). Clinicians should aim to identify and emphasize the potential benefits of physical exercise, thus adaptively shifting the individual's perception of the potential value of adopting a more physically active lifestyle. The identification of perceived barriers to participation in physical exercise is extremely important in order to reduce or overcome potential obstacles. Participation in exercise will continue as long as the exercising behavior is reinforced. Reinforcement of behavior occurs when its perceived positive consequences are judged as outweighing the perceived negative consequences of performing that behavior (Kazdin, 1994). Reinforcing events can range from physiological adaptations, such as enhanced cardiovascular fitness, to psychosocial rewards, such as, reduced feelings of depression and increased social support. Perceived negative consequences such as pain/discomfort and poor task performance must be minimized to ensure that the behavior is not in any way experienced as punishing. Enjoyment is one of the most powerful reinforcers of a behavior and might be more important for mental-health benefits than any single modality of exertion (Sime, 1997).

The identification of specific, realistically obtainable goals is important in establishing a sense of meaning and direction for the individual. Goals should be set in such a way as to enhance intrinsic motivation. Intrinsic motivation is characterized by an inherent desire and curiosity to respond to the challenges associated with a specific behavior. Participation, performance, and adherence to physical exercise might be more readily optimized among those who are intrinsically motivated. Morris et al. (1995) suggest that intrinsically motivated individuals are involved in physical exercise for fun, personal mastery, and the positive experience that results from personal achievement, a sense of competency, perceived control, and positive self-regard.

3.3.1 Physical activity for mental health promotion: main features

The literature reports few definitive statements or recommendations on optimal physical activity quantity, intensity, or type. This is often attributed to the fundamental complexity of both "mental health" and "physical activity;" and more importantly, the complex relationship between them (Ekeland et al., 2005). No generic mechanisms have been established to explain the positive effects of activity on psychological improvement. The effects in individuals are likely to be more variable than those found with physiological or biomedical change and may depend on the subjective experience of the activity and the setting in which it takes place. More specifically, research on this association was seen as being still in the relatively early stage, particularly in relation to understanding the associations between particular types of physical activity and various dimensions of mental health. However, it is possible to identify some basic features of physical activity.

3.3.2 Frequency and duration

There appeared to be a general association between increased quantities of physical activity (a product of both the duration of each physical activity session and the frequency of the sessions) and enhanced mental wellbeing, although it should be noted though that only a limited number of studies have confirmed this general trend (Fox et al., 2007).

There is little consensus on optimal frequency of activity; Fox (2000), concluding that there is insufficient variance in the studies to assess the impact of frequency, noted that the conventional view has tended to work within outmoded physical activity guidelines and to associate activity with formal physical education and sport. An accepted, though not necessarily valid, norm of three sessions per week has therefore tended to be used. On the basis of updated guidance, a norm for frequency would clearly move to being active on "most days of the week."

Within the context of what appear to be formally delivered physical activity opportunities (that is, discrete "sessions" of activity typically 30-45 minutes in duration offered 3 times per week), significant effect was found in durations ranging from 60 to 180 minutes per week (Fox, 2000, Calfas et al., 1994).

In contrast, others opted to work within a context that avoided associating physical activity with formally delivered opportunities and favored a broader "active living" definition. These studies suggested that 60 minutes of daily activity can result in potential mental health gain. Importantly, however, it is recognized that, compared to physiological benefit, for some individuals lesser levels may be sufficient for mental wellbeing gain: the quality of the physical activity experience may be as important as quantity (Hallal et al., 2006).

In summary, the reviews suggested that the optimal quantity of activity associated with mental health was generally in line with the existing physiologically oriented guideline of accumulating at least 60 minutes of physical activity per day (Parfitt et al., 2005). Significantly, relatively lower quantities of high quality physical activity may be sufficient for mental wellbeing gain.

3.3.3 Intensity

This area was relatively more difficult to define: in his study, Twisk (2001) concluded that there is evidence for a certain dose-response relationship or a particular threshold value from which guidelines can be obtained. Some reviews suggested that activity intensity ("gentle," "moderate," "vigorous," or "acute") or type (walking, running, aerobics, resistance training, weight lifting, low intensity exercise or psychosocial interventions), have no real impact on the end benefit (Larun et al., 2006; Fox et al., 2007). All had the potential to generally enhance mental health, and particularly to improve self-esteem and reduce symptoms of anxiety, depression, and stress. In contrast, Calfas et al. (1994), Fox (2000) and Leppämäki (2006) reported a differential effect in relation to activity intensity: some studies suggest that anxiety and stress are lower for those involved in high intensity aerobic activity compared to those involved in moderate intensity, flexibility type activity. Fox (2000) thus concludes that optimal activity intensity would be at least "moderately demanding." However, in relation to mood within the general population, Leppämäki (2006) proposed a contrasting situation identifying studies showing that high initial intensity activity could even inhibit formation of new exercise habits and harm mood.

3.3.4 Length of intervention

There was more agreement on the fact that longer-term programs have the potential to be more effective, though Fox (2000) notes that the time required for lasting change is still not known. Nevertheless, a minimum of at least 12 weeks with follow-ups at 6 months or more was suggested (Fox, 2000; Calfas et al., 1994). Dunn et al. (2005) studied the use of exercise in the reduction and remission of mild to moderate depression in a general population and concluded that the fundamental variability in the dose is related to the "general weekly energy expenditure" (that is, a function of both intensity and frequency).

3.3.5 Physical activity type

A significant contribution in this area was the recognition of variance in opportunities and individual preference. For example, Bailey (2005) observed that it is important to acknowledge that sporting activities are not a homogenous, standardized product or experience, and different individuals' experiences of the same activity will be subject to wide variations, as will the effects. Despite research work undertaken using a variety of activity, this domain offers little specific guidance. There is a belief that all types of activity have the potential to enhance mental wellbeing and that much will depend on individual preference. A relatively small number of reviews (Fox, 2000; Larun et al., 2006) made more specific assertions in this area, offering a number of tentative (and not necessarily consistent) pointers: running, walking, aerobic dance, and circuit training show indications that they can be effective; activities such as swimming, flexibility training, martial arts and expressive dance have generally failed to indicate significant change; weight and resistance is superior to endurance exercise in improving body image and self-esteem; physical fitness and aerobics programs produce superior results to motor skills and sports programs; rhythmic aerobic forms of activity (walking, jogging, cycling, swimming or dancing) appear to be most appropriate and effective in those who have previously been inactive; co-operative exercise settings produce particularly strong effects; group recreational sports and activities are also likely to bring social and mood benefits; resistance exercise may have a relatively immediate effect of body perception and can therefore promote self-concept; while sports and vigorous activity can promote mental wellbeing only for those who already prefer this type of activity.

3.3.6 Physical activity for patients with serious mental illness: some indications

Physical activity has the potential to enhance the quality of life for people with serious mental illness, improving not only physical health, but also psychiatric and social disabilities. In the general population, adherence to physical activity programs drops off sharply after six months (Dishman et al., 1996). It is unrealistic to expect adherence rates to be any better for individuals with serious mental illness, which often face substantial illness-related barriers to physical activity that healthier individuals do not face. However, existing research suggests that exercise is well accepted by people with serious mental illness (Martinsen, 1995) and is often considered one of the most valued components of treatment (O'Kelly et al., 1998). In order to realize an effective exercise program, some indications should be considered.

Both structured, supervised, facility based exercise programs and lifestyle physical activity interventions that encourage participants to incorporate physical activity in their daily lives may be effective. *Structured exercise programs* are appealing because it is easier to ensure safe and appropriate levels of physical activity in a supervised setting and because adherence can be more easily verified. Disadvantages include potentially costly space, equipment, and staffing. *Lifestyle interventions* have a positive effect on risk factors for cardiovascular disease, and they may be more effective than structured exercise interventions in increasing levels of physical activity (Moreau et al., 2001). Their flexibility, lower cost, and easy integration into daily schedules might be particularly appealing: walking is one of the easiest, safest, and most inexpensive types of exercise to promote. *Individual tailored interventions* (or for specific groups), taking into account the participant's features such as age, gender, cultural background, and health status, are more effective in increasing levels of physical activity than more generic interventions (Segar et al., 2002). Interventions that focus on more moderate-intensity activities, such as walking, tend to be more successful (Dishman et al., 1996). Although more vigorous activities do improve cardio-respiratory fitness and speed weight loss, the dropout rate from such programs may be higher than with less intensive interventions. Participants need to *set goals* and *self-monitor* achievement in order to successfully change their behavior. Unfortunately, self-monitoring of physical activity, particularly lifestyle interventions, is difficult. Participation in a structured exercise program, such as a regularly scheduled group class, may be easier to recall. Several inexpensive and effective ways to help participants self-monitor their physical activity are available, like daily paper logs, and objective monitoring devices, including pedometers and heart rate monitors (Strath et al., 2000). Interventions that incorporate objective physical activity assessment are more effective than interventions that rely on participants' self-report alone (Dishman et al., 1996). Feedback is a critical component of self-monitoring and self-regulation in lifestyle change: feedback that is fine grained enough to clearly document gradual physical activity improvement can be a powerful motivator (Cameron et al., 2003). *Group interventions* are generally less expensive than *one-on-one interventions*. However, individualized attention and tailored goal setting play an important role in behavior change among people with serious mental illness. Participants need personal acknowledgment of their efforts: providing certificates of participation and holding social sessions to mark milestones can help to recognize participants' efforts. Successful achievement of and recognition for small incremental increases in physical activity gradually builds *self-efficacy*, and self-efficacy is one of the most important predictors of adherence to a physical activity program (McAuley et al., 2000). Enthusiastic, knowledgeable, and supportive exercise leaders are fundamental. Because of a number of psychological issues, including hypersensitivity about their bodies, which may be due to weight gain and life experiences with trauma, it is very important to have skilled exercise leaders who are willing to provide support to help participants overcome a number of self-esteem barriers.

Physical activity programs for individuals with serious mental illness should be integrated into mental health services. An alternative but less desirable approach would be to refer these individuals to a primary care physician or other health care provider for management of cardiovascular disease risk factors, including promotion of physical activity.

There are three important reasons for integrating the promotion of physical activity into mental health services. First, individuals with serious mental illness have frequent contact with their mental health service providers: changing health behaviors can be difficult, and frequent reinforcement can play a critical role in success-

Principles to create an effective setting for physical activity

A. Variety is important: the ability to experience a range of activity types that include a balanced 'intertwined program' between its three primary components (endurance, flexibility, and strength training), and the choice between individual or group activity (Lotan et al., 2005).

B. Requirement for ease of access to high quality and safe activity opportunities and facilities, preferably based in local communities (Lotan et al., 2005; Dykens et al., 1998)

C. Individually determined realistic goals (Dykens et al., 1998; Biddle et al., 2005)

D. Emphasis should be placed on enjoyment and immediate pay off, rather than stressing longer-term health gains (Twisk, 2001)

E. The orientation of physical activity should be toward positive experiences, decreased pressure ,and success based on a sense of accomplishment, rather than simply winning (Bailey, 2006)

F. Activity should be based on a "peer model," fostering participation in activities young people enjoy with family and friends (Lotan et al., 2005)

G. Physical activity should attempt to develop core psychological competencies such as general competence, control, autonomy and self-efficacy (Bailey, 2006)

H. Physical activity should attempt to develop physical activity competencies & skills which in turn are associated with increase in self esteem, confidence, peer acceptance (Bailey, 2005)

I. Interventions should be conscious of theories and strategies for dealing with "relapse" or with young people opting out of activity. These strategies include decisional balance and stage-based models of change (Schomer et al., 2001).

J. Physical activity interventions should be delivered via high quality teaching & coaching and (local) leadership (Bailey, 2005). Fox (2000) suggests that this particular principle may be particularly critical to the promotion of self-esteem and social and moral development.

K. At a general planning level, there is a need for physical activity opportunities to be based on a "whole system/multi-sector approach," including education, health, local authorities and community sectors (Biddle et al., 2004)

ful long-term adoption of regular physical activity. Second, barriers specific to mental illness can be more appropriately addressed by individuals who have been trained to be sensitive and supportive around these issues. Finally, physical activity may play a role in successful mental health recovery. However, primary care physicians can play an important role in collaboratively identifying behavioral goals, reinforcing efforts to reach behavioral targets, and addressing barriers to physical activity. Particularly when people with serious mental illness have co-morbid physical health problems, the involvement of medical staff can ensure that the promotion of physical activity reinforces other efforts to improve an individual's overall health and well-being (Piette et al., 2004).

Textbox 3.1 summarized the principles to create an effective setting for physical activity.

3.4 SUMMARY: CLINICAL IMPLICATIONS OF PHYSICAL ACTIVITY AND INDICATION FOR EXERCISE SETTING

Fostering good mental wellbeing and preventing mental health problems are increasingly being seen as a crucial role for public health and health improvement. Policies on mental health incorporate both mental health improvement (that is, promotion, prevention, and support) and treatment (that is, implementation of mental health legislation and mental health services), and are also reflected in a range of associated areas such as education, enterprise, and lifelong learning. The past 15 years have seen the development of considerable literature that broadly suggests physical activity has the potential to contribute toward an enhancement in mood, self-perception and self-esteem; the prevention of the development of mental health problems such as depression; and to the alleviation of symptoms resulting from mental health problems. The controversies surrounding the available data on the effects of physical activity on mental health have led to confusion among clinicians about when and how to use exercise as part of the treatment regimen for an affected person. However, several clinically relevant points can be distilled from the research and deserve mention (see Textbox 3.2).

The transition from a physically inactive to an active state is often accompanied by alterations in affect and perceived stress. Regular assessment of mood states can serve to identify potential dropouts, who are often characterized by maladaptive alterations in affect. A successful transition from a sedentary to a physically active lifestyle requires that the process of change is experienced as discrete, emotionally energizing, and free from injury and excessive overload (Schomer et al., 1994). Unlike pharmacological interventions, the use of exercise as a therapeutic means of alleviating symptoms of de-

pression, anxiety, and low self-esteem is seldom associated with adverse consequences or side effects.

The link between exercise abuse and body-image concerns, especially among women, should be appreciated and anticipated where necessary (Davis, 2000). The mood-altering effects of physical exercise might also lead to the development of compulsive behaviors, and practitioners need to be aware of this possibility. Clinicians must ensure that exercise is not used as a substitute for counselling when counselling is required (Sime, 1997).

Regular participation in physical activity is associated with a variety of psychological benefits; exercise could thus be used (both as an adjunct to and in place of alternative therapies) as a means of enhancing psychological well-being and absolute health.

Many of the reviews speculated about the relative contribution of activity in itself against the broader social activity environment that might be significant in promoting mental wellbeing (Mutrie et al., 1998; Penedo et al., 2005).

TEXTBOX **3.2**

Exercise and mental health: clinically relevant points

A. Regular physical activity may play an important role in alleviating symptoms of depression and anxiety.
B. Both aerobic training and strength/flexibility training appear equally effective for treating depressive and anxiety symptoms.
C. Emphasizing physical activity itself rather than resultant cardiovascular fitness seems more effective in improving mental health symptoms and mood.
D. Physical activity appears as effective as psychotherapy for the treatment of mild-to-moderate depressive symptoms.
E. Individuals diagnosed with clinical depression with more severe symptoms or the need for psychological care manifest the greatest improvement in mood following increased physical activity.
F. No evidence has conclusively shown that physical activity prevents the onset of depression, but exercise may diminish the likelihood of individuals with mild depressive symptoms to develop major depressive disorder.
G. Physical activity adherence rates among depressed individuals are similar to other healthy populations, but simple, inexpensive exercise suggestions may improve overall compliance.
H. State anxiety improves with acute exercise, but the response of trait anxiety to chronic exercise is less clear.
I. Physical activity improves the symptoms of panic disorder without significant risks but is often avoided due to concerns about exercise triggering a life-threatening event.
J. Staleness resulting from overtraining and excessive exercise should be treated with prompt activity reduction and monitoring of the patient's depressive symptoms.

Psychopharmacological **drugs** and **physical activity**

4

Luciano Antonio Fiorellini Bernardis

4.1 INTRODUCTION

The purpose of this chapter is to highlight the main effects of some psychopharmacological drugs on several physical and biological functions of the human body. Psychoactive drugs interact with specific sites or receptors found in the nervous system to induce changes in psychological or physiological functions.

The structure of the nervous system can be schematized in the following three points:
1. an afferent branch (sensitive), that collects the information coming from both the external and the internal world;
2. an efferent branch (effector), that organizes the reactions and guides the muscular (voluntary, cardiac, and involuntary) and endocrine system;
3. a system that elaborates data from these branches producing "answers" with the function of maintaining homeostasis. A part of the elaboration implies mental activity, partly conscious and partly non conscious (thoughts, sentiments, emotions, dreams, memories). Another part of the elaboration involves changes in the organism so the adaptation (homeostasis) can be realized through the automatic nervous system.

These systems are related continuously, influencing one each other.

According to this scheme, an occurrence that at any point modifies this circuit changes and determines the deriving biological and mental functions. Given the complexity of mental/nervous action it is very difficult to consider and forecast how and how much it can be influenced by a determined occurrence. It is reasonable to think that it is possible to influence mental activity operating through apparently distant systems, like muscles, and through the inducements that movement has on the other systems such as the endocrine and immune system and on the releasing of neurotransmitter agents such as endorphins and neuropeptides. To assist our knowledge on how one can realize and control these inducements, we will examine the use of physical activity as a proper psychoactive therapy (see Chapter 3), controlled and guided by experts in the field, and not only as a separate, recreational or rehabilitative activity. It is well-known that the majority of people with mental health problems assume one or more psychoactive drugs, often for long periods, sometimes throughout their whole lives. In this venue, we will try:
- to schematize some possible consequences of the use of psychoactive substances on the overall behavior of persons;
- to give useful information to those who use physical activity as a therapeutic aid for people affected by mental illnesses.

4.2 ADVERSE DRUG REACTIONS

Adverse Drug Reactions (ADRs) are defined in Europe as harmful and unintentional reactions to a drug that has been administered in the adequate doses. In addition, the European Guidelines (Eudralex) include adverse reactions when the administered drug is off-label and/or when doses are higher compared to those reported in the provided indication (for medical indication, overdose, abuse). In the USA the FDA (Food and Drug Administration) is more broad-minded and define ADRs as any adverse reaction associated with the use of a drug, even those not clearly correlated and independent of correct dose or not, suspension or abuse. Every suspect adverse reaction should be

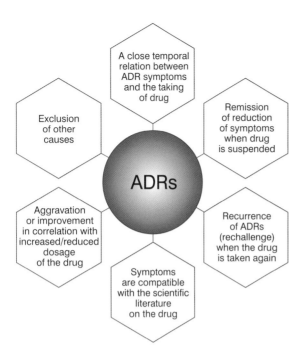

Figure 4.1 - Adverse drug reactions (ADRs).

reported by psychiatrists to the appropriate authorities.

It must be considered that ADRs can depend on some specific factors, these are described in Figure 4.1.

Risk factors that should be considered in patients with psychiatric disorders are:

- age;
- association with other drugs;
- combination with other illnesses;
- duration of the treatment (and of the illness);
- gender;
- ethnicity;
- previous adverse reactions;
- low therapeutic index of the drug (e.g. lithium salts).

Exercise science specialists and psychomotor therapists should consider some specific characteristics of persons with mental health problems in the implementation of physical activity into the rehabilitation program:

- the illness severity (intense symptomatology);
- the chronic course (persistent symptomatology);
- taking many drugs (4 drugs represents the risk threshold for ADRs). A recent review

shows that in the USA, 40% of the elderly population are prescribed 5 or more different drugs, 12% of them 10 or more (Williams et al., 2004);

- the greater part of persons with mental health problems are treated as outpatients, having no regular medical controls for pharmacotherapy.

With regards to physical activity, it must be considered that physical activity can improve and prevent but also provoke and worsen certain ADRs (see Chapter 3). Consequently, it is important to pay attention to possible side effects and to prevent and avoid negative consequences due to potential negative combination of exercise and unfavorable effects of drugs.

4.3 MAIN ADVERSE REACTIONS DUE TO PSYCHOTROPIC DRUGS

Below this paragraph a schematic list of the main adverse reactions (ADRs) that can be associated with the use of substances that act upon the Central Nervous System (CNS) is shown.

- Cognition:
  - sedation;
  - alteration of understanding;
  - Medication-Induced Movement Disorders (MIMDs).
- Lack of coordination:
  - ataxia;
  - convulsions, seizures;
  - dizziness, vertigo.
- Abnormalities of sensation:
  - loss of sensation;
  - paresthesia, disesthesia.
- Headache.
- Abnormalities/alterations in heart rate and/or blood pressure.
- Abnormalities in psychopathology:
  - mood: depression, excitement, anxiety;
  - motivation/volition;
  - sleep (hypersomnia/insomnia/parasomnias).

The algorithm of Naranjo (Naranjo, Shear & Lanctôt, 1992) should be considered for the first evaluation of signs and symptoms that could be associated with ADRs. It is synthetically reported in Table 4.1.

Table 4.1 - The algorithm of Naranjo

Signs and symptoms	Yes	No	I don't know
A close temporal relation between ADR symptoms and the taking of the drug			
Remission/reduction of symptoms when drug is suspended			
Recurrence of ADRs (rechallenge) when the drug is taken again			
Symptoms are compatible with scientific literature on the drug			
Aggravation/improvement in correlation with increase/reduction of the dosage of the drug			
Exclusion of other causes			

4.4 MEDICATION-INDUCED MOVEMENT DISORDERS

Medication-Induced Movement Disorders (MIMDs) cover all movement problems arising from pharmacological action on the neurotransmitter systems involved in movement. Abnormalities of movement, and spontaneous movements in particular, were described in association with mental illnesses before the advent of antipsychotic substances, but with the development of antipsychotic drugs we noticed the growing presence of MIMDs, until the recent introduction of new substances (the second generation antipsychotics, SGAs) that sensibly reduced these side effects.

The neurobiological mechanisms implicated in MIMDs are not always clear. Most cases arise from a blockage in the dopaminergic transmission, primarily at the level of D2 dopamine receptors in the extrapyramidal tract. Other important areas of the central nervous system (CNS) are involved: cortical motor areas, cerebellum, cortical, and subcortical areas are implicated in motivation, volition, and organization of movements. Longer lasting is the blockage in dopaminergic transmission: in this case there will be a stronger risk of movement problems caused by drugs. The first generation antipsychotics (FGAs; i.e. haloperidol) present a higher risk of producing movement disorders compared to the SGAs, which block in a less intense way the dopamine receptors, or can act as a dopaminergic system modulator (i.e. partial agonism of aripiprazole). Also important is the action of the drug on other receptors, above all the serotoninergic and cholinergic systems.

The DSM IV-TR lists seven categories of MIMDs (table 4.2).

4.4.1 Neuroleptic-induced parkinsonism

Neuroleptic-induced parkinsonism is very similar to the idiopathic primary Parkinson's disease and it shows the typical triad of rigidity, bradykinesia and tremor. The pathophysiology of this disorder results from a block of dopaminergic transmission and dopamine depletion in the nigro-striate areas (extrapyramidal symptoms, or EPS).

Muscular hypertonus causes *rigidity* with two particular presentations when you move the patient's arms or legs: continuous-elastic movement ("lead pipe") or discontinuous muscle motion ("cog-wheeling").

Table 4.2 - Categories of Medication-Induced Movement Disorders (DSM IV-TR)

Signs and symptoms
Neuroleptic-induced parkinsonism
Neuroleptic malignant syndrome
Neuroleptic-induced acute dystonia
Neuroleptic-induced acute akathisia
Neuroleptic-induced tardive dyskinesia
Medication-induced postural tremor
Medication-induced movement disorder NOS

Bradykinesia: all the spontaneous and automatic movements are minimized with typical masked face, abnormalities of walking (the arms do not have the normal automatic oscillation and the patient moves with short steps) and slowed speech.

Tremor: at rest, at a typical frequency of 3-6 Hertz (tongue, hands-fingers like "making pills," head, legs, jaw). It could be symmetrical or unilateral.

Women are more susceptible than men (about 2:1). The incidence of onset is higher over 40 years, and it increases over 60 years; it is more frequent in the first 3 months of cure or when the cure is modified. There are no clinical differences from the primary Parkinson's Disease.

Treatment includes: reduction of dose or medication cessation, a switch to lower-potency D2 blocking agent, and the use of antiparkinsonism medication (e.g. anticholinergic, amantadine).

4.4.2 Neuroleptic malignant syndrome

This is a severe condition with onset in response to antipsychotic drug agents that is typically characterized by elevated body temperature and muscle rigidity. Other symptoms are dysphagia, incontinence, changes in level of consciousness ranging from confusion to coma, blood pressure instability, and elevation of plasma level of creatine phosphokinase and liver enzymes. The onset can be rapid or gradual. The postulated mechanism is a hypodopaminergic state induced by dopaminergic blocking agents or abrupt discontinuation of dopaminergic agonists such as antiparkinsonism medication. Neuroleptic malignant syndrome is a life-threatening condition and needs intensive medical intervention. It is important to recognize the initial symptoms for early identification and treatment.

4.4.3 Neuroleptic-induced acute dystonia (NIAD)

Dystonia is the slow and lasting contraction of different muscle areas leading to involuntary movements and abnormal positioning of body muscles: neck and head (torticollis); eyes, deviated in different directions (oculogyric crisis), jaw muscles (trismus), tongue protrusion, impaired breathing, speaking, swallowing, trunk (opisthotonus) and limbs.

The patient feels a great discomfort, sometimes painful, with a state of alarm. NIAD can occur within minutes after taking a high-potency FGA (often injectable) but usually occurs a few days after the beginning of treatment or after modification of dosage. Recent use of cocaine (depletion of dopamine), non-compliance in long-term therapies, family history of movement disorders, black heritage, young age, and male gender increase the risk of NIAD. The exact mechanism of NIAD is not clear, but it could depend on the rapid saturation/desaturation of D2 receptors.

Treatment: severe NIAD which compromises breathing needs immediate treatment in emergency areas. In other cases, anticholinergics and benzodiazepines are useful.

4.4.4 Neuroleptic-induced acute akathisia

Akathisia is a very unpleasant and ill-defined feeling of muscle tension with restlessness, swinging of the legs, rocking from foot to foot, and lifting of the feet as if marching in place. The patient is unable to stand or sit in a relaxed way for a long time, and he feels the urge to move incessantly. This looks like an emotional state of instability and so akathisia can easily be confused with symptoms of anxiety or agitation and treated as a mental disorder. It usually starts within 2-4 weeks after the beginning of antipsychotic treatment, or after changing the treatment dose. It can also happen with various antidepressants, more often with selective serotonin reuptake inhibitors (SSRIs), because of the influence of serotoninergic action on the dopamine system. The pathophysiology is unknown. It's important to consider the correlation with high doses and rapid dose escalation, and with the potency of drugs. It happens more commonly with the FGAs. Akathisia seems related to gender (female more than male), age (older people), negative symptoms, and mood disorders.

The first choice of treatment for akathisia is a dose reduction or a switch to another, less potent drug. Benzodiazepines, anticholinergic, and beta-blockers can also be useful to reduce akathisia.

4.4.5 Neuroleptic-induced tardive dyskinesia

Neuroleptic-induced tardive dyskinesia is characterized by slow and continuous (athetoid) or fast and jerky (choreic, like a dance) involuntary movements of different parts of the body. It can be involved in the face with chewing, tongue protrusion and twisting, smacking, or puckering; or in the trunk and limbs with movements that resemble of dancing. It develops after several months of therapy with dopamine blocking agents. It starts slowly and lightly (often first in the tongue, lips, and jaw) but gradually becomes an important cause of inability involving most of the muscular districts. It occurs within 4 weeks after the discontinuation of a long term therapy with antipsychotics. The FGAs cause tardive dyskinesia more often than SGAs. The most accepted hypothesis is that this is due to dopamine receptor hypersensitivity after long-term blocking by antipsychotic agents. There is also recent evidence for genetic vulnerability.

Risk factors are age (older than 55 years), gender (female more than male), comorbidity with mood and anxiety disorders, dementia, Parkinson's, and other neurological illnesses.

The first choice of treatment is the switch to an SGA. Clozapine shows a greater rate of improvement in tardive diskynesia symptoms. To stabilize and assure favorable outcomes in clinical conditions, it can be useful to gradually discontinue the antipsychotic medication. It is necessary to avoid a sudden and total interruption of medication because the dyskinesia can become worse. Sometimes the use of Vitamin B6 improves the symptoms. In some cases antidepressant agents and lithium can improve tardive diskinesia, probably by positive influence on mood and anxiety. The symptoms of tardive diskynesia are triggered and/or worsened by both psychological and biological stress factors, and by muscular fatigue. Symptoms generally improve with muscular and emotional relaxation.

4.4.6 Medication-induced postural tremor

Postural tremor typically begins after starting antipsychotic, antidepressant medication and mood stabilizers (lithium, valproate). Stimulating agents (caffeine, theophylline, dopaminergic agonists) can also develop a postural tremor. This fine tremor, which has a typical frequency of 8-12 Hz, most often affects limbs and fingers, but also tongue, mouth, head and neck. The distinction of this feature from neuroleptic induced Parkinsonism (slower 3-6-Hz, at rest) and true Parkinson

(worsened with movements) is necessary. The treatment depends on the type of implicated medication. With the use of mood stabilizers physicians will check drug plasma level of lithium or valproic acid and define if the tremor is dose related. Stimulant medications can induce a hyper-adrenergic condition that can be countered by reducing the dose of the stimulant agent, or by using beta-blockers or benzodiazepines. Anxiety, emotional factors, stress, and fatigue worse, the postural tremor, and relaxing techniques could improve the symptoms.

4.4.7 Medication-induced movement disorder NOS

This category includes all the disorders that are not classified in the preceding list.

4.5 MEDICATIONS AND WEIGHT GAIN

Often psychotropic drugs cause a weight gain. Three of the most considered hypotheses to explain weight gain in psychiatric illnesses are:
- life style alteration (induced by the disorders, the stigma, the environment, the social disability) with decreased physical activity levels and food-intake alterations;
- hyperphagia as an offset to psychological affections;
- drug neurobiological profile.

Antihistaminergic activity (as antagonism on H1 and H3 receptors) is related to weight gain; this can be caused by an increase in the amount of food ingested or by a metabolic dysregulation.

Serothoninergic action can produce an increasing appetite, above all with a great need for hypercaloric and high-carbohydrate food; but on the other hand it can reduce hunger and help to resist bulimic behaviors (i.e. fluoxetine and sertraline at high dosage). Tryciclic drugs with multi-combined actions, such as anticholinergic, noradrenergic, serothoninergic and anti-hystaminergic, often support hypercaloric hyperglucose food intake (craving) and are very frequently associated with weight gain (even at low dosage). Antipsychotic agents (both first and second generation antipsychotic medications – FGAs & SGAs) elevate the risk for dyslipidemia, hyperglicemia, type II diabetes and weight gain. However,

Abnormal eating behaviors

1. Hyperphagia with the search for sensation of gastric fullness (volume eaters)

2. Hyperphagia as compensation for intense emotional states (emotional eaters) or vacuum, boredom, loneliness (nibbling)

3. Hyperphagia related to stressful situations (stress-related hyperphagia)

4. Compulsion to take certain foods, often carbohydrates, chocolate, high calorie foods (craving), with problems in control and related feelings of nervousness and restlessness

5. Taking large amounts of food quickly and uncontrollably (binging).

elevation of the cardiometabolic risk profile depends on the drug-specific receptor profiles. Physical activity plays an important role in reducing elevated cardiometabolic risk profiles. It promotes caloric consumptions, reduces weight and balances body composition, and promotes healthy lifestyle and social relationships. It represents an important tool for the patient's recovery, opposing adverse effects of the drugs and negative influence of mental illness on lifestyle. Furthermore, research suggests that during exercise (particularly endurance) body activity produces endogenous psychostimulant substances (antidepressants, painkillers, anti-fatigue) belonging to the category of endorphins or endogenous opiates (Dinas et al., 2011). These bodily endorphins can positively influence the psychological life of the individual, but at the same time can be one of the mechanisms involved in the phenomena of compulsive search for physical activity (e.g. compulsive runners, hyperactivity in anorexia nervosa) with the characteristic of addiction (Hausenblas et al., 2002; Johnston et al., 2011). Some recent studies have explored the possibility of identifying a suitable dose of physical activity to achieve a desired effect and control over mental functions, particularly in depression and anxiety disorders (Dunn, Trivedi, Kampert, Clark, Chambliss, 2005).

In the absence of specific-related organic diseases, overweight and obesity can result from the main forms of abnormal eating behaviors (see Textbox 4.1). These behaviors may be symptoms of mental disorders, but also the result of side effects from drugs used for psychiatric and non-psychiatric care.

4.6 ENDOCRINE SYSTEM AND PSYCHOTROPIC AGENTS

The central nervous system and the neuroendocrine system interact with feedback mechanisms for maintaining homeostasis in different environmental situations.

Psychoactive drugs often have actions on the neuroendocrine system and hormonal substances affecting the mental system. This may lead to modifications of the adaptive responses of the body during physical activity. The psychomotor therapist or the exercise science expert should therefore pay close attention to personalizing physical exercise.

4.6.1 Hypothalamic-pituitary-adrenal axis

The hypothalamus produces and releases CRH (Corticotrophin Realizing Hormone), which stimulates the pituitary gland to produce and release ACTH (adrenocorticotropin hormone), which stimulates the adrenal glands to release glucocorticoid hormones, primarily cortisol. Glucocorticoids inhibit by negative feedback the upstream release of CRH and ACTH.

This circuit is typically triggered by stress that has an influence on emotions, affects, behaviors, the immune system, and the autonomic nervous system. Physical activity can also put the body under stress; the ability to react adequately to the stress induced by exercise depends on the proper functioning of the circuits described above.

An altered function of the hypothalamic-pituitary-adrenal axis (HPA) (hyperactivity) has been suggested as a cause of reduced tolerance to fatigue, impaired performance and low-slow response to stimuli.

A hyperactivity of the HPA axis is hypothesized in depression, psychosis, posttraumatic stress disorder, eating disorders, Alzheimer's disease, and chronic fatigue syndrome.

Antidepressant drugs appear to act on the HPA axis with a reduction and stabilization of its activity.

4.6.2 Hypothalamic-pituitary-thyroid axis

The hypothalamus produces TRH (Thyrotropin Releasing Hormone), which stimulates the pituitary gland to release TSH (Thyroid Stimulating Hormone), which causes in the thyroid the production and the releasing of thyroid hormones (thyroxine and triiodothyronine T3 and T4). A retraction of T3 and T4 adjusts upstream TRH and TSH.

This circuit is mainly involved in the regulation of the metabolism. Reduced activity of the Hypothalamic-pituitary-thyroid axis (HPT) results in a reduction of metabolism in general, slowing both physical and mental processes. An increase of HPT axis causes an exaggerated activation of the metabolism with negative effects on mental and physical health.

Demonstrations of alternation of the HTP axis are mental disorders such as anxiety, depression, psychosis, cognitive impairment, and anorexia.

Drugs frequently affect the HPT axis, in particular lithium salts. Rapid and/or significant changes in weight, basal body temperature, mental activity, physical activity, and heart rate may indicate an alteration of HPT function, and require appropriate endocrinological assessments.

4.6.3 Growth hormone

The hypothalamus produces both a releasing factor (Growth Hormone Releasing Hormone, GHRH) and an inhibiting factor (somatostatin) of growth hormone that is produced and released by the pituitary gland. Many biological, psychological and environmental factors influence the circuit of growth hormones (GH). Research attributes an important value to physical exercise in regulating production and release of GH.

4.6.4 Prolactin

Prolactin is produced in the anterior pituitary gland under inhibitory control by dopaminic neurons located in the tubero-infindibolar part of the hypothalamus. The effect of antipsychotic agents on these neurons explains the elevation of prolactin, which often occurs during antipsychotic treatment. This increase in prolactin is frequently asymptomatic but sometimes produces breast tenderness secreting milky liquid in female.

Prolactin inhibits its own secretion by a short-loop feedback circuit to the hypothalamus.

A lot of factors can influence the prolactin release: serotonin, estrogens, norepinephrine, histamine, cortisol, Corticotrophin Realising Hormone (CRH), glutamate, oxitocine, and opioids.

Elevated and prolonged plasma level of prolactin is a risk for the development of cancer and osteoporosis, and is also related with reduced libido, hypoglicemia, irritability, anxiety, and stress intolerance.

4.7 CONCLUSIONS

An increasing body of evidence suggests that physical activity is an appropriate intervention to improve physical and mental health in people with mental illness. Physical activity is shown to be effective in reducing side effects of psychotropic drugs and can be a favorable instrument to contain the use of prescribed drugs and to limit negative side effects.

The psychomotor therapist and/or the exercise science specialist are more and more recognized in clinical and non-clinical contexts, offering their contribution, side by side with psychiatrists, psychologists and other therapists, to sustain the patient's recovery.

To reinforce motivational mechanisms, socializing, and reaction skills that go together with physical activity, it is necessary that physical activity meets patients' psychological and physical needs. Professionals have an obligation to mantain knowledge about the collateral effects of drugs on physical and psychological conditions of patients involved in these activities. Based on this knowledge, they have to modify their approach to prevent unfavorable effects of drugs. In addition, it is very important to gain information about withdrawal symptoms before and after each exercise session.

For these patients, physical activity may be an incisive way to gain consciousness of their body's limits and, at the same time, rediscover bodily resources to face the disease.

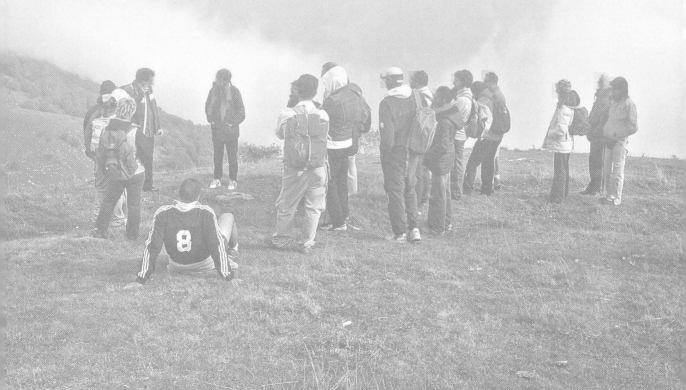

Section 2

Physical activity and exercise in the approach of **mental health problems**

The role of exercise
in the generation and regulation of **stress**

5

Markus Gerber, Uwe Pühse

5.1 INTRODUCTION

Today, many individuals encounter psychosocial stress on a regular basis. The regulation of stress is a complex biopsychosocial phenomenon comprised of several appraisal processes and coping mechanisms. The present chapter considers this complexity and provides a comprehensive overview of the role of exercise in stress generation and regulation. The definition of stress is articulated in relation to the mechanisms that affect health. Additionally, this chapter presents literature concerning the bivariate association between exercise and stress. A review of field studies tested the likelihood of exercise to serve as protection against the adverse health effects of stress. These findings suggest that various mechanisms may underlie the stress-protective potential of exercise, as discussed in the final section of this chapter.

5.1.1 What is stress?

Stress has several unique definitions throughout the scientific literature. Typically, researchers distinguish between reaction-oriented, stimulus-oriented, and cognitive-transactional stress models (Schwarzer, 2000; Steptoe & Ayers, 2004). Modern stress research has its roots in reaction-oriented stress models. Scholars like Cannon (1929) and Selye (1946) define stress as a dependent variable or a physiological, psychological, or behavioral response to a stressor. Selye defines stress as an unspecific reaction of a living organism to any form of demand. Based on animal models, he observed that certain stressors lead to specific reactions (e.g. blood vessel constriction in cold temperatures). Simultaneously, these stressors result in more general adaptations, regardless of the nature of the stressor (e.g. size reduction of the thymus gland, enlargement of the adrenal

cortex). He therefore proposed a general adaptation syndrome suggesting that many diseases have a common endocrinological basis. Alternatively, stress is defined as an independent variable within stimulus-oriented stress models. Under this definition, stress is seen as an external factor that disturbs the internal homeostasis of an organism. Field studies have investigated stress in various environments, such as experiences in war, living in remote areas, imprisonment, and exposure to natural disasters. Critical life events have also captured scientific attention (Holmes & Rahe, 1967), including major problems related to family, partnership, friendship, finances, living conditions, work, and leisure. Other researchers have been more interested in minor but more frequent stressors, which are commonly referred to as daily hassles (i.e. minor disputes and pressures). Reaction- and stimulus-oriented models show that the risk for various chronic diseases increases with elevated exposure to stress. These models fall short, however, in explaining the individual differences in the perception of and reactivity to stress (Gerber, 2008). In an attempt to overcome this shortcoming, stress has also been defined as a cognitive transaction between internal and external demands involving several subjective appraisals (Hobfoll, 1998; Lazarus & Folkman, 1984). This cognitive transaction model is useful in explaining why students often perceive the stressfulness of an exam very differently. These differences are not only based on the objective importance of an exam (e.g. finals are usually more stressful than prior examinations), but depend to a great extent on internal factors. Internal factors include the following: (a) subjective relevance of an exam (e.g. perceived importance of the exam that will affect employment prospects after graduation), (b) personal aspiration level (e.g. perfectionism), (c)

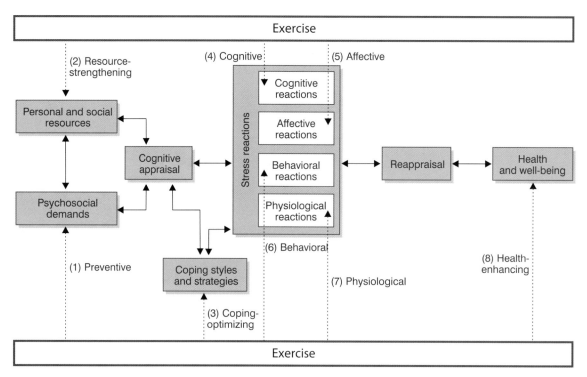

Figure 5.1 - Possible influences of exercise on the stress-health relationship (adapted from Fuchs & Klaperski, 2012).

past experiences (e.g. success or failure on previous exams), (d) personality traits (e.g. test anxiety), or (e) external pressures (e.g. parental expectations). Moreover, while individuals evaluate the subjective importance of a stressor in the initial appraisal process (primary appraisal: "What is at stake?"), the stressfulness is influenced by one's perceived problem solving resources (secondary appraisal: "Do I have the personal and social capacities to successfully deal with this stressor?").

Each individual has a different frame of reference when they are faced with stress. Therefore, it is not surprising that some people are more resilient to stress than others. Additionally, determining whether perceived stress has negative or positive consequences depends on one's coping abilities. The cognitive-transactional stress theory differentiates between problem- and emotion-oriented coping. Problem-oriented coping aims to reduce or eliminate a problem (e.g. preparing for an exam, seeking social support from classmates). Emotion-oriented coping regulates emotional responses to a stressor (e.g. positive self-talk, seeking diversion). Finally, the coping response is followed by a third appraisal, generally labeled as reappraisal. During this process, an individual

evaluates whether his or her efforts to reduce the effects of a stressor were successful. If relief is not achieved, the problem may evolve into a chronic source of distress that yields negative consequences for the individual's well-being. Figure 5.1 provides a schematic overview of the cognitive-transactional stress process. As a heuristic model, the main criticism raised against cognitive-transactional stress theory is that it is too complex and thus, too difficult to test. The reciprocality of the (primary and secondary) appraisal processes and the dynamic interrelationships between appraisals and coping have proven especially problematic.

5.1.2 Prevalence and impact of stress

Researchers have developed a multitude of instruments to assess different sources of stress for various populations of people (Grant, Compas, Thurm, McMahon, & Gipson, 2004; Schwarzer, 2000). Nevertheless, since a valid and reliable gold standard assessment of stress is missing, it is difficult to establish the prevalence of stress in the general population. The situation is further complicated since the most frequently used instruments (e.g. the Perceived Stress Scale) (Cohen, Kamarck, & Mermelstein, 1983) have no cut-off criteria that delineate between moderate or high levels of stress. In epidemiological surveys and field studies, however, a considerable percentage of participants typically report high levels of stress (Cohen & Williamson, 1988; Zuzanek, Robinson, & Iwasaki, 1998). For instance, a study within the Swiss working population indicated that 27% of all employees perceived stress often or always (Ramaciotti & Perriard, 2001), whereas 56% of the participants perceived stress at least sometimes.

Nevertheless, evidence regarding the negative association between stress and health is abundant. Data suggest that high stress levels correlate with increased risk for cardiovascular diseases, cancer, brain functioning, diabetes mellitus, psychosocial complaints, depression, and suicide (Steptoe & Ayers, 2004; Uchino, Smith, Holt-Lunstad, Campo, & Reblin, 2007). Furthermore, stress has been associated with increased alcohol consumption, smoking, bullying, and delinquency (Byrne & Mazanov, 2003; Hoffmann & Gray Cerbone, 1999; Natvig, Albrektsen, & Qvarnstrøm, 2001; Park, Armeli & Tennen, 2004).

In summary, many people perceive their lives in today's society as highly stressful. Åstrand (2004) states that "the last century has been characterized by enormous advances in almost all aspects of human achievements" and "a person born at the beginning of the 20th century and still alive has witnessed more of technical evolution than occurred during the preceding millions of years of the homo sapiens family." This technical evolution has contributed to material welfare in most Western countries, however this requires individuals to adapt to new circumstances and technologies within increasingly shorter periods of time. Additionally, factors that have merged over the last couple of decades now make working life more stressful than before. Increasing numbers of jobs are being merged together, longer working hours, more robust managerial styles, greater job insecurity, heavier workloads, and less job control with more work impinging on family and personal life, are all likely to influence employee work experiences and affect well-being and health (Cooper, 2003). Given the negative health outcomes and (monetary) costs associated with stress, preventing and reducing stress is a significant public health issue taking high priority on global agendas (Leka, Griffiths, & Cox, 2003).

5.2 HOW DOES STRESS AFFECT HEALTH?

During the last few decades, several mechanisms have described how stress may lead to impaired health. First, researchers have suggested that physiological responses play a vital role in stress. In line with this idea, studies have demonstrated that greater stress reactivity in response to laboratory stress is associated with a higher risk for cardiovascular diseases (Chida & Steptoe, 2010; Schneider, Jacobs, Gevirtz, & O'Connor, 2003; Schwartz et al., 2003). Second, the impact of stress on health may be due to psychological mechanisms. For instance, perceived stress and repeated failure to cope with stress could result in reduced self-efficacy and learned helplessness (Seligman, 1975). Similarly, high job demands and external pressures may lead to external motivation and alienation because one's basic psychological needs (e.g. competence, autonomy, relatedness) are no longer satisfied (Deci & Ryan, 2000). Third, stress may negatively affect an individual's health behaviors. For instance, people exposed to stress might be more prone to smoke and drink (Steptoe, Wardle, Pollard, Canaan, & Davies, 1996), and they may have less energy to engage in healthy behaviors (Brand, Gerber, Pühse, & Holsboer-Trachsler, 2010). Sonnentag and Jelden (2009) showed that after a stressful workday, police officers were more inclined to engage in sedentary behaviors than exercise, even though they believed that exercise would contribute more to recovery than passive behaviors.

5.2.1 Stress resilience factors: can exercise be one of them?

As outlined above, there is considerable variability in how stress affects individuals' well-being. At the end of the 1970s, researchers began examining stress resilience factors. For example, Kobasa (1979) showed that hardiness is a mindset that facilitates successful coping with stress. Some years later, Antonovsky (1987) proposed a high sense of coherence as a stress resilience resource. Since these seminal publications, a wide array of demographic factors as well as psychological and social resources have been labeled as protection against stress-related symptoms (Cohen & Edwards, 1989; Grant et al., 2006). Scholars have also emphasized that exercise might moderate the stress-health relationship (Gerber & Pühse, 2009). Figure 5.1 illustrates that the association between exercise, stress, and health is indeed complex and involves several mechanisms. The following paragraphs reveal the paths necessary to inspect the existing evidence regarding the impact of exercise on the relationship between stress and health.

5.3 EXERCISE AND THE PERCEPTION OF STRESS

Cross-sectional studies have generally shown that individuals with high exercise levels perceive less stress (e.g. Aldana, Sutton, & Jacobson, 1996; Kouvonen et al., 2005; Nguyen-Michel, Unger, Hamilton, & Spruijt-Metz, 2006; Wemme & Rosvall, 2005). This finding has often been interpreted as support for the preventive function of exercise (path 1 in Figure 5.1). In these studies, however, the question of whether exercise is the independent or dependent variable is not clear. Longitudinal research has indicated that the relationship between exercise and stress is reciprocal. On the one hand, perceived stress decreases over time if individuals engage in regular exercise (Jonsdottir, Rödjer, Hadzibajramovic, Börjeson, & Ahlborg, 2010; Schnohr, Kristensen, Prescott, & Scharling, 2005). On the other hand, individuals reduce their exercise levels if they encounter increasingly high levels of stress (Oaten & Cheng, 2005; Steptoe et al., 1996; Stetson, Rahn, Dubbert, Wilner, & Mercury, 1997). Using cross-lagged panel analyses, Lutz et al. (2007) and Gerber (2008) both observed a weak negative path between stress and exercise, whereas exercise did not predict subsequent stress. These findings show that stress and exercise are interdependent, but that stress might have a stronger impact on exercise behavior than exercise does on stress perception.

To determine the influence of exercise on stress perception, Fuchs and Klaperski (2012) have systematically reviewed intervention trials and programs with at least two training sessions, nonclinical samples, study designs with a control group, and measures of perceived stress as outcome variables. The authors concluded that out of eight randomized controlled trials, four supported that exercise has a stress-reducing effect. However, only one study was able to demonstrate a significant Time x Group interaction. In all other studies, either the control group reduced their scores as well, or no information was provided

about the Time x Group interaction (e.g. only post-test scores were reported). From the three studies without randomized group assignment, one investigation provided full support and two investigations showed partial support for a stress-reducing effect of exercise.

Finally, Lutz et al. (2010) found that the influence of stress on exercise behavior depends on the individuals' stages of change as defined by the Transtheoretical Model (TTM: Prochaska & Velicer, 1997). Women in maintenance stage were able to uphold their exercise levels in times of increased stress, whereas exercise levels dropped considerably among participants in the contemplation and action stages. The authors assumed that the self-regulatory resources of irregular exercisers might be depleted faster compared to individuals in a more habitual stage. In conclusion, this finding suggests that individuals' stages of change should be taken into consideration when exercise is proposed as a stress management strategy.

5.3.1 Exercise, stress resources and coping

Several studies have shown that exercisers possess more personal and social resources than nonexercisers, which supports the notion that exercise strengthens resilience resources (path 2 in Figure 5.1). For example, significant associations were observed between exercise and self-esteem (Ekeland, Heian, & Hagen, 2005), optimism (Kavussanu & McAuley, 1995), hardiness (Kobasa, Maddi, & Puccetti, 1982), and social support (Tietjens, 2001). The association between exercise and both optimal coping styles and coping strategies is unknown (path 3 in Figure 5.1). Antonini et al. (2004) examined whether the type of sport (weightlifting, running, swimming, triathlon) is associated with athletes' coping styles. Nevertheless, since the adequacy of coping cannot be judged in general, but depends on the combination of stressors, personal values, cultural influences, and environmental constraints that are involved, the practical significance of the different coping strategies anyhow remains questionable.

5.3.2 Does exercise buffer the negative effects of stress?

Beyond the bivariate relationships between exercise and stress, researchers have examined whether exercise protects against stress-induced symptoms of ill-health. Since the initial work of Kobasa et al. (1982), more than thirty field studies have been executed on this topic. A literature review showed that stress-buffering effects occurred in about half of the existing studies with non-clinical samples (Gerber & Pühse, 2009). Moreover, significant stress-buffering effects were also observed in clinical populations (Gaitanis, Tooley, & Edwards, 2005; Ginis et al., 2003). While these studies show that exercise protects against stress-related diseases, they do not provide information about the underlying mechanisms (Gerber, Holsboer-Trachsler, Pühse, & Brand, 2011; Gerber, Kellmann, Hartmann, & Pühse, 2010).

5.3.3 Exercise and cognitive, affective, and behavioral stress reactions: emerging relationships

Stress is often accompanied by negative cognitive processes that lead to an exacerbation of the perceived level of impairment (Brand et al., 2010). Such dysfunctional cognitions include excessive rumination or maladaptive attributions. For instance, individuals often continue to think about their problems even after the stressor is gone. In fact, a recent study with young adults showed that the relationship between perceived stress and disturbed sleep was fully mediated by dysfunctional cognitions such as rumination and focusing (Brand et al., 2010). Additionally, highly stressed individuals may feel a gradual loss of control over their lives. Following Seligman (1975), learned helplessness is a mindset that facilitates the development of depressive symptoms. It is particularly prevalent among individuals who internally attribute failure to stable traits such as lack of competence, while external influences are often overlooked (e.g. Klein, Fencil-Morse, & Seligman, 1976; Zimmerman, Coryell, Corenthal, & Wilson, 1986). To our knowledge, however, no research exists as to whether or not exercise is able to interrupt negative thinking cycles from stress (path 4 in Figure 5.1).

With regard to the affective reactions to stress, coping consists of problem- and emotion-oriented approaches. While problem-oriented coping is generally more productive, emotion-focused coping might be helpful in situations when the stressor cannot easily be changed (e.g. noise or heat at the workplace, high job demands). Most exercise

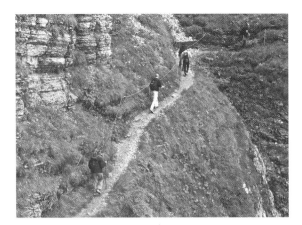

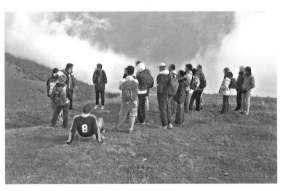

Figure 5.2 - Walking. Organizing long walks in natural environments help people to improve aerobic capacity and it is an effective low cost strategy to enhance health. Teaching an easy way to practice regular exercise could be a practical approach in changing people's lifestyles.

psychologists have considered exercise to be an emotion-oriented coping strategy (Berger, 1996; Rostad & Long, 1996). In support of this notion (path 5 in Figure 5.1), prior research has shown that mood states generally increase after acute bouts of exercise, particularly if initial mood states were low (Ekkekakis & Acevedo, 2006).

Finally, the influence of exercise on behavioral reactions to stress has not been investigated yet (path 6 in Figure 5.1). Future studies should determine whether exercise during periods of high stress helps to maintain sleep quality, decrease smoking, or increase the likelihood of healthy eating.

5.3.4 Exercise and physiological stress reactions

The largest body of literature focuses on the relationship between exercise and physiological stress reactions (path 7 in Figure 5.1). The relevance of this body of research is based on the notion that high physiological stress reactivity and slow stress recovery are associated with a variety of physical and mental diseases (Alexander et al., 2009; Chida & Steptoe, 2010; Gold, Zakowski, Valdimarsdottir, & Bovbjerg, 2003), whereas exercise has the potential to prevent many of these conditions (Sallis & Owen, 1999; Steptoe & Butler, 1996).

Physiological stress reactions are regulated by the autonomous nervous system and the neuroendocrine system. A stress-induced activation of the sympathetic nervous system simultaneously results in a series of changes in the cardiovascular system, the respiration and lung function, as well as in the renal and gastrointestinal systems (Cacioppo et al., 1998; Tsigos & Chrousos, 2002). For instance, stress results in increased blood pressure, increased heart rate, a dilation of the lungs and an increased blood flow to the muscles. At the same time, the secretion of adrenalin triggers an increase of blood sugar to supply the organism with the necessary energy for a "fight-or-flight" reaction (Birbaumer & Schmidt, 2006; Tsigos & Chrousos, 2002). With regard to the neuroendocrine stress reaction, stress causes the secretion of the corticotropin releasing hormone (CRH), which is transported to the pituitary gland. Consequently, the release of the adrenocorticotrope hormone (ACTH) in the general circulatory system is initiated. Afterwards, the ACTH is transported to the adrenal gland, where it stimulates the secretion of cortisol. Because most cells of the human body have glucocorticoid receptors, cortisol provokes a multitude of reactions in the human body.

The idea that exercise training results in a blunted physiological stress reaction is based on Selye's "cross-stressor adaptation hypothesis." Advocates of reaction-oriented stress models assume that exposure to a sufficiently intensive and prolonged stimulus provokes specific and unspecific adaptations. It is believed that regular exercise results in reduced stress reactivity, particularly when physical stressors are present (in the sense of a specific adaptation). Above that, an adaptation to a cognitive or psychological stressor is expected as well (Sothmann, 2006; Sothmann et al., 1996). Given this background, studies have shown that exercise can be regarded as a stressor that results in a strong increase of epinephrine and norepi-

nephrine (Dishman & Jackson, 2000; Kjaer, 1992; Péronnet & Szabo, 1993). Furthermore, previous research showed that increased levels of fitness result in a blunted increase of plasma norepinephrine concentration during physical exercise (Dishman & Jackson, 2000; Péronnet & Szabo, 1993). However, a reduced increase was only found if the absolute exercise intensity was considered (i.e. fixed watts on an ergometer test), whereas no difference occurred for the relative intensity (i.e. fixed heart rate with variable watts) (Kjaer, 1992; Sothmann, 2006). As a consequence, Péronnet and Szabo (1993) speculated that the reduced reactivity may not be based on functional changes of the sympathetic nervous system, but simply reflect improved levels of fitness. Similar findings were observed with regard to the neuroendocrine system. Hence, acute bouts of exercise resulted in increased plasma concentrations of ACTH and cortisol. During submaximal exercise, few weeks of exercise training were associated with a reduced secretion of ACTH and cortisol. Again, a reduced secretion was only observed for the absolute, not the relative exercise intensity level (Dishman & Jackson, 2000; Hand, Phillips, & Wilson, 2006; Kjaer, 1992; Sothmann, 2006).

A large number of investigations have been conducted concerning a cross-over effect on cognitive and psychological stressors, including a wide variety of different samples, study designs, and measures. To provide an example, Sinyor et al. (1988) conducted a mediation, music, and aerobic exercise program with three groups of university students. After completion of the 10-week training program, the participants were exposed to two subsequent laboratory tasks (mental arithmetic under noise pollution, Stroop task). The Stroop task is a stressor protocol specifically designed to elicit stress reactions in a laboratory setting (MacLeod, 1991). It is based on the principle of "inhibition" and the fact that colors as visual information are preferred to the cognitive processing of the meaning of words (e.g. the natural reaction would be to say "blue" if an individual sees the word "green" in blue font). Sinyor et al.'s study showed that trained subjects responded with a decreased reactivity in some outcomes (e.g. skin conductance), whereas no Time x Group effects were found in the majority of the variables (e.g. heart rate, epinephrine, norepinephrine).

Meanwhile, the international body of literature has been summarized into several narrative and quantitative reviews. In a meta-analysis, Crews and Landers (1987) found an effect size of .48 indicating that about two-thirds of the trained participants had a lower stress reactivity compared to the mean of the untrained individuals. However, this study was strongly criticized because the authors did not distinguish between different outcomes and also included studies with questionable validity. This criticism was addressed by Forcier et al. (2006) in another meta-analysis with more conservative selection criteria (i.e. they restricted their meta-analysis to cardiovascular outcomes). In summary, they found a significant negative relationship between fitness and attenuated heart rate and systolic blood pressure reactivity. The general consensus among scholars, however, is that the literature regarding the association between fitness and stress reactivity is inconclusive (Boutcher & Hamer, 2006; Dishman & Jackson, 2000; Péronnet & Szabo, 1993; Sothmann, 2006; Sothmann et al., 1996). For instance, Jackson and Dishman (2006) included a total of 73 studies (409 effect sizes) in their meta-regression analysis. A strength of this analysis is that only studies that used a maximal or submaximal fitness test and contained stressors without a physical component were included. Unexpectedly, the effect size indicated that trained individuals react with a slightly increased response to cognitive and psychological stressors (ES = .08). Moreover, the effect size did not vary substantially between cardiovascular outcomes and other measures such as epinephrine, norepinephrine, or cortisol.

The findings of the existing meta-analyses are more coherent regarding the relationship between exercise and stress recovery. Along with Jackson and Dishman (2006) who found that trained individuals recover faster from laboratory stressors (ES = -.27), the findings of two other meta-analyses (Forcier et al., 2006; Schuler & O'Brien, 1997) allude to similar results. Nevertheless, Jackson and Dishman only found evidence for an accelerated cardiovascular recovery, whereas no differences were found for epinephrine, norepinephrine, ACTH, or cortisol.

Following Jackson and Dishman (2006), previous research did not provide convincing evidence that increased fitness is associated with attenuated stress reactivity and faster stress recovery. Particularly, randomized controlled trials were unable to show a significant impact on both stress reactivity and recovery. Moreover, the underlying mechanisms of an altered stress response are not completely understood. Most studies used heart rate and blood pressure as the only outcome variables, and the analysis of haemodynamic, vascular, and endocrine changes was neglected.

Since the most recent meta-analyses, some interesting findings have been published. Of particular importance are two investigations carried out by Rimmele et al. (2007; 2009), who used the Trier Social Stress Test (Kirschbaum, Pirke, & Hellhammer, 1993) to induce stress. Dickerson and Kemeny (2004) argued that the TSST would trigger particularly robust stress responses due to its social-evaluative character. The TSST was a simulated job interview. After a brief preparation, the candidate must present himself as the perfect candidate for a job opening to three members of a management team. The candidate is told that the managers are trained to evaluate non-verbal behavior. After completion of the job-interview, the candidate must solve a mental arithmetic task (counting down from 1024 in steps of 13). After five minutes, the task ends and the TSST protocol is completed. In their first study, Rimmele et al. (2007) compared 22 male elite athletes and 22 "untrained" men. The findings indicated that the TSST evoked a lower cardiovascular (heart rate), endocrine (salivary cortisol) and emotional response (state anxiety) among elite athletes. These results were then confirmed in a second study (Rimmele et al., 2009). However, although significant differences between elite athletes and untrained males were observed in their cardiovascular, endocrine, and emotional responses, an attenuated cortisol and state anxiety response was not found in amateur athletes compared to untrained individuals. In summary, these findings showed that only high fitness levels resulted in an adaptation of the endocrine stress reactivity. Similar findings were reported in a recent study including female participants (Klaperski & Fuchs, 2011).

In another line of research, scientists were more interested in the effects of acute bouts of exercise on stress reactivity and recovery. Hamer et al. (2006) have argued that the stress-buffering function of exercise may occur only during a limited time (refered to as 'post-exercise window'). Thus, they assumed that the stress reactivity between exercisers and non-exercisers might be similar if the stress task takes place outside this window (which would explain the inconclusive results presented above). Meanwhile, the acute effects of exercise have been tested in various studies. For example, Hobson and Rejeski (1993) assigned 80 young women with low to moderate fitness levels to four different groups that exercised for either 0, 10, 20, or 40 minutes. After a short period of rest, the participants completed the Stroop task. The results showed that women who exercised 40 minutes displayed a lowered systolic and diastolic blood pressure compared to the non-exercising controls. In contrast, 10 and 20 minutes of exercise did not result in a blunted reactivity.

In a literature review, Taylor (2000) analyzed 14 studies that were published between 1988 and 2000. He observed that the length of the exercise episodes (10 to 120 minutes) and the intensities of the exercise protocols (18 to 80% of VO_{2max}) varied considerably. Furthermore, various outcome measures were used to test the laboratory stressor responses. Despite these methodological differences, Taylor (2000) concluded that only four studies did not show an attenuated stress reaction after an acute bout of exercise. In another qualitative review, Boutcher and Hamer (2006) drew the same conclusion. Most insignificant results were observed in studies with low intensity levels (below 60% of VO_{2max}) and with a short exercise duration (below 20 minutes). Additionally, Hamer, Taylor, and Steptoe (2006) have reviewed the results of randomized controlled trials that used blood pressure as a dependent variable with meta-analytic methods. In summary, of the 15 studies found, ten yielded a reduced blood pressure reactivity after exercise with a mean effect size of .38 for systolic and .40 for diastolic blood pressure.

5.4 SUMMARY AND PRACTICAL RECOMMENDATIONS

Over millions of years of evolution and natural selection, the human being has developed stress reactions particularly suited to deal with short-term, physical stressors encountered by humans living in the wilderness (fight-or-flight response). Today, however, most stressors are chronic and psychosocial in nature. Coping with this kind of stress presents a big challenge and requires a considerable adaptation from the human being. Fight or flight responses are seldom appropriate to solve psychosocial stress and the autonomous stress reactions are often irrelevant, with the resultant over-arousal or exhaustion leading to stress-related diseases (Hong, 2000).

The previous paragraphs have shown that exercise can influence the relationship between stress and health through several mechanisms. The empirical evidence suggests that there is a negative cross-sectional relationship between exercise and stress, but this relationship can be interpreted in various ways. First, exercisers might be less prone to experiencing high stress. Second, stressed individuals might reduce or stop their exercise participation due to high stress. Longitudinal research has pointed toward reciprocal influences between stress and exercise. Moreover, about 50% of all studies testing exercise-based stress-buffer effects showed a significant interaction between exercise and stress on health. Essentially, exercisers were less likely to develop poor health symptoms during high stress exposure. To explain this result, researchers have proposed cognitive, affective, behavioral and physiological mechanisms. However, while research on the cognitive and behavioral mechanisms is scarce, the physiological stress reaction research is conflicting. In light of these inconsistent findings, it is difficult to recommend any definitive prescribed course. To discuss the practical implications of the findings, the following questions will now be addressed: What kind of exercise is most suitable for stress regulation? How much exercise is needed for stress regulation? How can we help individuals to maintain their exercise levels in periods of high stress? Is more exercise simply better than no exercise? Is there more that individuals can learn about stress through their exercise experiences?

What kind of exercise for which type of person? No clear patterns emerged from the literature regarding the question as to what kind of exercise is best suited for any particular group of people. Berger (1996) argued that exercise should be pleasing and enjoyable, aerobic or facilitating rhythmical abdominal breathing, free of interpersonal competition, closed, predictable, and temporally and spatially certain. Nevertheless, empirical evidence for this assertion is not given. For instance, Fuchs and Klaperski (2012) found that both aerobic exercise and weight training programs have the potential to reduce stress. In contrast, evidence exists that exercise must have a certain intensity level (at least 60% of VO_{2max}) to alleviate stress. Fuchs and Klaperski (2012) have further shown that leisure exercise is more suited

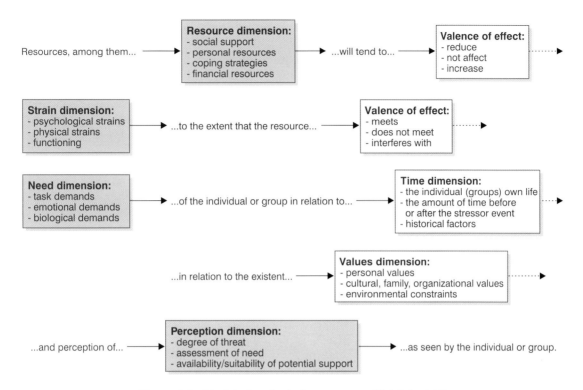

Figure 5.3 - Model of ecological congruence (Hobfoll, 1998).

to stress management than exercise as part of workplace health promotion.

Because a multitude of different stressors exist and because the generation and regulation of stress depends on individual appraisals, it seems suitable to recommend personalized exercise. In his Conservation of Resources Theory (COR), Hobfoll (1998) has formulated several principles that should be taken into consideration. Hobfoll argues that stress occurs when (a) resources are threatened with loss, (b) resources are actually lost, or (c) there is a failure to adequately gain resources following significant resource investment. One tenet of COR theory implies that resources are limited and should be invested deliberately. More stress will arise when there is a misguided investment of resources. Another tenet posits that resource loss is more salient than resource gain and that those who lack resources are likely to adopt a defensive posture to guard their resources. These tenets indicate that even though stressed individuals know the health benefits of exercise, it can be difficult to motivate them to engage in such. Consequently, Hobfoll (1998) proposed the model of ecological congruence in which he suggests that resources may fit, be fitted to, or not fit

stress demands dependent on individual, social historical, and maturational factors (Figure 5.3). In line with this notion, Fuchs and Klaperski (2012) have argued that not every type of exercise is suited to reduce stress. If the main stressor is social isolation, then social exercise and team sports may have the highest potential impact. If an individual lacks self-efficacy to successfully solve problems, exercise activities with mastery experiences such as golf, tennis, or a half-marathon are appropriate. If an individual has difficulties relaxing and is prone to engage in dysfunctional cognitions, aerobic exercise such as jogging might be the wrong choice. Rather, he or she should participate in activities that leave little time for rumination and demand full concentration (e.g. climbing) or involve social interaction (e.g. volleyball). In contrast, if the goal is to provoke anxiolytic and antidepressant effects, endurance training may evoke positive outcomes.

Dose and response? Information is scarce regarding the amount of exercise needed to reduce stress. Recent studies about reactivity and psychosocial stressors have shown that differences exist only between elite athletes and untrained controls, which suggests that substantial amounts of training are required to produce a blunted stress reactivity. On the other hand, studies have consistently shown that acute bouts of exercise result in an attenuated stress reactivity. Researchers assume that a lowered stress reactivity only occurs during a certain post-exercise window, therefore running during lunch breaks on a regular basis seems like a highly effective stress regulation strategy. Moreover, Taylor (2000) suggested that acute bouts of exercise should last at least 20 minutes and involve intensities of at least 60% of VO_{2max}.

Volitional skills? Individuals who are exposed to stress often have difficulties maintaining regular exercise participation. Researchers have shown that self-regulatory resources are limited and that exercise is a coping strategy requiring high self-control (Gailliot & Baumeister, 2007; Muraven & Baumeister, 2000). While Sonnentag and Jelden (2009) found that police officers are less likely to exercise after stressful workdays, Lutz et al. (2010) showed that only individuals who have developed stable exercise habits remained active under high stress. Because stress constitutes an obstacle for regular exercise involvement, volitional planning might help individuals to stay active. Coping planning can be defined as a prospective self-regulatory strategy that represents a mental simulation of challenging and overcoming anticipated action obstacles (Sniehotta, Schwarzer, Scholz, & Schüz, 2005). Typically, people who engage in coping planning attempt to identify personal risk situations (i.e. in which self-regulatory capacity is limited) and design detailed (emergency) plans, which are immediately accessible (if need be).

Experiential learning? The final question is whether or not the effect of exercise depends on the learning experience. While functional effects of increased exercise participation were strongly supported in prior studies, COR theory suggests that exercise is only a suitable stress management strategy when it fits with the individual's life circumstances. In our opinion, exercise offers special opportunities to learn about stress. For instance, exercise provides participants with opportunities to experience what stress means (imbalance between internal or external demands), and to develop the resources for problem solving. Likewise, exercise participants can experience stress symptoms (e.g. state anxiety, increased heart rate), discuss negative coping strategies (e.g. dysfunctional cognitions, negative self-talk), provide examples for good problem solving (e.g. testing problem solving cycles), develop mental skills (e.g. reframing, visualization), acquaint themselves with relaxation techniques (e.g. progressive muscle relaxation), seek social support (e.g. team tasks), and/or learn time and behavioral management skills (e.g. formulating concrete plans to learn a specific motor skill). Based on an experiential learning approach, we are currently evaluating the effects of a physical education-based coping training with vocational students (Gerber, Hartmann, Lang, Lüthy, & Brand, 2010). Prior research has shown that stress is an important issue for many adolescents (Jeannin et al., 2005), but that today, youth are not willing to seek professional support (Steiner & Gest, 1996). Since exercise does not have the stigma of psychiatric treatment (Larun, Nordheim, Ekeland, Hagen, & Heian, 2006), learning stress management through the physical dimension might be an acceptable and appealing approach for many adolescents and adults. In our opinion, the development of exercise therapy programs, in which participants do not only engage in exercise but also learn behavior skills to maintain regular exercise and obtain a deeper understanding of the factors involved in the generation of stress is a promising avenue for future research.

The role of exercise in **alcohol dependence recovery**

6

Attilio Carraro

6.1 WHAT ALCOHOL IS

Alcohol (ethanol is the most commonly ingested) is a clear, volatile, and very soluble organic compound that oxidizes easily, is rapidly absorbed and distributed in the body, and crosses the blood-brain barrier quickly, affecting brain centers for balance and coordination, judgment and reasoning, emotional control, level of alertness and socialization. The peak blood concentration is usually reached in 30-90 minutes and the absorption is faster when consumption occurs rapidly or on an empty stomach. Most of the alcohol consumed is metabolized in the liver by the cytochrome enzyme, the remainder is excreted unmodified by the kidneys or lungs. The body metabolizes about 15 ml of alcohol in one hour, equivalent to a moderate drink (e.g. 330 ml of beer or 140 ml of table wine).

Alcohol is a central nervous system depressant; the degree to which the function of the CNS is impaired is directly associated with the concentration of alcohol in the blood. The stages of alcohol intoxication vary from a subclinical stage (0.01-0.05 g of alcohol/100 ml of blood, with behavior almost normal), to a stage of confusion (0.18-0.30 g/100 ml, characterized by disorientation, mental confusion, dizziness, exaggerated emotional states, disturbances of vision, increased pain threshold, diminished muscular coordination, staggering gait, apathy), to the coma (0.35-0.50 g/100 ml, with complete unconsciousness, depressed or abolished reflexes, subnormal body temperature, incontinence, impairment of circulation and respiration, possible death) (Garriot, 2008).

It is important to note that many of these symptoms are exacerbated if alcohol intoxication is concurrent with fatigue and that several medications could increase the effects of alcohol.

6.2 MALADAPTIVE PATTERN OF ALCOHOL USE

Alcohol is the most widely available and culturally accepted psychoactive substance in the world. It is estimated that 90% of people in western countries consume alcohol at some point in their lives, with alcohol related problems arising in approximately 30% of drinkers. The high prevalence of abuse and dependence makes the evaluation of alcohol misuse an essential component of any psychiatric or medical assessment, and nearly all clinical problems may be related to the effects of alcohol abuse, addiction, intoxication, or abstinence (Kaplan & Sadock, 2001).

According to the American Psychiatric Association (DSM-IV-TR), a maladaptive pattern of alcohol use, leading to clinically significant impairment or distress, is defined by three (or more) of the following, occurring at any time in the same 12-month period:

1. Tolerance, as defined by either of the following:
   - a need for markedly increased amounts of alcohol to achieve intoxication or desired effect;
   - markedly diminished effect with continued use of the same amount of alcohol.
2. Withdrawal, as manifested by either of the following:
   - the characteristic withdrawal syndrome for alcohol;
   - alcohol (or a closely related drug) used to relieve or avoid withdrawal symptoms.
3. Alcohol is often used in larger amounts or over a longer period than was intended.
4. There is a persistent desire or unsuccessful efforts to cut down or control alcohol use.
5. A great deal of time is spent in activities necessary to obtain alcohol, use alcohol, or recover from its effects.

6. Important social, occupational or recreational activities are given up or reduced because of alcohol use.
7. Alcohol use is continued despite knowledge of having a persistent or recurrent physical or psychological problem that is likely to have been caused or exacerbated by alcohol.

Despite the fact that alcohol abuse and alcohol dependence are often used interchangeably, there are important differences between the two conditions. Diagnostically, alcohol dependence overrides the diagnosis of alcohol abuse. Dependence is a more complex and chronic condition and is generally considered to be an alcohol-related illness with physiological symptoms. Unlike alcohol abuse, the diagnosis of dependence addresses symptoms of alcohol tolerance and alcohol withdrawal.

6.3 THE DIMENSIONS OF THE PROBLEM

Alcohol abuse and dependence represents a growing global concern for public health. Alcohol dependence is related to premature death and avoidable diseases, is a major risk factor for neuropsychiatric disorders, cardiovascular diseases, cirrhosis of the liver and cancer, and is associated with several chronic diseases (e.g. HIV/AIDS and tuberculosis).

Abuse contributes significantly to unintentional and intentional injuries (e.g. road traffic accidents and falls) and, during pregnancy, can lead to severe neurological impairments of the child (WHO, 2009).

In Europe alcohol consumption shows a positive association with health care expenditure (Christiansen et al., 2007). Moreover, Europe is the heaviest drinking region in the world, with over 20% of the population of 15 years and older reporting heavy episodic drinking (defined as 50 g alcohol on one occasion) at least once a week (WHO, 2010). Data suggest an association of early onset drinking with health problems and mortality (Clark et al., 2001; Ahlström & Österberg, 2004/2005). The highest level of abuse is reached by men at 20-24 years and by women at 18-19 years. 25% of deaths between 15 and 29 years of age are attributable to alcohol, which is the first factor for disability, chronic disease and premature death in young people.

6.4 ALCOHOL CONSUMPTION AND SPORT PARTICIPATION

Despite the common perception of sport as a protective factor for risk behaviors, several studies (for a systematic review see Martens, Dams-O'Connor, & Beck, 2005) report a positive relationship between drinking in problematic ways and the participation in sport or physical activities. The problem is particularly evident during late adolescence and early young adulthood (Brandl-Bredenbeck, 2006), when psychoactive substance use represents one of the most prominent topics in the context of risk behaviors (Musselman & Rutledge, 2010). There is data indicating that young athletes engage more frequently in heavy episodic drinking and experience more negative alcohol-related consequences than non-athletes, and that a higher level of exercise in university students is associated with more, not less, alcohol consumption (Moore & Weerch, 2008). Binge drinking ranges from 25% to 50% for athletes, compared with 16% to 43% for non-athletes (McDuff & Baron, 2005). It appears team membership, and not physical activity per se, is the key element of this relationship. Excessive levels of alcohol consumption have been found in athletes at different levels of qualification and in different sports when socializing with sporting team mates compared to drinking on social occasions with other groups (Black, Lawson, & Fleishmann, 1999).

Alcohol use among athletes is associated with bad general health and negative athletic performance consequences. Moreover, injury rates among regular drinking athletes are higher (about twice) than among nondrinking athletes (O'Brien & Lyons, 2000).

Athletes seem aware of this situation college athletes, for example, cite alcohol as the most negative substance pertaining to performance and health, and mention different reasons (social, coping, hedonistic and performance related) to drink (Lorente et al., 2003; McDuff & Baron, 2005; Musselmann & Rutledge, 2010).

Because alcohol continues to be the most frequently consumed drug among athletes and habitual exercisers, the recommendation reported in 1982 by the American College of Sports in on the use of alcohol in sports is still relevant today: "Serious and continuing efforts should be made to educate athletes, coaches, health and physical educators, physicians, trainers, the sport media, and the general public regarding the effects of acute ingestion upon human performance and on the potential acute and chronic problems of excessive alcohol consumption."

On the other hand, there is evidence indicating that exercise-related activities are associated with positive outcomes in the treatment of substance abuse disorders (Weinstock, Barry, & Petry, 2008) and that a regular program of activity leads to a significant reduction in alcohol consumption for subjects who are heavy social drinkers (Murphy, Pagano, & Marlatt, 1986).

6.5 THE EFFECTS OF ALCOHOL ON PHYSICAL PERFORMANCE

Alcohol ingestion negatively impacts physical performance in a number of different ways. Alcohol consumption decreases the use of glucose and amino acids by skeletal muscles, adversely affects energy supply, and impairs the metabolic process during exercise (El-Sayed, Ali, & El-Sayed Ali, 2005). Well known additional negative effects are dehydration, dysregulation of body temperature (particularly during prolonged exercise), mood instability, and sensory motor system dysfunction, with worsening of psychomotor skills and reduced balance (Rosenbloom et al., 2007; Wober et al., 1999). Alcohol is also poor nutritionally; although it provides 7 calories of energy per gram, it does not improve energy availability or muscular work capacity and does not replace expended carbohydrates. Moreover, alcohol is often associated with weight gain caused by its "empty calories." These effects are mainly due to alcohol slowing the rate of metabolism (zero order kinetics) and its toxic interference with carbohydrate metabolism.

Several effects of alcohol ingestion have been recognized:
- consequences on the citric acid cycle (increased NADH, reduced NAD and consequent letup of the cycle and consequently of the aerobic metabolism);
- effects on lactate/pyruvate ratio (hyperlactatemia);
- negative consequences due to dehydration (2% of body weight dehydration significantly reduces aerobic performance);
- effects on available carbohydrates (reduced levels of muscle glycogen and blood glucose);

- effects on testosterone (alcohol can radically decrease serum testosterone levels);
- adverse psychological effects (migraine, depression, decreased sensitivity to external stimuli, delayed reaction time, reduced mental acuity, decreased hand-eye coordination).

6.6 EXERCISE INTERVENTIONS IN ALCOHOL DEPENDENCE TREATMENT

In 1974 Maletzky and Klotter wrote in the American Journal of Psychiatry: "Alcohol abusers are body abusers." This sentence represents the need to consider the body (or better, the relation between mind and body) as an epicenter in alcoholism treatment, with exercise interventions playing an important role in alcohol misuse rehabilitation and recovery.

In addition to the excessive consumption of alcohol, alcohol addicted people are frequently observed to have a high level of tobacco consumption (greater compared to the corresponding non-alcoholic population), bad nutritional status, and the presence of various organic damages due to abuse, including muscle weakness, joint instability and disturbances in the conduction of nervous impulses. Moreover, as reported in the previous paragraphs, acute ingestion of alcohol has detrimental effects on psychomotor skills (reaction time, eye-hand coordination, precision of movement, general coordination) and causes problems of thermoregulation during prolonged exercise. All these conditions make an exercise-based intervention for alcohol dependence recovery a useful but very delicate operation.

Despite the evidence for a psycho-physical approach to alcohol related problems, intervention studies which focused on exercise as an adjunctive treatment for alcoholism are very limited in number. Research suggests promising results, but scientific evidence is still limited and there is the need for more empirical indications to include extensively the use of exercise in alcohol rehabilitation programs.

A schematic review of papers published from 1980 onward is reported in Table 6.1. Eleven studies were found which analyzed the role of exercise as an adjunct to alcohol misuse treatment programs: four were randomized controlled trials (Murphy, Pagano, & Marlatt, 1986; Anstiss, 1991; Donaghy, Ralston, & Mutrie, 1991; Vedamurth-

Table 6.1 - Studies on exercise-interventions with alcohol addicted people

Study	Experimental design	Participant's Gender	Clinical setting	Type of exercise	Duration Frequency	Length of treatment	Outcome measures and outcomes
Tsuke & Shohoji (1981)	Single group pre-post	25 M	Japan, inpatient	Basketball	60 min 3/week	10 months	BP, vital capacity, waist/chest circumferences, skinfold, flexibility, strength, coordination ↑ fitness and coordination ↓ neurological disturbances
Sinyor et al. (1982)	Quasi-experimental control at different centers	58 M, W	Canada, inpatient	Stretching, calisthenics, walking/running, strength, cross-country skiing	60 min daily	6 weeks	VO₂ max, skinfold, BP, drinking report ↑ fitness and abstinence rates in experimental group at post-test and at 3 month follow-up ↓ body fat in fitness program participants
Murphy et al. (1986)	RCT 3 groups (running, meditation, control)	31 M	USA, undergraduate student high-volume-drinkers	Running	30 min 3–4/week	8 weeks	VO₂ max, daily self-reported journals, expectancy questionnaires ↑ VO₂ max in running group ↓ alcohol consumption in the 3 groups, with significant lower level in running group, no significant differences by group at follow-up
				Meditation (Carrington techniques)	Not stated; 3/week as a group, plus 20 min 2 times per day individually		
Palmer et al. (1988)	Quasi-experimental at different time points	27 M, W	USA, inpatient	Walking/ jogging ACSM guidelines	20–30 min 3/week	4 weeks	VO₂ max, Zung depression scale, STAI, TSCS No change in fitness and self-concept in experimental group ↓ anxiety and depression
Anstiss (1991)	RCT 2 groups (high and low intensity)	166 M, W	England, inpatient	Cycling high intensity and below training zone	Not stated; Daily	4 weeks	Unspecified fitness tests, BDI, STAI ↑ fitness in both groups ↓ depression in both groups No difference between groups in VO₂ max, BDI, STAI, drinking behaviors, increased dropout in high intensity exercise group
Donaghy et al. (1991)	RCT 3 groups	37 M	Scotland, outpatient	Aerobic and non-aerobic ACSM guidelines	30 min 3/week	8 weeks	VO₂ max, BDI, Leeds Scale, strength and flexibility ↑ strength in the 2 exercise groups, changes in fitness in aerobic group only ↓ anxiety and depression

Table 6.1 - Studies on exercise-interventions with alcohol addicted people

Study	Experimental design	Participant's Gender	Clinical setting	Type of exercise	Duration Frequency	Length of treatment	Outcome measures and outcomes
Ermalinski et al. (1997)	Quasi-experimental 2 treatment groups	90 M	USA, inpatient	Aerobic, stretching and body-mind components	30 min 5/week	6 weeks	↑ training effect and LOC in exercise group ↓ craving in exercise group No difference between groups in depression and self-esteem
Ussher et al. (2000)	Multiple case study	5 M, W	England, outpatient	Supervised exercise class (aerobic and strength) plus group-based physical activity counseling	75 min 9 sessions plus independent exercise	6 weeks	Field diary and self-reported measures. ↑ fitness, strength, self-image, body image, independence, integration, ↓ body weight, depression, smoking
Carraro et al. (2002)	Single group pre-post	65 M, W	Italy, inpatient	Aerobic, strength, stretching and body-mind components	60 min 3/week	6 weeks	EUROFIT test battery, Rosenberg self-esteem scale, DBQ, PACES ↑ fitness, coordination, self-esteem, enjoyment no changes in decisional balance
Vedamurthachar et al. (2006)	RCT 2 groups (yoga, control)	60 M	India, inpatient	Yoga (Sudarshana Kriya)	60 min Alternate day	2 weeks	BDI, plasma cortisol, ACTH, prolactin ↓ depression, cortisol, ACTH ↑ prolactin in both groups, significantly higher in experimental group
Brown et al. (2009)	Pilot study	19 M, W	USA, outpatient	Moderate intensity aerobic exercise, plus group behavioral training component	20-40 min 1 + 1 group behavioral training/ week	12 weeks	Physical activity screen, SCID-P, TLFB, breath analysis, cardiorespiratory fitness, body composition. ↑ cardiorespiratory fitness, alcohol abstinence ↓ body mass index, no differences at 3-month follow-up

Notes: BDI = Beck Depression Inventory; BP = blood pressure; CDT = carbohydrate deficiency transferring blood analysis; CES-D = Centre for epidemiological study on depression scale; DBQ = Decisional Balance Questionnaire; LOC = locus of control; M = man; MMPI = Minnesota Multiphasic Personality Inventory; PACES = Physical Activity Enjoyment Scale; PSPP = Physical Self Perception Profile; RCT = Randomized Controlled Trial; SCID-P = Structured Clinical Interview with Psychotic screen; SPE = Self efficacy for Physical Exercise; STAI = Spielberg State Anxiety Inventory; TLFB = Time–Line–Follow–Back; TSCS = Tennessee Self-Concept Scale; VO_2 max = estimated maximum oxygen consumption; W = woman.

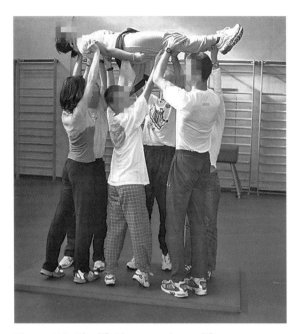

Figure 6.1 - The lift. The group has to lift up one member from the ground over their heads, stretching their arms, carrying the person tightly. This is a very exciting situation in which people deal with their force, their weight, trust in the others, and their sense of collaboration. In groups it is possible to realize what is impossible alone.

acher et al., 2006), three were quasi-experimental studies (Sinyor et al., 1982; Palmer, Vacc, & Epstein, 1988; Ermalinski et al., 1997), two were single group pre-post studies (Tsuke & Shohoji, 1981; Carraro, Mioni, & Pessa, 2002), one was a case study (Ussher et al., 2000) and one a pilot study (Brown et al., 2009). Studies investigated both inpatients and outpatients, one of them (Murphy et al., 1986) regarded heavy drinking in college students.

The majority of the studies described group-based exercise programs, including different aerobic activities (mainly walking, running and biking), strength training, calisthenics, team sports (basketball), yoga, or meditation. Three of them (Murphy et al., 1986; Ussher et al., 2000 and Brown et al., 2009) included home-based exercise programs. Frequency varied from once a week to daily; the length of treatment was from two weeks to ten months, with no clear rationale in the selection of the timescale. Only two studies (Palmer et al., 1988 and Donaghy et al., 1991) referred clearly to the American College of Sport Medicine guidelines on the frequency, duration and intensity of exercise. Various measures were used to test fitness, psychological, and behavioral modifications. The most frequently used fitness outcome was estimated VO_2 max; other physical measures were strength (mainly handgrip), flexibility, and coordination. All the studies which analyzed physical fitness, except Palmer et al. (1988), reported positive training effects. Psychological outcomes regarded above all depression and anxiety, with a general decrease in the level of depression and anxiety observed at the end of the treatment. Only limited attention has been devoted to evaluating the part of exercise in facilitating abstinence, reduced craving, and prevention of alcohol relapse. For this reason, and due to the small number of RCTs and follow-up studies, it is currently difficult to make firm conclusions about the role of exercise in alcohol rehabilitation and recovery.

6.7 POTENTIAL MECHANISMS OF ACTION

Different potential mechanisms of action for exercise in alcohol-related problem rehabilitation and recovery have been individuated (Brown et al., 2009; Donaghy & Ussher, 2005; Read & Brown, 2003). Exercise may:

- *provide pleasurable states without the use of the substance and constitute a positive non-drinking alternative.* Exercise may provide similar pleasurable effects to those experienced by means of alcohol consumption, it may mediate the activation of opioid systems induced by alcohol, which effects alcohol's reinforcement properties and contributes to excessive substance use (Froelich, 1997). Moreover, physical exercise, particularly when performed as a group activity, may be an opportunity for experiencing enjoyable recreational activities for persons with alcohol related problems (Murphy et al., 1986, Carraro et al., 2002) and can serve as a substitute behavior for drinking. Exercise may help to educate alcoholic patients in changing their habits, adopting a positive lifestyle with physical activity as a key component of this change;
- *reduce depressive and anxiety symptoms.* Alcohol misuse is frequently comorbid with depression and anxiety (Baigent, 2005). As indicated in different parts of this book, a consistent amount of research reports positive effects of

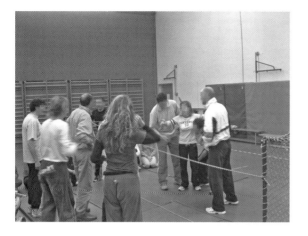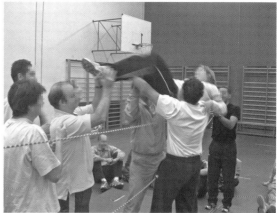
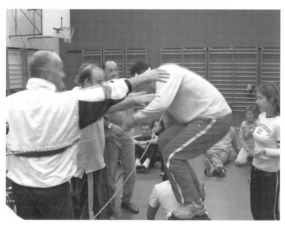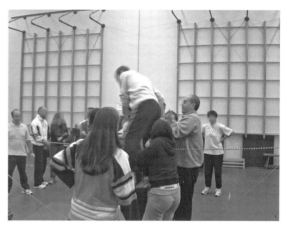

Figure 6.2 - The electric rope. Group has to organize to pass over the "electric rope," one person at a time. At each passage the rope is moved higher.

exercise in reducing depressive and anxiety symptoms and in acute improvement of mood (Physical Activity Guidelines Advisory Committee, 2008). This has also been shown in alcohol treatment exercise program (Palmer, Vacc, & Epstein, 1988; Palmer et al., 1995; Vedamurt-achar et al., 2006), and is associated with improved drinking outcomes;

- *increase self-efficacy.* Self-efficacy (the belief in one's ability to master particular skills) is classically viewed as a cognitive mechanism that affects behavior. The acquisition of exercise skills can be linked to increased levels of self-efficacy that may generalize to other areas such as implementing coping strategies necessary to maintain abstinence in the long-term;
- *decrease stress reactivity and improve coping.* Alcoholics can drink because of their deficiency in basic coping skills necessary to cope with

stressors associated with daily living (Keyes, Hatzenbuehler, & Hasin, 2011). Exercise can reduce stress reactivity (see Chapter 5) and could take the place of alcohol as a primary coping mechanism;
- *decrease urges to drink.* Reduction in the urge to drink has been identified as one of the most important objectives in alcoholism treatment. Single bouts of moderate intensity exercise seem to produce positive effects, decreasing alcohol urge in the short term (Ussher et al., 2004);
- *provide social support.* Group-based physical exercise may help to increase social support, to create supportive networks for recovery and to enhance the adherence to a program. Group participation allows members to experience meaningful interactions that do not involve alcohol consumption.

6.8 SUGGESTIONS TO ORGANIZE A GROUP-BASED EXERCISE PROGRAM IN A CLINICAL SETTING

The treatment of patients with alcohol-related problems is usually structured in three stages: *detoxification*; *rehabilitation and assessment*; *maintenance*.

1. *Detoxification* includes emergency treatment and screening (usually given at general medicine hospital departments or in specialist centers).
2. *Rehabilitation* and *assessment* cover primary care and the structuring of a therapeutic path (often organized in psychiatric clinics or specialist residential centers).
3. *Maintenance* after the therapy includes home-based treatment and is mainly oriented to prevent relapse (self-help groups – e.g. Alcoholics Anonymous – can play a fundamental role at this phase).

The treatment model that was originally most widespread was the *Minnesota Model*, ideated and implemented since 1950, a key element of which was the involvement both of professionals (physicians, psychologists, educators, social workers) and of inactive alcoholics (Anderson, McGovern, & Dupont, 1999). Today, the general trend is toward the implementation of multimodal programs, less rigid than the original *Minnesota Model* and capable of dealing more flexibly with the multiple problems that alcohol dependence entails.

In addition to offering specific treatment programs, the creation of residential rehabilitation centers can be particularly significant in reducing the frequent "revolving door" situation, characterizing patients that are cyclically hospitalized in general medicine hospital units due to periodical deteriorations of their organic and/or psychological conditions.

Exercise, as an integral part of a multimodal alcohol recovery program, can have positive effects mainly during the stage of rehabilitation and assessment (Donaghy, Ralston & Mutrie, 1991; Read & Brown, 2003; Sinyor et al., 1982). As of today there is a very limited number of studies providing evidence on the benefits of exercise in the prevention of relapses (see Table 6.1).

In our experience, we found that physical exercise, adapted sports activities, games, and relaxation are well accepted parts of a residential program, that can play important roles in the recovery of people with alcohol dependence (Carraro et al., 2002).

Three dimensions should be considered when to including exercise in a residential program oriented to rehabilitate people with alcohol related problems: a psycho-physical area, a social area, and an educational area (Table 6.2).

To better achieve positive results, there are various organizational aspects to consider, including:

- *the selection of the proposed activities* (in terms of movement situations, exercise, games, …). Close to specifically problem-oriented activities, it could be appropriate to include activities with which participants are familiar and that can easily be continued after the term of the residential program, in an everyday environment;
- *the selection of the instruments to use* (e.g. fitness and exercise machines, free weight exercise equipment, unconventional equipments) *and the settings* (indoor, outdoor, combination). Fitness and exercise machines (e.g. treadmills, exercise bikes, strength machines) facilitate and speed up the approach to the activities, re-

Table 6.2 - Objectives and areas for an exercise program with alcoholics

Objectives		
Psycho-physical area	*Social area*	*Educational area*
The body and the perception of the body: • rebuilding acceptable fitness; • to favor positive bodily feelings; • improving self-efficacy and self-esteem	Relation with others and communication: • respect the rules of behavior; • respect the rules of games	Changing lifestyle and elaborating suitable physical behaviors

ducing executive errors, but limit the range of options. Other equipment can permit a more creative approach and can facilitate group communication. The inclusion of outdoor activities can stimulate participants to be more active in their free time as well, and can easily continue at home after discharge;

- *the typology of exercise* (aerobic, strength, combination). The great majority of papers on alcohol and exercise, and more generally on exercise and psychiatric disorders, describes the effect of moderate intensity aerobic exercise. The rationale for this situation is not always clearly explicated. Certainly, the prescription of aerobic exercise, almost always performed on fitness machines (usually exercise bikes or treadmills) reduces the number of intervening variables to consider and make it easier to determine the amount of work, but on the other hand, aerobic exercise only limits the variability of the proposed activities and might not be the best strategy to cope with some problems frequently observed in patients with alcohol related problems (e.g. deficit in balance, reduction of coordination and loss of muscle strength);

- *intensity and duration*. Programs should be tailored on the basis of organic and psychological conditions, as well as individual characteristics and habits. It is necessary to avoid excessive intensity that could discourage participation, cause unnecessary tiredness and negative feelings, and that could require prolonged recovery time hindering subsequent exercise sessions. Evidence suggests that adherence rates for exercise can be improved with moderate versus high intensity (Perri et al., 2002);

- *weekly frequency*. It should be related to typology, intensity and duration of the exercise and to the length of the treatment. Weekly frequency should be selected to enable participants to experience skill improvements and positive changes in their fitness condition, meaning that the shorter a program is, the more sessions there should be per week;

- *group composition and exclusion criteria*.

Group-based treatment programs for alcoholics often involve patients with very different organic and psychological conditions, of different ages, with different fitness levels and various physical activity habits. Moreover, the number of patients who say they have had traumatic accidents in the past is usually very large. All these conditions require great attention in determining inclusion and exclusion criteria, and could make the selection criteria in creating a group a critical operation. In our experience, we preferred to maintain groups with rolling admission, characterized by the simultaneous presence of patients at different stages of the treatment. There is no gender or aged-based selection process, so people of very different ages may come together in the same group. Though it may complicate matters from a "technical" point of view, open groups can help to enrich the experience and to facilitate communication, favoring the onset of cooperative and support group dynamics, that are key points in the recovery from alcohol-related pathologies;

- *providing information on the activity*. Providing information regarding the physiological and psychological benefits of exercise and the proper organization of the activity (instruments, warm-up and cooldown procedures, facilities) is an important part of the program, that can orient participants to continue with the practice after their discharge from the hospital.

6.9 CONCLUSION

Exercise, particularly when group-based, can be a valuable instrument to include in a multi modal program to treat alcoholism. It permits the patient to cope with a number of problems related to alcohol abuse and to reduce individual resistance to take part in the recovery process.

Exercise can be an enjoyable experience giving easily perceived benefits, based on the respect of clear and simple rules, that contributes to the reduction of perceived barriers in abstaining from alcohol, and which sustains a positive change in lifestyle.

Physical activity in the treatment of people with schizophrenia

7

Davy Vancampfort, Jan Knapen, Ruud van Winkel, Marc De Hert

7.1 CHARACTERISTICS OF SCHIZOPHRENIA

Schizophrenia is one of the most severe mental illnesses. The Diagnostic Statistical Manual-IV (DSM-IV) criteria (American Psychiatric Association, 2000) for schizophrenia includes positive and negative symptomatology severe enough to cause social and occupational dysfunction over a period of at least 6 months. Positive symptomatology reflect an excess or distortion of normal functions and manifest themselves in symptoms such as delusions, hallucinations, and disorganised speech and behavior. Negative symptoms reflect a reduction or loss of normal functions, consisting of symptoms such as affective flattening, apathy, social withdrawal and cognitive impairments. The lifetime prevalence is estimated at 1% with a typical onset during adolescence and early adulthood (Lieberman, Stroup, & Perkins, 2006). The peak incidence of onset is between 20-24 years in men and 25-29 years in women (Kirkbride et al., 2006). Schizophrenia is perhaps the most debilitating psychiatric disorder (Rossler, Salize, van Os, & Riecher-Rossler, 2005). According to the Global Burden of Disease Study, schizophrenia accounts for 1.1% of the total DALYs (disability-adjusted life years), and 2.8% for men and 2.6% for women of YLDs (years lived with disability) (World Health Organization, 2008). Schizophrenia is listed as the 5th leading cause of DALYs worldwide in the age group 15-44 years (World Health Organization, 2008).

7.2 RATIONALE FOR PHYSICAL ACTIVITY IN SCHIZOPHRENIA

People with schizophrenia have a 20-25 year reduced life expectancy compared to the general population (Osby, Correia, Brandt, Ekbom, & Sparen, 2000), primarily due to premature cardiovascular disease (CVD) (Brown, 1997; Casey et al., 2004; Newcomer, 2007; Capasso, Lineberry, Bostwick, Decker, & St Sauver, 2008). They have nearly twice the normal risk of dying from CVD (Brown, 1997; Casey et al., 2004; Saha, Chant, & McGrath, 2007; Capasso et al., 2008). This has led to a growing concern about physical illness in the course of schizophrenia in recent years, specifically CVD risk (Casey et al., 2004; Hennekens, Hennekens, Hollar, & Casey, 2005; Carney, Jones, & Woolson, 2006; Leucht, Burkard, Henderson, Maj, & Sartorius, 2007; Fleischhacker et al., 2008; von Hausswolff-Juhlin, Bjartveit, Lindstrom, & Jones, 2009). Large population-based studies have identified key modifiable risk factors for CVD, including obesity, smoking, hyperglycemia, hypertension, and dyslipidemia (Wilson et al., 1998; Luepker, Evans, McKeigue, & Reddy, 2004). Metabolic syndrome (MetS) brings together a series of the abnormal clinical and metabolic findings that are predictive of CVD risk (Expert Panel on Detection and Evaluation of High Blood Cholesterol in Adults, 2001; Alberti, Zimmet, & Shaw, 2006; Grundy et al., 2005). The criteria for MetS are summarized in Table 7.1.

People with schizophrenia are known to have a two-to-threefold increased relative risk for MetS compared to healthy individuals (De Hert, Schreurs, Vancampfort, & van Winkel, 2009; De Hert, Dekker, Wood, Kahl, & Müller, 2009; Meyer & Stahl, 2009). In part, the worse cardio-metabolic profile in people with schizophrenia is attributable to the use of antipsychotic agents, which can have a negative impact on some of the modifiable risk factors (Fleischhacker et al., 2008; De Hert et al., 2009). However, over recent years it has become more apparent that in schizophre-

Table 7.1 - Working criteria for the metabolic syndrome

Criterium	ATP-III	ATP-III-A	IDF
Waist (cm)	M>102, F>88	M>102, F>88	M≥94, F≥80
Blood pressure (mmHg)	≥130/85	≥130/85	≥130/85
HDL (mg/dl)	M<40, F<50	M<40, F<50	M<40, F<50
Triglycerides (mg/dl)	≥150	≥150	≥150
Glucose (mg/dl)	≥110	≥100	≥100

Note: ATP = Adult Treatment Protocol (Expert Panel on Detection and Evaluation of High Blood Cholesterol in Adults, 2001), ATP-A = Adult Treatment Protocol-Adapted (Grundy et al., 2005), IDF = International Diabetes Federation (Alberti et al., 2006), M = male, F = female..

nia, an unhealthy lifestyle including smoking, poor diet, and sedentary behavior is associated with adverse cardio-metabolic effects (Correll, Frederickson, Kane, & Manu, 2006; De Hert et al., 2009). People with schizophrenia are less physically active than healthy controls. Total energy expenditure is more than 20% lower than the minimum recommendations of the American College of Sports Medicine and the American Heart Association (Sharpe, Stedman, Byrne, Wishart, & Hills, 2006), and only 25% meet the minimum public health recommendation of 150 minutes a week of at least moderate-intensity activity (Faulkner, Cohn, & Remington, 2006). On weekdays they spend less time with strenuous activities than healthy individuals, and during leisure time a greater proportion of people diag-

nosed with schizophrenia are not involved in sport activities (Roick et al., 2007). Only about 30% can be classified as being regularly active relative to 62% of a non-psychiatric comparison group (Lindamer et al., 2008).

The course and outcome of schizophrenia is difficult to predict (Di Michele & Bolino, 2004). Although in the past most attention was given to reducing psychopathology, other outcome parameters such as cognitive and occupational performance, emotional stability, quality of life, and psychosocial functioning are increasingly recognized for their importance. Instead of merely reducing symptoms, current treatment must strive for more ambitious goals such as remission and recovery (Juckel & Morosini, 2008). Physical activity (PA) interventions may have an important complementary role in this process (de Haan, 2009). Furthermore, the observation that regular PA over the long term is strongly associated with a reduction in all-cause mortality in active subjects compared to sedentary persons (Lollgen, Bockenhoff, & Knapp, 2009) is particularly interesting in this high risk-group.

7.2.1 **Physical health benefits**

Good physical health is a realistic goal in the multidisciplinary treatment of people with serious mental illness, and lifestyle programs that consider smoking cessation, diet and PA are essential (Bradshaw, Lovell, & Harris, 2005; Richardson et al., 2005). Two systematic reviews investigating physical health parameters in people with schizophrenia concluded that PA is associated with modest weight loss (Faulkner, 2005; Vancampfort, Knapen et al., 2009).

The consensus in the general population that

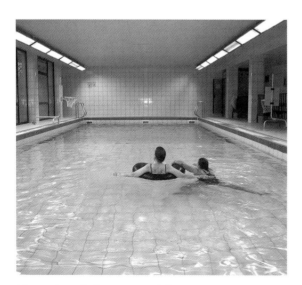

Figure 7.1 - Swimming pool. Water activities can represent useful tools in the rehabilitation of psychiatric diseases.

PHYSICAL ACTIVITY AND MENTAL HEALTH – A Practice-Oriented Approach

moderate weight loss is associated with a reduction in CVD-risk factors is likely to also be observed in people with schizophrenia. After PA, people with schizophrenia demonstrated significantly reduced systolic and diastolic blood pressure, baseline fasting glucose concentrations, insulin resistance, circulating levels of triglycerides, and total serum cholesterol, while the ratio of low density lipoproteins to high density lipoproteins also decreased significantly (Vancampfort, Knapen et al., 2009). An important observation is that the functional capacity, as measured by the 6-minute walk test, improved in several studies (Beebe et al., 2005; Marzolini, Jensen, & Melville, 2009). The 6-minute walk test reliably reflects daily life activities (Enright, 2003).

Poor motivation as a consequence of negative symptoms (avolition, anergia and anhedonia) which are inherent to the symptomatology (Archie, Wilson, Osborne, Hobbs, & McNiven, 2003; Centorrino et al., 2006; Duraiswamy, Thirthalli, Nagendra, & Gangadhar, 2007) and side-effects of medication (Carter-Morris & Faulkner, 2003; Centorrino et al., 2006) are often perceived as important barriers to PA participation. Adherence to PA therefore is the most important predictor of outcome (Vancampfort, Knapen et al., 2009). Without support of physical therapists, people with schizophrenia exercise only sporadically (Centorrino et al., 2006) and drop-out rates in PA programs may raise up to 90% after six months (Archie et al., 2003). However, with the application of motivational strategies, attendance rates can increase up to 90% after six months (Wu, Wang, Bai, Huang, & Lee, 2007). Group-based attendance seems to be superior to individual home-based PA (Marzolini et al., 2009).

7.2.2 Mental health benefits

Psychopathology

Three systematic reviews indicate that PA can be a useful adjunct for the multidisciplinary treatment of both negative and positive symptoms (Faulkner & Biddle, 1999; Faulkner, 2005; Vancampfort, Knapen et al., 2009). In particular, delusions, confusion and hallucinations as positive symptoms decrease, and emotional insensitivity, apathy, anhedonia and attention from the cluster of negative symptoms may significantly improve (Acil, Dogan, & Dogan, 2008).

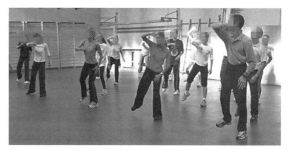

Figure 7.2 - Gym with music. Group-based activity with music can be very stimulating in motivating people to be physically active.

Psychosocial parameters

Improvements in global mental health (Marzolini et al., 2009) and increases in perceived physical and psychological quality of life (Duraiswamy et al., 2007; Acil et al., 2008) can be observed after 10 to 12 weeks. Furthermore, PA offers an oppor-

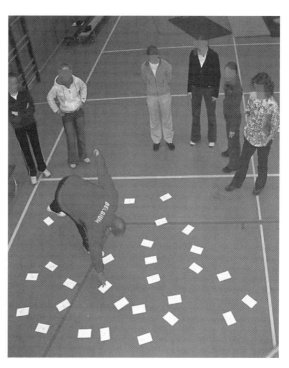

Figure 7.3 - Post-it game. A number of post-its numerated in ascending order are scattered on the ground. Participants line up on the field border. At the start signal, they have to touch as quickly as possible all post-its on the ground, in the requested order (increasing, decreasing, singular, plural, etc...). The challenge is to ameliorate the total time required to complete the task. The team has to collaborate to find the best strategy to facilitate each performance.

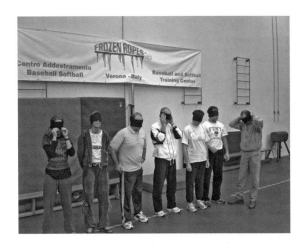

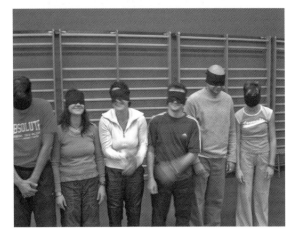

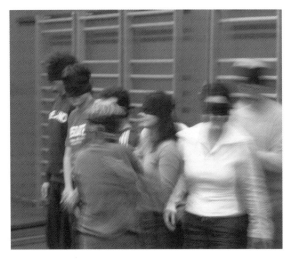

Figure 7.4 - Partner in voice. Paired blindfolded participants form two frontal lines. Only by means of partner's verbal indications, each participant has to join his/her partner in the frontal line. This game increases selective attention in discriminating sound stimuli and encourages confidence in partner.

tunity for social interaction (Carter-Morris et al., 2003; Fogarty, Happell, & Pinikahana, 2004; Duraiswamy et al., 2007). Recently, it has been demonstrated that acute bouts of aerobic PA and yoga are equally effective in decreasing state anxiety and psychological distress and increasing subjective well-being (Vancampfort, De Hert et al., 2009). These observations may offer interesting treatment perspectives in dealing with co-morbid substance abuse (Mueser, Yarnold, & Bellack, 1992; Kumari & Postma, 2005; Green, Drake, Brunette, & Noordsy, 2007). Although different motivations exist to use these substances, it has been suggested that the mentioned unhealthy behaviors may in part be attempts to alleviate or to cope with unpleasant affective states and feelings of anxiety (Gregg, Barrowclough, & Haddock, 2007) or are a way to cope with side-effects of antipsychotic medication. The limited benefit of such efforts supports the need to provide other, more healthy methods to regulate the variability of subjective well-being.

7.2.3 Cognitive benefits

In one study, people with schizophrenia reported an improved cognitive status in terms of memory and concentration after PA (Hasson-Ohayon, Kravetz, Roe, Rozencwaig, & Weiser, 2006). The same has been observed more rigorously in the general population (Hillman, Erickson, & Kramer, 2008; Angevaren, Aufdemkampe, Verhaar, Aleman, & Vanhees, 2008). Beneficial effects on cognition occur even more so for those processes requiring greater executive control (i.e. processes involved in scheduling, planning, monitoring, and task coordination) (Dishman et al., 2006). In particular, these functions are related to daily activities and community functioning of patients with schizophrenia (Aubin, Stip, Gelinas, Rainville, & Chapparo, 2009).

7.3 PRACTICAL IMPLICATIONS FOR PHYSICAL ACTIVITY INTERVENTIONS IN SCHIZOPHRENIA

Given the physical and mental health benefits of regular PA participation, PA should be integrated within the multidisciplinary treatment of schizophrenia. Nevertheless, people with schizophrenia have low access to physical health care, which moreover is often of poor quality (Newcomer, 2005; Nasrallah et al., 2006; Leucht et al., 2007; Fleischhacker et al., 2008). Therefore, attention should be given to making PA facilities easily accessible and available. Screening for risk factors should be undertaken and baseline physical fitness investigated while specific cardio-metabolic comorbidities need to be taken into account by using the PA recommendations for chronic somatic diseases (Pedersen & Saltin, 2006). In offering PA, therapists should provide their patients with a supportive environment. Opportunities for social interaction and exchange are important. Group-based programs can provide consistent support and help build initial motivation by helping participants understand how PA will benefit them. As participants become more physically active, such programs can help them address barriers that may arise. Specific barriers that a physical therapist needs to take into account in patients with schizophrenia are:

- avolition, anergia, and anhedonia, which limit patients' ability to experience pleasure and positive reinforcement during PA which in turn limits the ability to generate the same level of internal drive or intrinsic motivation as peers in the general population;
- pervasive cognitive impairment which limits the ability to sustain focus on a strategy or goal, the ability to integrate situational context or previous experience into ongoing processes;

TEXTBOX **7.1**

Practical suggestions for physical therapists

- Do not require patients to set any goals about their physical behavior when they enter the program. Rather, first attempt to engage them in the PA program itself. One factor that deters patients from commitment to PA is low self-efficacy based on a long history of failure in achieving goals. Consequently, attempt to enhance a sense of efficacy by building the experience of success into the program.

- Afterwards, together with the patient, identify small and concrete steps that the patient is comfortable with.

- Rather than attempting to make a broad shift in the decisional balance about being physically active or not, attempt to identify one or two specific consequences that have a strong impact on the patient and that can serve as a prompt for change.

- Provide patients with choices and options about the type of PA (e.g. yoga or aerobic exercise) that best fit with their current preferences.

- Structure the time schedule and content of the PA program.

- Use intensive individual flip charts with concrete information about the exercises.

- Prompt patients as many times as necessary. Repeat the exercises within and across the PA sessions.

- Acknowledge the individual PA responses. These individual responses should be taken into consideration when (re)designing and (re)delivering the PA program. Modalities of the program resulting in beneficial effects should be repeated while those having adverse or even effects should be stopped.

- When group sessions are planned, careful patient assessment is imperative in order to prevent inadvertent stress and worsening of symptoms. Excessive affective expression, confrontation, and probing within a group setting can be overly stimulating and stress inducing to the patient with schizophrenia. Management of these patients in a group setting requires a skilled physical therapist who can set limits and structure the group environment.

- marked social impairment which limits the communication of personal thoughts, feelings and bodily sensations;
- psychotic symptoms (delusions, hallucinations, disordered thinking and bizarre behaviors) which may impede the patients' efforts;
- medication side-effects which may cause disturbances in balance and coordination.

These limitations suggest the very anchors by which physical therapists traditionally have navigated PA sessions need adjustment in applications of PA for people with schizophrenia. However, based on the scientific literature presented, some suggestions can be made; they are described in Textbox 7.1.

7.4 SUMMARY AND GUIDELINES FOR PHYSICAL ACTIVITY INTERVENTIONS IN SCHIZOPHRENIA

An increasing body of evidence suggests that PA is a feasible and effective intervention in improving physical and mental health in people with schizophrenia. Current scientific literature indicates that identifying an optimal dose or intervention strategy for PA programs for both cardio-metabolic parameters and positive and negative symptomatology in people who have schizophrenia is not (yet) possible. Rather, the individual responses and compliance to PA need to be taken into account. PA programs should be adapted to the patients' previous experiences, their attitude toward PA, their personal preferences and objectives, and their individual physical abilities. Physical therapists should provide people with schizophrenia with options about the type and content of their program. Until there is more clarity related to an optimal PA dose or strategy, current guidelines for the general population should be used. If improving the cardio-metabolic fitness in patients with schizophrenia is the major aim, the recent guidelines of the American College of Sports Medicine and the American Heart Association for weight loss and prevention of weight regain in the general population (Donnelly et al., 2009) should be applied to people who have schizophrenia. According to these guidelines, moderate-intensity PA between 150 and 250 min. a week will provide modest weight loss and is effective to prevent weight gain. Greater amounts of PA (>250 min. a week) can be associated with clinically significant weight loss.

When promoting general health, the guidelines of the American College of Sports Medicine and the American Heart Association can be applied (Haskell et al., 2007). Moderate-intensity aerobic (endurance) PA for a minimum of 30 min. on five days each week or vigorous-intensity aerobic physical activity for a minimum of 20 min. on three days each week is needed. Combinations of moderate- and vigorous-intensity activity can be performed to meet this recommendation. For example, a person can meet the recommendation by walking briskly for 30 min. twice during the week and then jogging for 20 min. on two other days. Moderate-intensity aerobic activity, which is generally equivalent to a brisk walk and noticeably accelerates the heart rate, can be accumulated toward the 30-min. minimum by performing bouts each lasting 10 or more min. Vigorous-intensity activity is exemplified by jogging, and causes rapid breathing and a substantial increase in heart rate. In addition, individuals should perform activities that maintain or increase muscular strength and endurance a minimum of two days each week.

Life in movement: a **physical activity program** involving schizophrenic participants in **community settings**

8

Kátia E.L. Borges, Filipe A.S. Moura-Lima

8.1 INTRODUCTION

According to the World Health Organization (WHO), schizophrenia is on the world's top ten list of the most disabling conditions, and it is, together with bipolar disorder, the most common condition confronted by Brazilian mental health professionals (World Health Organization, 2009; Brazil's Health Ministry – SUS, 2009).

Studies indicate that approximately 1.5% of the world's population may develop schizophrenia related disorders (American Psychiatric Association, 1990; Sadock, Sadock, & Ruiz, 2009; World Health Organization, 2009). There is considerable controversy about the prevalence of schizophrenia in developed countries as compared to those on the developmental periphery. Some studies indicate that the differentials are significant, whole others are skeptical regarding the range of incidence (World Health Organization, 2002; Thirthalli, J. & Jain S., 2009). Furthermore, there is controversy about the data concerning the ratio of patients who show full remission in developed as opposed to less developed countries. There is a trend for higher rates of remission in peripheral countries attributed to environments where there is more family support and less stressful lifestyles (Jablensky et al., 1995; World Health Organization, 2009).

Brazil is a country of nearly 8.5 million Km² with a population of 190 million inhabitants. It is composed of 26 states, 5560 cities, and one federal district. The enormous contrasts existent in Brazilian society are evidenced by the Human Development Index (HDI). According to the HDI, Brazil occupies the 79th place in the world. This ranking depicts it as a low-middle income country. Nevertheless, Brazil's economy is acknowl-

edged as a large one by the World Bank (World Bank, 2008). Belo Horizonte is the capital of the state of Minas Gerais and its population is approximately 2.5 million. Public health care, provided by the Unified Health System (SUS) covers all inhabitants (Instituto Brasileiro de Geografia e Estatística, 2004).

Table 8.1 presents the number of users with psychiatric diagnostic register at SUS in Belo Horizonte in 2010, the percentage of these users enrolled in the day care and the percentage of users diagnosed with Schizophrenia participating in the day care activities.

CAPS structure is organized in two complementary sections: The Center of Reference in Mental Health and the Community Centers. The first provides day and/or night hospital care and the second provides activities such as arts, handcrafts, gardening, and physical activity. The service users' participation in the program is voluntary (Greco & Carvalho, 1994; Silva & Bastos, 2005).

The Life in Movement Program (LMP) started in 1997 at the Federal University of Minas Gerais through the School of Physical Education, Physiotherapy and Occupational Therapy – in partnership with Belo Horizonte's City Hall. The Mental Health Department aimed to establish and devel-

Table 8.1 - SUS users with psychiatric diagnostic in Belo Horizonte

Total of users (n.)	4352
Users in Day Activity Centers (%)	18.54
Users with Schizophrenia (%)	50.6

Table 8.2 - LMP: participants' profile

Data	Value in %
Age	
15-24 years old	13.2
25-34 years old	20.9
35-44 years old	32.6
45-54 years old	18.6
55 years old or more	14.7
Gender	
Male	51.9
Female	48.1
Marital, social and educational status	
Single	69.0
Married	20.2
Lives with parents or husband/ wife	76.0
Incomplete Elementary School	58.9
Self supported	68.2*
At least 1 psychiatric hospitalization	70.0

*From these 68.2%, 79.5% receive retirement or pension of approximately US$270.00 per month.

op a Community-Based Physical and Recreational Activities Program.

The idea behind this program came from the belief that overcoming functional and psychological limitations that disable or reduce social access can best be remedied by psycho-physical-social approaches, in the context of rehabilitation psychiatry (Borges, 1998).

LMP's main objective is to encourage CAPS users to be physically active and more independent.

It consists of four phases, ranging from a basic approach related to the participants' functional body development in a process of self-differentiation in phase 1 to the participants' active and competitive participation in sports and more demanding activities in phase 4.

Table 8.2 shows the profile of schizophrenic participants in the LMP[1] (Borges, 2005).

_____
[1] sample = 128 with diagnosis from F20 to F29 – ICD–10.

8.2 SCHIZOPHRENIA AND PHYSICAL ACTIVITY: THE LIFE IN MOVEMENT PROGRAM EXPERIENCE

Physical activity has been recommended as an adjunctive treatment for schizophrenic patients based on its physical and psychological benefits, and due to the potential that this kind of activity has for implementing habits and lifestyle changes (Beebe, Tian, Morris, Goodwin, Allen, & Kuldau, 2005).

Facing the physical health issues, it is already known that a high number of these patients present weight gain, high obesity profiles, diabetes, cardiovascular risk factors, metabolic syndrome, cigarette, alcohol and/or hard drug abuse, and other physical conditions that are related to sedentary lifestyles (Gothelf et al., 2002; Morgan, 2005; Richardson, Faulkner, McDevitt, Skrinar, Hutchinson, & Piette, 2005; Sharpe, Stedman, & Byrne, 2006; Mauri, et al., 2006; Faulkner, Cohn, Remington, & Irving 2007).

Furthermore, the everyday use of antipsychotics by this population has been identified as one of the variables which induce increased body weight, diabetes and other co-morbid medical diseases (Connolly & Kelly, 2005; Richardson et al., 2005; Scheen & De Hert, 2005, 2007).

There is some scientific agreement that modifications of sedentary lifestyles, poor nutritional habits, cigarettes, alcohol, and/or hard drug dependence are essential in preventing co-morbid diseases and resultant high mortality rates (Meyer & Broocks, 2000; Morgan, 2005; Sorensen, 2006; Faulkner, Cohn, Remington, & Irving, 2007).

Physical activity has been associated with psychological benefits for schizophrenic patients, mainly as related to depression and anxiety control; as well as improved self-confidence, body image and the perception of well-being (Meyer & Broocks, 2000; Richardson et al., 2005; Faulkner, 2005; Borges, 2005). However, if it is possible to affirm that regular physical activity can prevent and treat cardiovascular risk factors and other physical diseases related to the sedentary profile in schizophrenic patients, affirming that physical activities can bring benefits to their psychopathological condition requires caution.

Further research needs to be conducted to better understand the relationship and impact of physical exercise on severe psychopathology. In addition, more study is needed regarding the role that severe psychopathology plays on body control and learning motor capacity (Hannaford, Harrell, & Cox, 1988; Connolly & Kelly, 2005; Ellis, Crone, Davey, & Grogan, 2007; Gaudiano, Weinstock, & Miller, 2008).

Recent statistical data reveal that 46% of schizophrenic patients are not involved in sport activities compared to 33.5% of general population. Another important datum is that 30% of this medical population is considered physically active compared to 62% of the non-psychiatric group (Roick, Fritz-Wieacker, Matschinger, Heider, Schindler, Riedel-Heller et al., 2007; Lindamer, McKibbin, Norman, Jordan, Harrison, Abeyesinhe et al., 2008).

In the last research conducted by CAPS, approximately 36.8% of their schizophrenic population were interviewed regarding their level of motivation and participation in physical activities. The results showed that 76.6% stated the importance of regular physical activity and 65.5% indicated motivation to be enrolled in a physical activity program. However, 90.7% of them were not involved in sport activities and only 30.2% were practicing some kind of physical activity.

The main sport practiced by this small group was football (soccer), while walking was the main physical activity practiced among the more physically active CAPS clientele. According to 43.5% of users, walking was the main physical activity recurrently advised by their physicians (Borges, 2005).

Some evidence has been found that psychiatric patients encounter more barriers than the general population in terms of practicing physical activities on a regular basis. These barriers may in part explain why schizophrenics are typically less active than the normal population (Brown, Birtwistle, Roe, & Thompson, 1999; Gothelf et al., 2002; Sorensen, 2006).

The CAPS investigation into their clientele's contingent factors in sport and other physical activity identified three main factors (Borges, 2005):
- accessibility (deficit in the public infrastructure);
- social interaction (restricted sharing activities with relatives, friends and colleagues);
- dependence (restricted autonomy; dependence on family and submission to family routines).

The factors that render sport and other physical activity more available to the service users are:
- freedom (understood as the capacity of interacting and choosing activity without someone else's interference or control; the person's desire);
- competence (understood as the recognition of one's abilities and the efficiency in this domain);
- security (understood as the recognition of belonging to a specific group; self-confidence).

One factor that should be taken into consideration relative to these issues is the schizophrenic's persistent vulnerability to the disruptive impact of positive symptoms (hallucinations, delusions and racing thoughts) on his or her ability to integrate perceptions (Fernandes da Fonseca, 1997; Martinsen & Stanghelle, 1997; Dalgarrondo, 2000; Sadock, Sadock, & Ruiz, 2009).

Based on these CAPS data, and a literature review of physical activity programs for schizophrenic patients, what was eventually to become the long term Life in Movement Program was organized to provide practical meetings to achieve the following two goals: to prevent participants' recurrent psychotic crises and to help them return to a home-based program, augmenting their inclusion in local society.

The basic pedagogical scheme is presented in the first part of this chapter and the practical experiences of the program's intervention routines are discussed in the latter part. The theoretical-practice topics are based on and guided by specific issues mentioned in the international literature and on the basis of the CAPS actual experience.

8.3 THE RATIONALE

In the humanization process (universalization principle), falling victim to a severe mental disturbance is a condition of being in the world and it manifests itself by altering the reality and social interactions of the suffering individual. However, embracing the flows of desire allows stabilization of the symptoms, which in turn allows the search for meaning and enables *subjectivation* (principle of singularity). This will enlarge the socialization process (the discovery of the other as a principle of reality).

Thus, the program proposes to embrace the schizophrenic participant's flow of desire in its

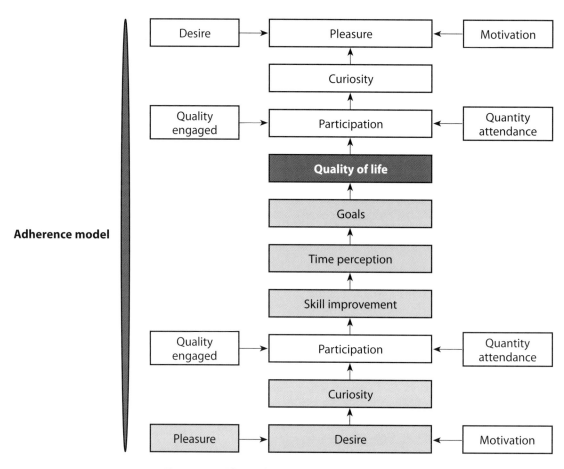

Figure 8.1 - The pedagogical platform used in LMP.

8.4 LMP – THE PEDAGOGICAL PLATFORM

Psychic integration is promoted when the experience of the imaginary is captured in the leisure environment of physical activity, such as those provided by dance and sport. When their content and form are coupled with professional care, the results can be quite positive. It is during these brief moments that the participant's desire emerges, and it is possible at that point to stimulate the individual's intrinsic motivation (Borges, 1995, 1998; Borges, Marques, & Silva, 2006, 2007).

These short moments allow the participant to enter the symbolic order which bars the imaginary order of their completeness. The entrance into the symbolic order allows the participant to look for difference and to confront pleasure and displeasure (figure 8.1)[2] (Lacan, 1986).

When this position is attained, it is then possible to talk and create pedagogical interventions based on participant's body-perception and body-image. When this subjective position is achieved by the participant, it is the proper time to deliver motor and physical activities that stimulate the transformation of body experiences into life experiences. At this point, it is important to give special attention to how the participant verbally and physically expresses the construction of their

---

[2] The spatial vectors (the arrows) are designed to explain this scheme. It represents the idea of a continuing process of potential development when considering the human domains.

PHYSICAL ACTIVITY AND MENTAL HEALTH – A Practice-Oriented Approach

corporeity and to emphasize the importance of this construction on their own life history.

The objective of planning and delivering interventions based on this pedagogical platform is to stimulate the participant's curiosity for a better quality of life (Giannetti, 2002; Borges, 2005; Borges, Marques, & Silva, 2006, 2007).

As stated above, when the search for differences begins, it becomes pedagogically possible to assist the participant in developing their *curiosity*. The participant's enhanced curiosity enables didactic intervention on the *motivational base* of the participant. This intervention begins with an invitation to participants to simply come share a physical space with other participants. With frequent attendance, this simple presence can transform into actual participation. The participant's attendance has to be transformed into a habit of being which is present on a regular basis during physical activity.

Regular physical activity, established as a commitment, positively influences the individual's self-confidence. The frequent practice attendance habit and the resulting improved self-confidence make the participant physically and emotionally available to integrate into a group practice. In turn, together with the other participants' frequent practice attendance, the affective support of the group provides the conditions for the participants to develop and recognize their own basic motor abilities.

The improvement of self-confidence and self-recognition of basic motor abilities, as a result of both the frequent practice attendance and the *participation* in the construction of a cohesive group, provides the minimal conditions necessary for the development of appropriate interaction with other people in physical activity, dance, and sports.

At this point in a participant's practice development, it is important to organize practical interventions that will ensure the individual's group engagement momentum. For this reason, it is essential to maintain a balance between the activities that are developed in place and time under the control of the participants and the new places and schedules where practice will be developed. The achievement of the physical and psychic conditions above described allows pedagogical interventions based on the participant's volition to engage in physical activities. When a better group communication is achieved, it is time to stimulate

the valorization and the advance of specialized movements. Development of dance and sport *skills* creates the possibility of pedagogical interventions based on the participant's *temporal orientation*.

The intervention plans should be composed of games, educative sport activities, and dance. Sport rules need explanation, followed by short periods of dance and sport activities.

The inclusion of the participant's relatives and friends in practices is important because it can help validate the participant's abilities and skills. In addition, this intervention can and should emphasize the local cultural roots of the dance or sport that are included in the program. This also integrates the participant with their family's dance and sport routines and helps develop affective relationships between the participant and other family members. In this context, systematic motor and physical activities, games, dance, and sport practices should offer the participant activities where choices and decisions have to be made. When this motivational base is attained, two other transformations should occur in the intervention, one in the group of family and friends and the other in the participant's psychic process of judgment. At this point in the program, the participant's family members and friends should be prepared to fully assume their responsibility to change the family's physical activity routines so as to include the participant. On the other hand, the participant should be prepared to define the physical activity, dance and/or sport objectives and *goals* to be shared with friends and family members. These, in turn, serve as the guidelines for reforming the participant's sedentary lifestyle habits.

The capacity to define these goals is associated with the participant's capacity to establish a standard of competence that should be integrated into the participant and his family's social discourse. The participant should be stimulated to establish a standard of participation that gives them singularity in the social participation.

The intervention in the psychic process of judgment is accomplished through the technical and tactical challenges presented to the participant during their dance and/or sport practices.

As mentioned before, the objective of this pedagogical scheme is to stimulate the participants' curiosity and motivation to develop a better quality of life.

The concept of quality of life proposed by the World Health Organization associates the personal perception of one's own aspirations and interests in life with the values established by the social system in which the participant finds themself (Lehman, 1996; Huxley, 1998; Giannetti, 2002; World Health Organization, 2009). In this way, the concept of quality of life highlights the interconnections that exist between the values, interests, motivations, and personal definitions (subjective dimension) with the system of values established in the cultural context of the community in which the participant lives (objective dimension).

For this reason, one of the most important challenges faced by the Life in Movement Program is the development of the participant's intrinsic motivation toward this kind of activity. Its specific goal is to assist the person to modify their sedentary lifestyle, poor nutritional habits and addiction dependence (Borges, 1997, 1998; Borges, Marques, & Silva, 2003, 2006, 2007).

8.5 THE LIFE IN MOVEMENT INTERVENTIONS PLATFORM

The structure of the LMP intervention is presented in Figure 8.2.

8.5.1 Pedagogical methods

Underlying LMP's current structure, several theories and teaching techniques have been studied, reviewed, and adapted to suit to the reality of the participants and of the program (Donadia, 2007). Some of these theories and techniques will be described below.

The Applied Behavior Analysis has been used over the past forty years. Some of the techniques used by Reid, O'Connor, and Lloyd (2003) are the Discrete Trial Format and the use of Prompts and Reinforcement. The Discrete Trial Format figures as the basis of the Applied Behavior Analysis. It consists of 4 phases: 1) to solicit the participant's attention, 2) to give a command, 3) to wait for the participant's response and 4) to reinforce an adequate response.

Another technique used in this method is the Prompts. It consists of using external stimuli (physical, visual, verbal) to teach a determined response to a stimulus in a teaching situation. The professional is responsible for helping the partici-

pant respond adequately to determined stimulus (Loovas, Koegel, & Schereibman, 1979). In the Prompts technique, as the level of skills shown by the participant increases, the assistance diminishes by a corresponding degree.

Another pedagogical method used in LMP is Incidental Teaching, which has been adapted from Phonoaudiology. In this method, some objects are randomly placed in a space where the intervention will be conducted.

Then the professional must attempt to determine which objects captured the participant's attention. However, the participant cannot remain passive, but must request the object on the basis of their own volition.

Pivotal Response Training, which incorporates some of the Incidental Teaching principles, is also one of the pedagogical methods used in LMP. However, the main innovation it entails is that it focuses on central behaviors such as answering cues, self-initiative, and self-management.

In this method, the cues are important as to distinctions between size, color, size and shape. An example of a cue situation would be a professional asking the participant to get the big and soft green ball. Self-initiative consists in teaching and encouraging the participant to talk about the location of the objects, to ask for help when needed, and to make choices. As for the self-management, it is directly related to the time-space relationship, where the participant will have to manage the time necessary to perform a particular activity (Reid, O'Connor, & Lloyd, 2003).

8.5.2 The practical experiences

Scientific literature recommends that physical activity programs for this population should be performed on a regular basis, composed of moderate intensity aerobic exercise and/or anaerobic exercise, focused on the participant's motivations and their social partners' recognition (Faulkner & Taylor, 2005; Borges, 2005; Morgan, 2005; Skrinar, Huxley, Hutchinson, Menninger, & Glew, 2005; Faulkner, Cohn, Remington, & Irving, 2007; Martinsen & Raglin, 2007; Stuart, Biddle, & Biddle, 2008).

It is advisable to prescribe aerobic exercises from 50% to 60% Heart Rate Reserve for psychiatric patients and this level of effort should be maintained from 20 to 30 minutes. However, this general rule should be considered within the context

PHASE 01	
3 months - 12 meetings	

General Objectives (Based on Crouch, 1989):
   To increase the participant's constructive actions
   To develop the participant's functional body	

Motor Capacities and Abilities

General Contents	*Specific Contents*	
• Motor conduction • Motor adaption and re-adaptation • Learning motor capacity	• Posture • Expression • Mobility	• Coordination • Rudimentary basic abilities

Psychological Capacities and Skills

General Contents	*Specific Contents*	
• Psychological adaptation and re-adaptation • Emotional and cognitive learning capacity	• Attention • Memory • Orientation	• Affectivity • Self • Language

Social Capacities and Skills

General Contents	*Specific Contents*	
• Social adaptation and re-adaptation • Social learning capacity	• Frequency norms • Recognition of the other participant	• Social Attention • Communication

PHASE 02	
3 months - 12 meetings	

General Objectives:
   To increase the participant's explorative and experimental actions
   To increase the participant's motor scheme	

Motor Skills and Physical Capacities

General Contents	*Specific Contents*
• Motor control • Motor adaptation, re-adaptation and movement competence to a variety of stimuli • Learning motor capacity	• Motor Exploring • Motor Experimenting • Mobility • Coordination • Fundamental Skills

Psychological Capacities and Skills

General Contents	*Specific Contents*	
• Emotional control • Feelings adaptation, re-adaptation and control • Emotional and cognitive learning capacity	• Attention • Memory • Orientation • Affectivity	• Volition • Self Identity • Language

Social Capacities and Skills

General Contents	*Specific Contents*
• Social skill control in practice environment • Social adaptation and re-adaptation • Social roles • Social learning capacity	• Social Presence • Identification of the others participants • Social Attention • Communication

Figure 8.2 - LMP intervention structure.   (*continued*)

PHASE 03	

3 months - 12 meetings

General Objectives:
  To increase the participant's experimental and imitative actions
  To increase the participant's motor and physical actions

Specialized Movements and Physical Fitness

General Contents	Specific Contents
• Elaborated and combined movements • Competence in specialized movements for daily life, recreation, and sport pursuits • Practicing motor repertoire	• Motor Experimenting • Motor Imitation • Motor Original • Specialized Movements • Cardio respiratory endurance

Psychological Capacities and Skills

General Contents	Specific Contents	
• Emotional adaptation • Feelings exploration • Emotional and cognitive learning capacity	• Attention • Memory • Orientation • Affectivity	• Volition • Self Identity • Language • Judgement

Social Capacities and Skills

General Contents	Specific Contents	
• Open social practices experimentation • Social roles • Set social goals • Social learning capacity	• Share social space • Share materials and equipments • Share social time • Define social expectations	• Social Attention • Communication

PHASE 04	

3 months - 12 meetings

General Objectives:
  To increase the participant's original and product-centered actions
  To increase the participant's specialized sport movements

Sports and Physical Fitness

General Contents	Specific Contents
• Specialized Sport Skills • Specialized Physical Fitness Skills • Practicing Skills Repertoire	• Specialized Sports Movements • Specialized Physical Fitness Movements • Cardiorespiratory Endurance

Psychological Capacities and Skills

General Contents	Specific Contents	
• Emotional Experience • Sharing Feelings • Emotional and Cognitive Learning Capacity	• Attention • Memory • Orientation • Affectivity	• Volition • Self Identity • Language • Judgement

Social Capacities and Skills

General Contents	Specific Contents
• Social roles, • Setting social objectives and goals • Setting specific environment demanded objectives and goals • Social Learning Capacity • Social Inclusion	• Sharing inclusive Sport practices • Sharing inclusive Physical Fitness practices • Sharing social time • Defining social expectations, objectives and goals for an active life • Social Attention and Memory • Communication

Figure 8.2

of the patient's age, sport participation history and current physical condition.

Young participants and participants in good physical condition can be motivated to exercise at least 30 minutes between 2 to 4 times per week (Faulkner & Taylor, 2005; Morgan, 2005; Stuart, Biddle, & Biddle, 2008).

In a tropical city like Belo Horizonte, where the mean annual temperature during the winter month of July is 18 °C (64 °F) and physical activities occur outside between 8:00 am and 5:00 pm, it is suggested during aerobic and anaerobic practice to have small breaks for participants to drink some water. These breaks should be around every 15 minutes of time practice.

For this reason, in order to define the exercise schedule, some variables need to be taken into consideration, such as: the hour of day the session will occur, the specific CAPS hours, the season of the year, meal schedule, the participants' medication and impregnation quality. The participant's actual physical condition at the time is also an overarching variable (Borges, 1997).

Some technical marks have been investigated to serve as references on physical activity prescriptions on control of cardiovascular risk factors, and as part of the participants' evaluation on a program. Some of them are listed below (Meyer & Broocks, 2000; Rocha, 2001; Manson & Katzmarzyk, 2009):

- the formula based on individual age to define the Heart Rate (HR) has been used to control the aerobic and non-aerobic activity intensity;
- the Body Mass Index (BMI) to verify the cardiovascular risk factors;
- the Waist Circumference (WC) to verify the cardiovascular risk factors and limitations in physical functioning in everyday life.

In spite of the fact that estimation procedures, like HR, compromise research work, this is a practical formula for application in a community program.

In the same way, WC compared to BMI has a stronger correlation to Quality of Life (QoL) and is simple to use in community programs (Meyer & Broocks, 2000).

Excitatory symptoms – as excitement and poor impulse control – and the need for constant psychopharmacology to inhibit these kinds of symptoms on this populational group must be considered when prescribing physical activity (Dalgarrondo, 2000; Sadock, B., Sadock, V., & Ruiz, P., 2009).

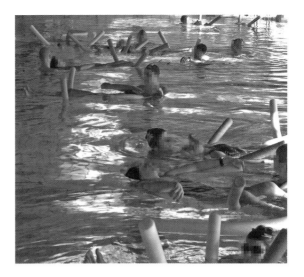

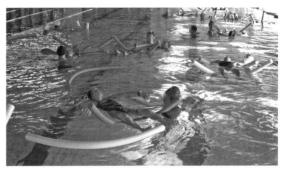

Figure 8.3 - Swimming group. Water is an ideal setting for relaxing activities and adapted games.

Since the Life in Movement Program is focused on functional improvement, quality of functional gestures, and sport performance, the evaluation of participants' motor behavior has been taken into consideration.

However, few motor tests have been considered scientifically reproductive and valid to this clinical adult group, and these are specifically, regarding hand-eye coordination (Moura-Lima, Borges & Probst, 2009).

As the motor behavior evaluation is made, it is important to give special attention to the participants' age, past history in sport, dance, or physical activity, and psychic and emotional condition.

For the reasons mentioned above, the marks on motor behavior in schizophrenic populations and their practical use in community programs needs to be better discussed.

Advisably, using 50% to 60% Heart Rate Reserve in aerobic exercise prescription to psychiatric patients may ensure the patient's systematic exercise practice and decrease cardiologic incidents during the exercise program, but it is considered a restriction on improving the individual training level and a limitation on understanding this variable as a therapeutic factor for schizophrenic patients.

Another factor that should be considered concerns program length.

Interventions based on modification in patients' daily habits is desirable to ensure long term habituation and long term physical health gains. It has been suggested to plan programs that last at least 14 weeks (Meyer & Broocks, 2000; Ellis et al., 2008). However, if the intervention is planned for adult participants with very low physical training profile, without any sport or physical activity history, in a low income community setting, and focused on stigma combat and social inclusion, 14 weeks is considered to be a very short time for implementing pedagogical actions to modify sedentary habits and influence social inclusion.

It has been verified that at least 6 months are needed to implement the base of such modifications (Simão, Monteiro, Saporetti & Borges, 2007).

Additionally, the Life in Movement Program experience has shown that family members' and friends' involvement in participants' physical activity routines also demand a longer period (Borges, 2006).

As mentioned before, the Life in Movement Program is organized by phases and each phase has short, medium, and long term plans to improve the participant's curiosity, functional motor abilities, specific sport skills, time perception, and leisure and physical activity/sport goals.

Currently, the program is working with the hypothesis of 3 months participant's frequency in each phase to achieve the next phase. Further researches need to be conducted to verify phases and program length.

8.5.3 Aerobic exercise

Aerobic exercise is also known to reduce risk factors related to sedentariness such as obesity and cardiovascular problems. Since these conditions are frequently observed in people with schizophrenia, it is also very important to encourage the participants to cycle, walk, or jog regularly (McArdle, Katch & Katch, 2007; De Hert, Schreurs, Vancampfort, Van Winkel, 2009).

In LMP, the participants walk for 10 to 15 minutes at a space outside the gym. As they exercise they are frequently asked about how they are feeling and about how they perceive that activity in terms of effort. Since there are not heart rate monitors available for everyone, they are taught to spot and count their heart rate at the wrist and neck.

During the first 6 weeks, the main concern is helping them develop good walking patterns and to focus on breathing as they walk. After the first six weeks (or earlier for participants who demonstrate good walking patterns), they walk or jog at 50-60% of Heart Rate Reserve in agreement with Knapen et al. (2008)

The 6-Minute Walk Test is performed at the beginning and end of the 3 month period to verify the adequacy of the training in for provoking the expected physiologic adaptations and improving functional capacity.

At the beginning and end of the 3 months the participants' BMI and Waist to Hip Ratio are calculated to compare pre and post values.

8.5.4 Strength and aerobic training

Mostly due to the development of exercise machines in the sixties and the bodybuilding movement of the eighties, more attention has been given to strength training variables and methods. However, regarding people with schizophrenia, the implementation rationale used for the general population does not seem to be the same (Marzolini, Jensen, & Melville, 2009).

The sedentary lifestyle of people with schizophrenia leads to a lack of previous experiences related to movements that require balance and motor coordination (Newcomer, 2005; Scheen & De Hert, 2005; Scheen & De Hert, 2007; De Hert, Schreurs, Vancampfort, & Van Winkel, 2009).

Added to this sedentary lifestyle, when considering schizophrenia, the body fragmentation and jeopardized time-space relation are hard obstacles to overcame (Lacan, 1986; Ey & Brisset, 1969; Müller, 1985).

The first and second conditions are respectively related to a compromised perception of the individual's body and to an absence of synchronicity between external and internal time (Lima, 1999).

These conditions make it even more challenging to teach the participants exercises, as they move and feel their body under the constraints of time. On the other hand, to put them in exercise situations that confront these conditions is important, since it gives them the chance to experience body and muscle perception on specific moments and place.

LMP has developed a practical approach in overcoming some of the difficulties of engaging participants in strength training programs.

It consists of group exercise sessions where the participants experience some of the movements performed at the gym without weights or with only their body weight. Three different exercises are performed in groups, organized as circuit training. They perform the movements for one minute, and the command to exercise is a song that is played. When the music stops there is a 90-second pause. During the pause, they are asked about the muscles that were worked and how they are feeling. During this practice, their attention is directed to their own body. They are invited to touch the moving articulations and working muscles, providing moments where they are conscious about themselves, enhancing their self-awareness.

Every time they perform exercises that isolate some parts of the body such as the arm curl, movements that use more parts of the body are carried out afterwards. An example would be to bend down, touch the floor, and stand up raising their hands.

After this initial process, they are directed to the gym and introduced to exercises that use preferentially large muscular groups with three or more articulations simultaneously. The exercises are executed in machines rather than with free weights in attempt to assure a good trajectory during execution.

As they perform the exercises they are encouraged to focus on their body and on the working muscles. At every moment they are invited to touch themselves where they feel the effort and to tell the professional responsible for the meeting about that feeling.

At this moment, there is no concern in terms of intensity. The emphasis is given in volume so that participants can learn and practice the movements, and feel the muscles they should focus on in that particular exercise. This deemphasis on intensity is also a measure of safety. Since they are not experienced enough, there is some danger of injury due to improper articulations.

8.5.5 Dance

The Brazilian folk dances have been used in LMP as a strategy of developing the participants'

perception of their bodies, their perception of time and space, and for creating socialization opportunities. According to Côrtes (2003), folklore is a the body of expressive culture, including stories, music, dance, legends, oral history, proverbs, jokes, popular beliefs, customs, and so forth within a particular population comprising the traditions of a determined culture. The study of folklore enables us to understand and reflect on the traditional knowledge disseminated in the society.

In LMP, a folk dance called *Dança do Pezinho* (Little Foot Dance), traditional to Rio Grande do Sul (Brazil's South Region) has been included in Phase 3 of the program because it is performed in pairs, stimulating contact with others, increasing chances of socialization by group participation, and for its simplicity.

The meetings are organized with two 1-hour sessions per week using the partial teaching method. This method has been chosen because of rhythmic difficulties presenting in some of the participants. The dance steps are taught one by one and practiced first without, then with music.

In order to stimulate the participants, several *Dança do Pezinho* videos are shown to them with the aim of illustrating the cultural context involved and to inspire the design of the outfit, which is made by them with the LMP's support.

During the meetings, the Observational Check List: Motor, Psychological and Social Performance in Dance Meetings and specific notes are used to register individual performances and to analyze whole pedagogical processes later on (Simões et al., 2007). The observations are based in 3 different categories: motor skills, psychic functions, and involvement with the group. The categories are sub-divided into:

1. *Motor skills*: motor exploring, motor experimenting, mobility and coordination;
2. *Psychic functions*: attention, memory, orientation, affectivity, volition, self identity, language;
3. *Involvement with the group*: social presence, identification of the others participants, social attention, communication.

8.5.6 Body expression

Hurtado (1991) defines expression as the process of symbolizing what is significant to our perception. So, to express is to manifest feelings and thoughts hidden by the person.

Body expression is understood by Tubino and

Tubino (2007) as an art expression derived from the dance, and is also present in sports, due to the gracefulness of sport gestures and movements.

Because of its technical, clinical, and pedagogical qualities, this kind of art activity is considered relevant to inclusion in physical activity programs for schizophrenic participants. Within this context, Amaral (2004) presents practical goals that are possible to be achieved with this group:
- personal development;
- body control;
- object control;
- cooperation;
- solidarity;
- creativity;
- group engagement;
- gesture and movement pleasure;
- anxiety control;
- aggressiveness control;
- communication ability.

To Mauerberg-deCastro (2005), part of these goals are possible to be achieved because body expression exercises facilitate body part recognition. It also puts the participants in situations where they can explore movement in different perspectives, plans, positions, directions, and intensity, and contrast their own body parts in terms of space and time, body-object relation, and sharing space with others.

In LMP the body expression activities are usually offered in Phases 1 and 2 of the program, and interventions are planned based on a list of 12 body expression activities. These activities were researched to investigate their motor, psychic functions, and social impact on schizophrenic participants. After the results of this study, the activities were divided into 4 topic groups and organized in the program as listed below (Monteiro, 2008):
- self-discover, self-articulation, movements;
- space, notion, combination;
- ball, I and the ball, the ball and my body;
- self recognition, interaction, I and the other.

These body expression activities can also be seen as an evaluation tool for observing the participants' body awareness as they join the program. For this reason, it is important to keep the body expression activities in the same order as offered on the first body expression meeting to compare the participant's body part recognition, space and time integration, body-object relation, and ability to share space with others.

On the LMP's weekly schedule, body expression activities take place once a week.

It is suggested to use the following didactic procedures to organize the activities: a) verbal cues and feedback from the participants; b) objects are randomly placed in a space where the intervention will be conducted. The verbal cues consist of naming parts of the body, positions, dimension, specific perspective plan, colors found in the meeting room, etc.

The Global pedagogical method has shown to be more consistent than the Partial method in conducting this kind of activity. No adaptation is made when offering the body expression activities, even if physical challenged are included in the group. They are stimulated to express themselves without any boundaries.

The participants' feedback regarding to the activities is collected by gathering and making notes about verbal comments, observations, and suggestions. Each participant is encouraged to share their comments with another participant or to all participants of the group. Social interaction has been an important part of this didactic methodology.

The LMP investigation about the impact of the 4 topic group activities in schizophrenic participants motor, psychic functions, and social development showed that these three domains receive equal impact.

8.5.7 Recreational games

To Edginton, Jordan, DeGraaf, and Edginton (1998), recreation is a pleasant activity, which can be used to recover social values. It involves voluntary participation, which can be focused on the development of social habits.

According to Li (1981) and Werneck (2000), recreational approach consists of helping individuals in environmental and relational stress control and in the recognition, analysis, and anticipation of daily situations that cause pressure for the individual on a social level and in recreational activities.

This author emphasizes that learning abilities, knowledge of community programs, and different ways of dealing with daily stress should be the aim

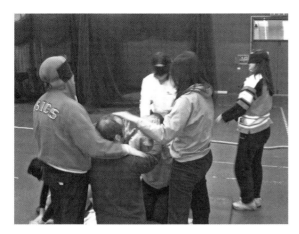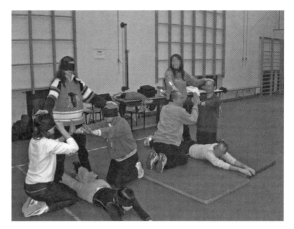

Figure 8.4 - Blindfolded sculptors. Participants are divided into two groups; a group of blindfolded sculptors and another group that has to build a sculpture by themselves. Blindfolded sculptors touching and handling the sculpture have to reproduce it. This contact play provides much stimuli in the social, emotional, and physical domains, improving collaboration and imagination.

of professionals and recreational programs for schizophrenic patients.

Recreational contents are part of activities offered by LMP. It is organized in 1-hour meetings carried out once a week. The interventions are planned around a list of 20 recreational games characterized as competitive and cooperative. These selected games were previously studied to identify the motor, psychic, and social function in schizophrenic LMP participants (Saporetti, 2008).

Participants' observations are structured and systematized under the concept of competence. This term is taken to mean the capacity to perform, control, and produce adequate results in a requested or spontaneous action. The observational check list is established with three categories: motor competence, psychic competence, and social competence. The following are the variables used in each category:
- motor: physical-motor, perceptive-motor, cognitive-motor;
- psychic functions: attention, memory, language;
- social: attitudes and values.

Every semester when scheduling the LMP's recreational interventions, it is suggested to organize, at least a second turn of the recreational games previously applied, to have a second systematized observation of the participants on the same cooperative and competitive activities.

The didactic applied to the recreational games uses the Partial pedagogical method, and the interventions are planned with aim to respect the participants' physical and motor ability levels, and the motivational, cognitive, psychological and social capacity of the participants.

It is suggested to use the following didactic procedures to organize the activities: demonstration, verbal instruction, and feedback from the participants. As a positive reinforcement it has been established that participants should be called by first name and stimulated to speak their own observations out loud when playing the games.

The impact category and the list of the 20 recreational games studied by the LMP are:
- Social and Psychic Functions: *Batata Quente, Passa Anel, Coelhinho Sai da Toca, Mímica, Adoletá, Uatatá, Desperta Memória, Escuridão da fantasia*;
- Social and Motor: *Estátua, Bate, vai e volta, Brincadeira de Advinhação, Trenzinho Maluco*;
- Social: *Quem é o Maestro, Cai no Poço*;
- Social, Motor, and Psychic Functions: *Jogo da Velha, Corre Cutia, Mãe da Rua e Nó Humano, Roubo do Rabo, Pega no Pulo*.

Every year, CAPS administrators organize a tournament that gathers all community centers' users, called Spring Tournament. Participation is voluntary. There are games such as Dodgeball, Indiaca, Indoor Soccer and Football (Corrêa, 1995; Ornelas, 1997; Borges, 1997).

8.6 ASSESSMENT AND EVALUATION EXPERIENCES

The integration of clinical, pedagogical, and scientific methods of assessment and evaluation has to be reached to develop program evidences on physical activity in this specific group.

Some instruments and protocols have been used to assess and to evaluate the Life in Movement participants. Some of the LMP assessment and evaluation experiences will be discussed on the following paragraphs (Lima, 1999; Rocha, 2001; Borges et al., 2003; Borges, 2005; Simões et al., 2008; Saporetti, 2008; Monteiro, 2008; Moura-Lima et al., 2009).

8.6.1 Semi-structured interview, questionnaire and check list instruments

In the interview planning, some extra time should be reserved for explaining the object, the objectives, the data confidentiality, the benefits, and the risks involved in the assessment. It may take longer or it may be necessary to go through this procedure more than twice, before the interview can be conducted.

It is suggested to state clearly to the interviewee that all doubts related to the object, the objectives, the data confidentiality, the benefits and the risks of the interview procedures can be explained during the interview. It is important to reserve a private and secure location to conduct the interview to guarantee the interviewer-interviewee confidentiality and security, and to raise the interviewee's attention to the questions. The interviewer has to be prepared to receive the interviewee's verbal consent to participate in the interview, but due to the psychic condition of the interviewee or their analphabetic condition, the participant may refuse to sign the Informed Consent Form.

On the first condition mentioned above, extra time should be taken to gain a better trust relationship with the interviewee, and on the second the interviewer can write down the name of the participant.

The LMP experience has demonstrated that questions about exercise routine, sport participation, recreation, and physical leisure activity is taken by the participants as a nostalgic issue. This nostalgia leads the participants to be talkative during the interviews; for this reason it demands more attention from the interviewer to consolidate the answers.

When more than one interview is needed to be conducted with the same participant, it is suggested that it be done by the same interviewer. Sometimes, there is a refusal by the interviewee to talk about specific topics to different professionals.

The number of instruments applied during the assessment process should be taken into consideration. Long interviews can be considered boring or be seen as privacy invasion by this clinical group.

Dividing the process is important to keep the interviewee's attention for all instruments applied. It is also important to consider their complaint about always being tested and to respect the interviewee's subjective position toward being asked and questioned about specific issues.

The assessment process may require two or three days in a row to be organized. However, the instruments sequence has to be maintained through all interviews applied in order to guarantee the reproducibility of the assessment procedures.

The LMP interview experience suggests that objective questions should be asked first before starting more subjective questions. It has been demonstrated that through this procedure it is possible to get deeper and more substantial answers.

In the interest of obtaining better answers, it is essential to define how many times one single question is going to be asked during the process and if it is necessary to change the question sequence during the interview to ensure the interviewee's capability to understand the questions. There is a tendency in this population group to present the answers located on the extreme of the answer chart.

It is recommended to write down the time spent on each interview. This procedure helps to plan the next interviews, if necessary.

Besides the linguistic, semantic, and cultural adaptations of foreign instruments to be applied in this community program, the implementation of a pilot project into this clinical group is suggested to guarantee the applicability of the instrument due to their low educational profile and poor exercise, sport, and physical activity experiences.

Regarding the assessment instruments in which the answer sheet is organized as check points, it is recommended to look at the instrument manual to verify if it is possible to transform the affirmatives into questions. This possibility could help in applying the instrument to analphabetic groups.

If affirmative, it is also important to define how many times the question is going to be asked and if the grammatical form used in the affirmative assures the same interpretation as a question.

In case of having to read some specific question emphasizing specific words, or if specific temporal marks demand the interviewee's attention, it is important to conduct a careful study of the instrument manual or its validation norms.

It has been very useful, when using this kind of instrument in the LMP, to change the order of the answers every three questions. This procedure helps capture the interviewee's capacity to understand the question.

Some specific findings:
- the more recently the participant has enrolled in CAPS service, the more difficulty they have in answering the questions and participating in LMP interviews;
- the interviews conducted just after collective workshops, such as music or text reading workshops, demand more time to engage the interviewee;
- the difficulty in hearing and intellectual deficit can present obstacles in the interview, special adaptations may be needed to ensure its successful realization.

8.6.2 Evaluation

In order to be well structured and to keep the pre-set goals in mind, physical activity programs must have assessment and evaluation tools.

To perform the physical and motor tests a statement is required from the participant's general practitioner or cardiologist clearing them to take part in the tests. Physical and motor test organization and execution demand some extra time from the professionals responsible for the evaluation. This extra time is important for explaining the tests' goals, procedures, the benefits and risks involved in the test, and to demonstrate how the tests should be performed. All professionals involved must be well synchronized to deliver the information in the clearest way possible and to demonstrate accurately.

It may be necessary to go through this routine more than three times, and sometimes it will have to be to be conducted one by one. For this reason, it is important to plan at least one or two extra meetings to assure the conclusion and the quality of the evaluation.

The motor test demonstration should follow the test protocols, but it is important to describe the motor tasks step by step and fragment the demonstration if necessary. However, in case of fragmenting, the last demonstration should be complete, in the way it is stated on the test protocol.

LMP's schedule during summer has to count on extra meetings, since summer is the rainy season in Belo Horizonte and most physical and motor tests are conducted outside.

Based on LMP participants' education levels and diagnoses, the physical, motor, and test-battery's simplicity and the few materials needed are important to facilitate the participants' tolerance throughout the evaluation process.

Other important aspects in these tests are related to the material cost and the community programs' funding. The cost of material and equipment is one of the most important variables to finding a test included in this kind of community program.

Since the educational level of LMP participants is low, the Informed Consent Form is usually read to them. If they agree with the conditions of the tests they sign it or have their name written for them by the professional responsible for the test.

Exercise for **depression** and **anxiety**: an **evidence based approach** and recommendations for **clinical practice**

9

Jan Knapen, Davy Vancampfort

There have been over 25 years of systematic investigation examining the relationship between physical activity, especially aerobic exercise and weight training, and depression and anxiety. In this chapter, we first present the findings of two recent meta-analyses in the area of physical activity and depression and anxiety. Potential mechanisms by which exercise may reduce depression and anxiety are described.

Depression and anxiety are associated with a high incidence of co-morbid somatic illnesses, especially cardiovascular diseases and type 2 diabetes. Positive effects of regular exercise on these diseases in individuals with depression and anxiety disorders are discussed. Finally, we offer evidence based recommendations for good clinical practice.

9.1 DEPRESSION

Depression is a common mental disorder that presents with depressed mood, loss of interest or pleasure, feelings of guilt or low self-worth, disturbed sleep and appetite, low energy, and poor concentration. The diagnostic criteria for major depressive disorder following the American Psychiatric Association (2004) are presented in Textbox 9.1.

TEXTBOX **9.1**

The American Psychiatric Association criteria for diagnosis of Major Depressive Disorder

Five (or more) of the following symptoms have been present during the same 2-week period and represent a change from previous functioning; at least one of the symptoms is either (1) depressed mood or (2) loss of interest or pleasure.

A. Depressed mood, nearly every day during most of the day

B. Marked diminished interest or pleasure in almost all activities

C. Significant weight loss (when not dieting), weight gain, or a change in appetite

D. Insomnia or hypersomnia (excess sleep)

E. Psychomotor agitation or psychomotor retardation

F. Fatigue or loss of energy

G. Feelings of worthlessness or inappropriate guilt

H. Impaired ability to concentrate or indecisiveness

I. Recurrent thoughts of death, recurrent suicidal ideation

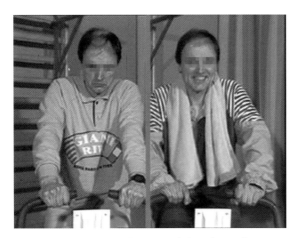

Figure 9.1 - Depressed man on bike. Physical activity can help people with depression regain physical energy and to ameliorate their mood. It can give people a new attitude toward facing ordinary activities.

Depression is a widespread and often chronic condition. Lifetime prevalence estimates for major depressive disorder are approximately 15% to 20%; 1-year prevalence estimates are 5% to 10%. Moreover, depression is characterized by high rates of relapse: 22% to 50% of patients suffer recurrent episodes within 6 months after recovery (World Health Organization, 2004).

In 2000, depression was the leading cause of disability as measured by Years Lived with Disability and the 4th leading contributor to the global burden of disease. The World Health Organization expects that by the year 2020, depression will reach second place in the ranking of Disability Adjusted Life Years calculated for all ages, including both sexes (World Health Organization, 2004).

The American Psychiatric Association (2004) describes several other mood disorders from which major depressive disorder should be distinguished. Dysthymic disorder is a mild but chronic depression, lasting at least two years but usually longer. People with dysthymia may subsequently develop an episode of major depressive disorder. Bipolar disorder (manic depression) is characterized by a chronic dysregulation of mood, with fluctuations between low mood (i.e. depression) and elevated mood (i.e. mania or hypomania). The American Psychiatric Association (2004) distinguishes two forms: bipolar type 1 with episodes of mania and type 2 with hypomanic episodes. Manic episodes are typically associated with be-

havioral activation (e.g. increased goal-directed activity, decreased need for sleep) and altered cognitive functioning (e.g. racing thoughts, distractibility, grandiose delusions). The symptoms of hypomania are less severe.

9.1.1 Exercise as intervention for depression and depressive symptoms: findings of the most recent meta-analysis

There is growing evidence that exercise may be an effective therapy for mild to moderate depression and a valuable complementary therapy to the traditional treatments for severe depression. Several meta-analyses examine the effect of exercise on depression; however, some meta-analyses have been criticized for including studies of poor methodological integrity and lacking analysis of moderating variables. The most recent meta-analysis of Rethorst, Wipfli, and Landers (2008) addresses this criticism by including only randomized control trials and analyzing moderating variables (i.e. population characteristics and exercise program characteristics). This meta-analysis examines the effects of exercise on depression/depressive symptoms in 58 randomized controlled trials (n = 2982). An overall effect size of -0.80 (large effect) indicates that participants in the exercise treatment had significantly lower depression scores than those receiving the control treatment or no treatment. Seventeen studies examined the effect of exercise on *clinically depressed individuals* (n = 547). Clinically depressed participants in the exercise treatment had significantly lower depression scores than those in no treatment or wait-list control condition (effect size = -1.03, large effect). Four studies compared exercise treatment with psychotherapy in clinically depressed people, resulting in an overall effect size of -0.26, indicating that exercise resulted in larger antidepressant effects than psychotherapy. However, this difference was not significant. Three studies compared exercise versus antidepressant medication and found an overall equal effect. Nine studies investigated the clinically significant improvement of exercise groups; six of the nine groups were classified as "recovered" at post-treatment and two groups as "improved," and only one group as "unchanged." Forty-one studies investigated effects of exercise intervention in *non-clinically depressed samples*, participants in the exercise condition had significantly lower depression scores than those in non-treatment control conditions (effect size = -0.59, medium effect). The overall effect size of -0.80 (large effect) of both clinically and non-clinically depressed samples provides strong evidence for the effects of exercise upon depression. To evaluate the efficacy of exercise in the treatment of major depression and depressive symptoms, it is useful to examine the criteria for grading treatment recommendations that have been refined by the American College of Chest Physicians Task Force (Guyatt et al., 2006). Based upon these criteria, a treatment that achieves Level 1, Grade A status receives the highest level of recommendation. In order for evidence to reach Level 1, Grade A status, the following criteria must be met: the evidence must come from randomized controlled trials with a large sample size; the results must be clear consistently; and there must be a high benefit-to-risk ratio. By including only randomized controlled trials with a cumulative sample of nearly 3000 participants, the results of this meta-analysis meet these criteria. In an earlier meta-analysis (Wipfli, Rehorst, & Landers 2008), the same authors also analyzed the moderating variables of exercise programs (i.e. duration, exercise type, frequency and intensity). Within the overall population, exercise interventions lasting 4-9 weeks resulted in greater improvements in depressive symptoms than interventions with shorter or longer duration. However, within the clinically depressed population, programs lasting 10-16 weeks resulted in greater effects than shorter interventions. The exercise programs that combined aerobic and resistance exercise resulted in greater effects than aerobic or resistance training alone. In the overall population, exercise with a frequency of 3 or 4 times per week resulted in a significantly larger effect than programs with 2 or 5 exercise sessions per week. Within the overall population, exercise bouts of 20-29 minutes resulted in larger effects than bouts of ≥45 minutes, while within the clinically depressed population, exercise bouts of 45-59 minutes resulted in greater effects than bouts of 30-44 minutes and of ≥60 minutes.

The aetiology of bipolar disorder is considered to be to primarily biological in nature (Barbour, Edenfield, & Blumenthal, 2007). Therefore, psychopharmacologic intervention is the gold standard treatment, paired with psychotherapeutic interventions (e.g. cognitive behavioral therapy). However, adjunctive therapies that target symptoms of the disorder and relapse prevention are also beneficial. The potential impact of exercise on mood fluctuation and stress adaptation responses in bipolar disorder has not been widely studied. Only two studies investigated the effects of walking; in the walking program of Edenfield (2007), 30 minutes 4 times per week for 4 weeks resulted in an increase in the use of adaptive coping strategies to stressful life events in bipolar patients. In the non-random controlled trial of Ng, Dodd, and Berk (2007), the walking group showed significantly lower scores than the non-walking group for the self-reported 21-item Depression Anxiety Stress Scales and all its subscales (i.e. Depression, Anxiety, Stress).

9.1.2 Summary and conclusions for clinical practice

The strong evidence for the effect of exercise upon depression supports its use in the treatment of major depression:

- clinically depressed individuals show greater improvements than non-clinically depressed people;
- within the clinically depressed population exercise treatment seems to be at least equally effective to antidepressant medication and psychotherapy;
- within the clinically depressed population, interventions lasting 10-16 weeks result in larger effects to interventions lasting 4-9 weeks; and exercise bouts of 45-59 minutes produce larger effects than bouts of 30-44 minutes and of ≥60 minutes;
- within the overall population (i.e. both clinically depressed and non-clinically depressed people) exercise programs that combined aerobic and resistance exercise resulted in greater effects than aerobic or resistance training alone; and programs with a frequency of 3 or 4 times per week show a significantly larger effect than programs with 2 or 5 exercise sessions per week;
- the impact of exercise in bipolar disorder has not been widely studied. Two studies report beneficial effects of walking programs on adaptive coping strategies to stressful life events, and symptoms of depression, anxiety and stress.

9.2 ANXIETY

Anxiety disorder is a blanket term covering several different forms of abnormal and pathological fear and anxiety. The anxiety response consists of several clusters of symptoms, including cognitive (worry, apprehension, fear of failure and future consequences), emotional (negative affect), behavioral (nervousness, exaggerated mannerisms, tics), and physiological (increases in heart rate, blood pressure, muscle tension, perspiration, stress hormone levels). The American Psychiatric Association (2004) recognizes a wide variety of anxiety disorders.

- *Generalized anxiety disorder*, one of the most common anxiety disorders, is characterized by the experience of excessive worry in a number of life domains (e.g. family, work) that is difficult to control. The worry is associated with insomnia, tension, and restlessness. People with *panic disorder* experience sudden, unexpected periods of extreme fear known as panic attacks. Some symptoms of panic attack include sweating, heart palpitations, feelings of choking, dizziness, and fear of dying.
- *Obsessive compulsive disorder* is typified by the presence of disturbing and uncontrollable thoughts (obsessions). To elevate these thoughts, individuals use repetitive behaviors (compulsions) in an effort to prevent or reduce distress or prevent some dreaded event or situation (e.g. excessive hand washing to prevent contamination).
- *Post traumatic stress disorder* arises in response to experiencing or witnessing a traumatic event. Although many people exposed to trauma temporarily experience stress-related symptoms, those with post traumatic stress disorder continue to struggle with intrusive thoughts and nightmares, as well as increased arousal (e.g. anger) and avoidance of reminders of the trauma.
- *Social phobia* is characterized by an intense fear of making mistakes or looking foolish in public. This fear often leads to avoidance of certain people, places, or social events.

The 1-year and life-time prevalence rates for all anxiety disorders are 10.6% and 16.6%, respectively (Somers, Goldner, Waraich, & Hsu, 2006). In addition, anxiety disorders are often accompanied by comorbid mental disease, including depression (at rate of 75%) and substance abuse (Wipfli, Rethorst, & Landers, 2008).

9.2.1 Exercise as intervention for anxiety disorders and anxiety symptoms: findings of the most recent meta-analysis

Wipfli, Rethorst, and Landers (2008) analyzed the results of 49 randomized controlled trials in the area "exercise and anxiety" (n = 3566). Forty six studies used subjects with anxiety symptoms (non-clinical population), three studies involved patients with anxiety disorders (clinical population). The overall effect size of both clinical and non-clinical populations was -0.48 (medium effect), indicating larger reductions in anxiety among exercise groups than no-exercise control groups. The clinical populations effect size (-0.52) was greater than the non-clinical population effect size (-0.40). Twenty seven randomized controlled trials (n = 1924) compared exercise treatment to other forms of therapy. The overall effect size of -0.19 was significantly different from zero, indicating that exercise is slightly better at reducing anxiety than other therapy forms. Exercise was more effective than stress management education, slightly more effective than group therapy, stretching and yoga, relaxation and meditation, and as effective as cognitive behavioral therapy. Only psychopharmacotherapy produced a very slight greater anxiety reducing effect than exercise. Because only randomized controlled trials were examined, the results provided Level 1, Grade A evidence for using exercise in the treatment of anxiety. The authors also analyzed the moderating variables of exercise programs (e.g. frequency, exercise type, acute versus chronic exercise). Exercise programs with a frequency of 3 or 4 times per week resulted in significantly higher effect sizes than programs with 1-2 or 5 exercise sessions per week. Compared to aerobic training, weight training and a combination of aerobics and weight training provided greater effects, however effect sizes of weight training and combined training were based upon only three trials. The American Psychiatric Association (2004) makes a distinction between anxiety as a state and anxiety as a trait. *State anxiety* is the acute (or short-term) emotional response that follows the appraisal of threat. *Trait anxiety* is the predisposition to interpret a variety of situations as threatening and to respond to them with increases in state anxiety. The assessment of anxiety in intervention studies usually follows this important theoretical distinction. Thus, studies of the effects of "acute exercise" (i.e. a single bout of exercise) typically focus on changes in state anxiety, whereas studies of the effects of "chronic exercise" (i.e. a program of exercise lasting for several weeks or months) typically focus on changes in trait anxiety. By analyzing the role of duration of exercise intervention as a moderating variable, Wipfli, Rethorst and Landers (2008) found significant effect sizes for both acute bouts and exercise interventions lasting 4 to 15 weeks (effect sizes varying from -0.39 to -0.59). The limitation of this meta-analysis is that the majority of studies used non-clinical anxiety individuals; only three studies employed patients with anxiety disorders (clinical population). However, the authors only included studies that were published before January 2006. We found four studies using patients with anxiety disorders published after that date.

Some of these studies have focused on individuals diagnosed with panic disorder. Such individuals experience recurrent, unexpected panic attacks. In addition, this disorder is accompanied by anticipatory anxiety regarding the occurrence of episodes of panic, worry regarding the possible implications of panic attacks, and associated behavioral change such as avoidance of anxiety-provoking stimuli. Before 2006, Broocks et al. (1998) compared aerobic exercise with pharmacotherapy (clomipramine) and placebo in 46 patients with moderate to severe panic disorder. At the end of the 10-week treatment period, aerobic exercise and medication significantly reduced panic symptoms compared to placebo, though clomipramine was superior to exercise. Recently, Ströhle et al. (2009) showed that acute bouts of aerobic exercise at mild to moderate intensity yield an antipanic and anxiolytic response in patients with panic disorder. Two studies investigated the potential impact of aerobic exercise in patients with obsessive compulsive disorder. Abrantes et al. (2009) examined acute benefits of a 12-week aerobic training program on depression, anxiety, obsessions, and compulsions among patients with obsessive compulsive disorder. After each exercise session, patients reported reductions in depression, anxiety, and obsessive and compulsive symptoms. At 6 months follow-up, improvements in obsessive and compulsive symptom se-

verity appeared to persist (Brown et al., 2007). In a randomized controlled trial, Merom et al. (2008) compared the effects of a home-based walking program added to standard cognitive behavioral therapy with educational sessions within patients with panic disorders, generalized anxiety disorder, and social phobia. After 10-weeks intervention, participants in the walking condition showed greater improvements in depression, anxiety, and stress than those in the educational control condition.

9.2.2 Summary and conclusions for clinical practice

There exists evidence for the impact of exercise upon both state and trait anxiety:
- patients with anxiety disorders show greater improvements than individuals with only anxiety symptoms;
- recent studies confirm beneficial effects of both acute bouts of exercise and exercise programs lasting 10-12 weeks in patients with panic disorder, obsessive compulsive disorder, generalized anxiety disorder and social phobia;
- exercise is more effective than stress management education, slightly more effective than group therapy, stretching and yoga, relaxation and meditation, and as effective as cognitive behavioral therapy. Only psychopharmacotherapy produces a very slight greater anxiety reducing effect than exercise;
- single exercise sessions at moderate intensity result in reductions in state anxiety; however, acute bouts of exercise at high intensity (i.e. above 80% of VO_2max) produce significant elevations in state anxiety (Knapen et al., 2009);
- exercise programs with a frequency of 3 or 4 times per week result in significantly higher effect sizes than programs with 1-2 or 5 exercise sessions per week.

9.3 POTENTIAL MECHANISMS OF ACTION

Several hypotheses that involve biochemical, physiological, and psychosocial mechanisms have been offered to account for the effect of exercise on depression and anxiety. Despite continuing research that demonstrates the positive effects of exercise on depression and anxiety, no single theory adequately explains how exercise leads to

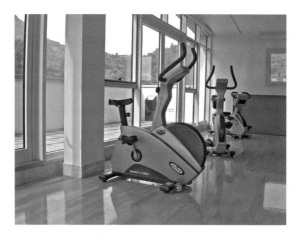

Figure 9.1 - Aerobic machines. Cycle ergometers, steps, and others machines aid the practice of aerobic training, which is recognized to significantly improve mental health in both the general and clinical population.

a reduction in depressive and anxiety symptoms. A plethora of physiological and psychological mechanisms have been proposed to explain the interaction between exercise and negative affect. The physiological mechanisms hypothesized include the central monoamines theory (i.e. exercise corrects dysregulation of the central monoamines and serotonin believed to lead to depression and anxiety), as well as the role of the hypothalamic-pituitary-adrenal (HPA) axis (Wipfli, Rethorst, & Landers, 2008; Rethorst, Wipfli, & Landers, 2008). In response to psychological stress experiences, depressed and anxious individuals exhibit an increased secretion of stress hormones from the HPA axis. Regular exercise leads to decreases in the amount of these stress hormones, resulting in lower levels of depression and anxiety. The central premise of these biochemical theories is that exercise acts on the same pathway that antidepressant medications target in the treatment of clinical depression and anxiety. Animal studies have observed increases in neuromodulators, like serotonin and norepinephrine, when the animals exercised. The increased production of neuromodulators caused by exercise is consistent with the target of antidepressant pharmacotherapy. In fact, exercise produces the same neuro-chemical changes that are often targeted by pharmacotherapy (Otto et al., 2007).

In addition to the physiological models, several psychological theories have been proposed to explain the effect that exercise has on depression and anxiety. A first theory, the Exercise and Self-Esteem Model of Sonstroem and Morgan (1989), focuses on the established association between depression and anxiety and negative self-evaluations, including lowered self-esteem and self-efficacy (Fox, 2000). In fact, prospective data suggest that negative self-evaluations may play a causal role in major depression and anxiety disorders. It has therefore been hypothesized that effective depression and anxiety therapies work by improving self-evaluations.

Indeed, different studies demonstrate that exercise training results in enhanced self-esteem, which is attributed to improved physical self-evaluations (such as exercise self-efficacy and body image). This enhanced self-esteem was accompanied by a decrease in depressive and anxiety symptoms, suggesting that that an enhancement of self-esteem may be responsible for the alleviation of depressive and anxiety symptoms (Blumenthal et al., 1999; Knapen et al., 2005). Several other psychosocial mechanisms have also been linked to depression and anxiety (Barbour, Edenfield, & Blumenthal, 2007). For example, a response style that favors distraction from negative emotions (as opposed to rumination or repetitive analytic focus on one's negative feelings) is associated with a more favorable prognosis for depression; exercise may create a break from these unproductive negative thoughts and may be a means of distraction. In addition, exercise may be a form of behavioral activation, which is an important component of cognitive behavioral therapy for depression and anxiety disorders. Other psychological theories focus on different constructs such as intrinsic motivation, self-determination, perception of control over physical and mental health, and exposure to anxiety-related physical sensations in cases of panic disorder or high anxiety sensitivity (Brosse, Sheets, Lett, & Blumenthal, 2002; Otto et al., 2007). In general terms, these models focus on a variety of mechanisms that partially explain the link between exercise and reduced depression and anxiety, such as improved accomplishments and self-confidence, improved self-esteem, positive distraction, social reinforcement, increasing positive coping skills available for use during stressful situations, and exposure in vivo. All these mechanisms seem to be very useful in clinical practice.

PHYSICAL ACTIVITY AND MENTAL HEALTH – A Practice-Oriented Approach

9.3.1 Summary and conclusions for clinical practice

The scientific evidence supporting the proposed physiological as well as psychological mechanisms is ultimately varied. There are probably several different mechanisms mediating the positive effects of exercise on depression and anxiety. Different mechanisms may work for different people and several mechanisms may operate interactively (Otto et al., 2007; Rethorst, Wipfli, & Landers, 2008). Thus, it is difficult to separate physiological mechanisms from psychological explanations. In an analysis of the possible mechanisms and their interactions, Biddle and Mutrie (2001) propose that for people just starting exercise programs, greater emphasis should be placed on the psychological mechanisms since the exerciser had not adapted, physiologically, to the exercise stimulus. In the maintenance phase, Biddle and Mutrie (2001) suggest that both psychological and physiological mechanisms are likely to be important, and in the final habituation phase, they suggest that emphasis be placed on the physiological mechanisms and the influence of behavioral conditioning.

Psychological models/mechanisms, such as the Exercise and Self-Esteem Model, distraction from negative emotions, behavioral activation, intrinsic motivation, self-determination, perception of control over physical and mental health, and exposure to anxiety-related bodily sensations provide therapists useful therapeutic strategies for clinical practice.

9.4 DEPRESSION, ANXIETY DISORDERS, AND PHYSICAL HEALTH

Depression and anxiety disorders are associated with a high incidence of comorbid somatic illness. Individuals suffering from major depression and/or anxiety disorders run a higher relative risk of coronary heart disease and type 2 diabetes compared to the general population (Huang, Su, Chen, Chou, & Bai, 2009). In general, depressed and anxious individuals exhibit a less active life-style and have reduced cardiorespiratory fitness in comparison with the general population (Zoeller, 2007). Strong evidence demonstrates that lack of physical activity is associated with an unhealthier body mass and composition, and a biomarker risk profile for cardiovascular disease and type 2 diabetes. In addition to this less active life-style, people with depression and/or anxiety disorders are more likely to smoke and have a higher risk for development of overweight and obesity (Zoeller, 2007). However, the association between cardiovascular disease, diabetes, and depression and anxiety disorders is bilateral, i.e. patients with anxiety and depression experience cardiovascular events more frequently, and patients with type 2 diabetes and cardiovascular diseases suffer more frequently from anxious-depressive disorder.

9.4.1 Summary and conclusion for clinical practice

- Depression and anxiety disorders are independent risk factors for cardiovascular disease and type 2 diabetes. Individuals suffering from both major depression and generalized anxiety disorder show the highest risk for cardiovascular disease.
- Exercise is extremely powerful in preventing cardiovascular disease and type 2 diabetes.
- Exercise is an outstanding opportunity for the treatment of patients who have a mix of mental and physical health problems, and is a holistic care option (Zoeller, 2007).

9.5 DEPRESSION, ANXIETY DISORDERS, AND COGNITIVE FUNCTIONING

Depression and anxiety disorders are associated with declined cognitive functioning. Being depressed and anxious is accompanied by slower information processing, psychomotor retardation, and poor memory functioning. There is growing evidence that exercise has a beneficial impact on cognitive function in older adults (Dishman et al., 2006). Positive effects of regular aerobic and resistance training on cognition have been observed in studies among subjects with and without cognitive decline (Erickson & Kramer, 2009; Liu-Ambrose & Donaldson, 200). The positive effects on cognition occur generally, with the largest effects being on cognitive speed, auditory and visual attention. Chronic exercise increases the expression of brain growth factors and may have neurogenerative and neuroprotective influences on the brain by stimulating the growth and development of new cells (Cotman, Berchtold, & Christie, 2007).

Exercise training not only improves negative affect and physical health in depressed and anxious individuals, but also produces "positive side effects" on depression and anxiety associated cognitive decline.

9.6 EVIDENCE BASED RECOMMENDATIONS FOR CLINICAL PRACTICE

In this last section, we offer some recommendations for physical fitness assessment and exercise prescription, and strategies for improving patient's motivation and adherence to exercise. (See also Textboxes 9.2, 9.3 e 9.4).

TEXTBOX **9.2**

Assessment of physical fitness and the perceived exertion during exercise

Direct measurement of maximal oxygen intake by way of a maximal exercise test is the most accurate indicator of cardio-respiratory fitness (American College of Sports Medicine, 2009). Maximal tests, however, have the disadvantage of requiring the subject's optimal motivation to work to "near exhaustion," and require the supervision of a physician and the use of expensive equipment. For depressed and anxious patients, however, submaximal measures are highly recommended for the reason that many patients have poor physical health, low levels of fitness and physical self-worth, limited experience with aerobic training, and less energy and motivation for heavy physical effort (Knapen, Van de Vliet, Van Coppenolle, Peuskens, & Pieters, 2003). Salmon pointed out that, especially in this population, physiological measurements studied in a laboratory could be influenced due to pre-test anxiety (Salmon, 2001). Patients with an increased trait/state anxiety, for example, might fear that maximal aerobic effort will provoke physiological reactions such as hyperventilation, tachycardia, dizziness, or sweating, which they associate with symptoms of panic attacks (Ströhle et al., 2009). These clinical considerations usually lead to the application of submaximal exercise tests in psychiatric settings. At the University Psychiatric Centre KU Leuven, Campus Sint-Jozef Kortenberg, the six-minute walk test (Vancampfort et al., in press) and the Franz ergocycle test (Knapen, Van de Vliet, Van Coppenolle, Peuskens, & Pieters, 2003) are most commonly used.

For patients with depression and anxiety disorders who often suffer from fatigue and low motivation, the rate of perceived exertion during physical activity is an important parameter when designing an appropriate exercise program (Knapen, Van de Vliet, Van Coppenolle, Peuskens, & Pieters, 2003). The fatigue and recovery time after an effort are not only dependent upon physiological stressors (intensity, duration, and frequency of the training stimulus), but also upon psychosocial factors. Psychological and social problems cause considerable stress. Generalized fatigue and lack of energy are typical symptoms of depressive syndrome. The exercise tolerance of anxious patients is reduced due to the fact that they are preoccupied with physiological reactions during effort such as palpitations, perspiration, and hyperventilation. These psychological factors cannot be ignored when developing a well-designed fitness program. The evaluation of degree of perceived exertion can be derived from the psychophysiological concept of Borg (Borg, 1998). The Borg 15 Graded Category Scale and the Borg Category Ratio 10 Scale quantify the sensations that the subject experiences during physical effort. The Borg 15 Graded Category Scale has a score range from 6 to 20 (15 grades), and the Borg Category Ratio 10 Scale from 0 to 10 (10 grades). Both scales show a linear relationship with heart rate during progressive incrementally exercise ($r = 0.94$ and $r = 0.88$, respectively). At the University Psychiatric Centre KU Leuven, Campus Sint-Jozef Kortenberg, we use the Borg Category Ratio 10 Scale because the longer Borg 15 Graded Category Scale requires a greater differentiation capacity.

PHYSICAL ACTIVITY AND MENTAL HEALTH – A Practice-Oriented Approach

Risk stratification for patients with comorbid somatic disease

Before initial treatment, the clinician should identify high-risk individuals, such as patients with a history of cardiovascular disease or diabetes (American College of Sports Medicine, 2009). These patients should be medically cleared before beginning physical activity. For the vast majority of people, the risk of sudden cardiac events is minimal, as long as they start at a realistic pace. Low intensity physical activity is related to a low risk. For example, a walking program at light to moderate intensity is safe for most patients. Intensity can be increased over time, and the patient and therapist should pay attention to symptoms such as chest pain or shortness of breath. The moderate training stimulus should be adapted to the training status and side effects of psychotropic medication (such as constipation, dizziness, dry mouth, nausea, sweating and tremor).

9.6.1 Physical fitness assessment and exercise prescription

Developing an exercise prescription for people with depression and anxiety disorders differs from the prescription used for healthy individuals. Therapists should be aware that several characteristics of depression and anxiety disorders (i.e. loss of interest, motivation and energy, generalised fatigue, a low self-worth and self-confidence, fear of movement, and social fear) and physical health problems interfere with participation in exercise.

Designing well-considered exercise programs for these patients requires:

a. assessment of physical fitness and the perceived exertion during exercise;
b. a risk stratification for patients with comorbid somatic disease;
c. an inventory of the perceived barriers and benefits toward exercise participation.

9.7 STRATEGIES FOR IMPROVING MOTIVATION AND ADHERENCE TO EXERCISE

Strategies can be based on the ideas of Motivational Interviewing following Miller and Rollnick (2002), and the Transtheoretical Model of Behavior Change (Prochaska & Velicer, 1997; Marshall &

Inventorying perceived barriers and benefits of exercise participation

Depressed and anxious patients accumulate a lot of barriers to participation in exercise such as a low self-worth and self-confidence, loss of energy, interest, and motivation; generalised fatigue, weak physical fitness and health condition, fear of movement, social fear, overweight and a low feeling of personal control concerning their own fitness and health, and helplessness and hopelessness. For these reasons, it is highly recommended to have a conversation before starting an exercise program concerning barriers and possible strategies that assist a patient in overcoming these barriers (e.g. problem solving, planning activity, seeking social support). Furthermore, giving information regarding both mental and physical health benefits of regular physical activity and determining which benefits are most salient to each patient is essential. For inventorying of perceived barriers and benefits, therapists may use a decision balance that helps patients to reflect the relative weight of the pros and cons of exercise participation (Marshall & Biddle, 2001).

Biddle, 2001). This model postulates that exercise behavior change involves progress through six stages: precontemplation, contemplation, preparation, action, maintenance, and termination.

Initial phase:
starting with supervised exercise

- Create exercise programs based on the patient's current preferences and expectations, the initial physical fitness assessment and the measurement of perceived exertion during exercise.
- Draw up an individual plan with the patient taking into account emotional, cognitive, and physiological components of depression and anxiety.
- Help the patient set realistic and achievable goals which lead to success experiences; this generally gives courage to persevere.
- Adapt the moderate exercise stimulus to the individual's physical abilities, training status, expectations and goals, side effects of psychotropic medication, exercise tolerance and perceived exertion.
- Follow the program with exercise cards and a logbook, and provide regular progress feedback to the patients.
- Avoid comparisons between patients.
- Emphasize the short-term benefits after single exercise sessions: improvements in mood and state anxiety, stress level, energy level, distraction of negative thoughts, the ability to concentrate and focus, and quality of sleep. Many patients are focused on the distant outcomes, such as weight loss and improved self-worth, so emphasizing short-term benefits can help patients adhere to exercise participation.
- Empathy, validation, praise, and encouragement are necessary during all phases but especially when patients struggle with ambivalence and doubt their ability to accomplish the change.

Second phase:
maintaining supervised exercise

- Focus on perceived fitness gains, achievement of personal goals, mastery experiences and sense of control over the body and its functioning.
- Use cognitive-behavioral strategies such as self-

monitoring, stimulus cuing, goal-setting and contracting.

- Once patients begin to feel better as a result of exercise, they are eager to continue their exercise if the therapist can help them attribute their improved mood to the exercise regimen. Improved mood as a result of increased physical activity may be obvious to the therapist, but the connection is not always obvious to the patient. Exercise can give patients a sense of power over their recovery, which in itself counteracts the feelings of hopelessness often experienced in depression and anxiety.
- Reinforcing the connection between mood and anxiety change and exercise is particularly relevant for patients with panic disorder. The prescription for exercise for panic disorder requires patients to engage in progressively more intensive exercise in order to elevate their heart rates so that they can become accustomed to sensations that will help them overcome their fear of panic.
- Self-determined motivation toward exercise is very important and results in adaptive exercise-related behaviors, cognitions, and physical self-evaluations. Therefore, it is important to make physical activity as self-determined as possible by focusing on the positive experiences of the activity itself, as well as helping to develop an identity of a physically active person.

Third phase:
follow-up after supervised exercise

- Follow-up contact is very important: discuss problem-solving around barriers, reinforce all progress toward change (even if initially very small progress), and encourage modification of goals as needed.
- Seek support of others such as family and friends.
- Use relapse behaviors/strategies: it is important to explain to patients that relapses are part of the process of change, and that responding with guilt, frustration, and self-criticism may decrease their ability to maintain physical activity. Relapse prevention strategies such as realistic goal setting, planned activity, realistic expectations, identifying and modifying negative thinking, and focusing on the benefits of single exercise sessions seem to be effective.

Eating disorders and physical activity: a complex relationship

10

Michel Probst, Johana Monthuy-Blanc, Milena Adamkova

The spectrum of eating disorders (ED) ranges from mild to severe. The severe form of this behavior results in the clinically recognized diagnoses of anorexia nervosa or bulimia nervosa. Anorexia Nervosa (AN) is characterized by a refusal to maintain a minimally normal body weight and by the distorted perception of one's body (weight, size, shape), the negative experience of their appearance as too fat and the intense fear of gaining weight, even when severely underweight (American Psychiatric Association [APA], 1994). Bulimia Nervosa (BN) is characterized by repeated episodes of binge eating followed by inappropriate compensatory behaviors such as self-induced vomiting, misuse of laxatives (or other medications), fasting or excessive exercise (APA, 1994). For the diagnostic criteria see DSM-IV (APA, 1994). However, it is important to note that a distorted attitude toward one's own body shape and weight is an essential feature of both disorders. Thus, there is a considerable diagnostic overlap between the two disorders and their natural histories tend to intertwine (Andreasen & Black, 1995; Fairburn, Cooper, & Shafran, 2003).

These diagnostic features could be accompanied by somatic, psychic, social, and behavioral disturbances (Andreasen & Black, 1995; Treasure & Szmukler, 1995; Becker et al., 1999). The most common somatic disturbances are presented in Table 10.1. The somatic complaints should be evaluated by a medical doctor before a training program is set up.

Furthermore, psychic symptoms are developed such as distorted body experience, sexual problems, attempts to prolong childhood and to escape the responsibilities of adulthood, perfectionism,

Table 10.1 - AN and BN patients: details of somatic disturbances

Somatic disturbances	Description
Cardiovascular	Bradycardia and tachycardia, hypotension, ventricular arrhythmia, cardiac failure and a variety of electrocardiographic changes, electrolyte disturbances, acrocyanosis
Gastrointestinal	Oral or dental abnormalities, benign enlargement of the parotid salivary gland, oesophagitis
Renal	Electrolyte abnormalities, pitting and peripheral oedema, hyper- or hypophosphatemia
Hematological	Pancytopenia with mild anemia
Skeletal	Osteoporosis
Endocrinal	Amenorrhea, hormonal abnormalities
Metabolic	Sensitivity of cold, sleep abnormalities, hypothermia, hypercholesterolemia
Dermatological complications	Atrophic dry skin, carotenodermia, lanugo hair

feelings of ineffectiveness, inflexible thinking, limited social spontaneity, overly restrained initiative and emotional expression, a strong control over one's environment, denial of illness, and mood changes with marked lability. Obsessive-compulsive features, both related and unrelated to food, are often prominent. The anorectic patient quickly develops a repertoire of behaviors in the pursuit of weight loss including caloric restriction, refusal to eat food, adoption of special diets or vegetarianism, calorie-obsession, hyperactivity, vomiting, and laxative abuse. Unusual eating rituals are frequently described. These behaviors create a vicious cycle with behavioral and psychological sequelae that perpetuate the disorder. In a social context, patients become isolated and many conflicts often arise with family members. Although AN and BN differ in behavioral features, patients with either one share an intense preoccupation with body weight and shape.

To conclude, it is important for all people who work with ED to realize that anorexia and related ED are serious disorders. Every person with an eating disorder has a different story to tell, a different background, and a different personality.

10.1 PHYSICAL ACTIVITY IN PATIENTS WITH EATING DISORDERS

10.1.1 Physical activity: healthy or unhealthy?

In general, physical activity results in both physical and psychological improvements in health and well-being, and more precisely, sports performance may lead to high self-esteem, healthy body image, and positive health status (Putukian, 1998). However, physically active girls and women participating in a wide range of physical activities may be at risk for developing AN and BN; for example the female athlete triad consisting of ED, amenorrhea and osteoporosis (Torstveit & Sungot-Borden, 2005). Thus, physical activity can also play a major part in unhealthy attempts to control weight and serves to alleviate anxiety in AN and BN patients. In some cases, the levels of exercise in relation to their BMI and in comparison with peers are too high. In other cases, they don't exercise enough and they develop a passive behavior. In bulimia nervosa, passivity and a lack of exercise are more frequently described.

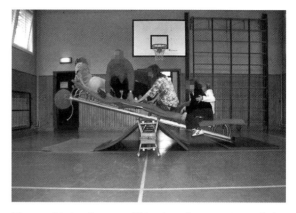

Figure 10.1 - Seesaw. This situation consists of the research of the balance state. Participants have to collaborate to maintain opposite sides of the seesaw as it leaves the ground: it requires the collaboration of everyone underling the importance of accord with others.

In the literature of ED, the amount and/or drive of physical activity has figured prominently as a secondary diagnostic symptom among patients with AN and BN (APA, 1994; Casper, 2006; Epling & Pierce, 1996; Mond et al., 2006). If early physical activity detection is important to avoid aggravate ED, it is very difficult to apply for two main reasons: terminology problems and cut-off problems. First, there is no single internationally accepted term and definition concerning physical activity in the eating disorder literature (see Epling & Pierce, 1996). Second, no guidelines discriminate the difference between normal and excessive exercise. Theoretical and practical questions arise when analyzing the behavior of over-exercise.

10.1.2 Varied terminology and objective vs. subjective measures

A survey of existing literature on physical activity and exercise in AN and BN patients revealed a large variety in activity related terminology: each term having slightly different criteria, and most including both behavioral and psychological features (see Table 10.2). In this chapter, the term "excessive physical activity" was chosen to describe the high amount of physical activity often observed in patients with ED.

Regardless of the different terms, the definition of unhealthy exercise appears to fall on two related dimensions: a quantitative dimension ("exces-

Table 10.2 - Activity related terms used in the literature of ED

Different terms	Authors
Compulsive exercise	Adkins & Keel (2005); Brehm & Steffen (1998); Brewerton et al. (1995)
Compulsive physical activity	Davis et al. (1989)
Diffuse restlessness	Kron et al. (1978)
Drive for activity	Casper (2006)
Elevated physical activity	Holtkamp et al. (2004); Klein et al. (2007)
Excessive exercise	Adkins & Keel (2005); Davis & Fox (1993); Davis et al. (1990); Davis & Kaptein (2006); Favaro et al. (2009); Peñas-Lledó et al. (2002); Shroff et al. (2006)
Excessive physical activity	Beumont et al. (1994); Davis et al. (1995)
Exercise addiction	Klein et al. (2007)
Extensive exercise	Davis et al. (1998); Fosson et al. (1987)
High level exercise	Davis et al. (1995); Davis et al. (1998); Solenberger (2001)
Hyperactivity	Davis et al. (1997); Kron et al. (1978); Hebebrand et al. (2003); Hillebrand et al. (2005); Vansteelandt et al. (2007)
Motor restlessness	Exner et al. (2000)
Overactivity	Feighner et al. (1972)
Restlessness	Casper (2006); Holtkamp et al. (2004)
Over-exercise	Seidenfeld et al. (2004); Sudi et al. (2004)

sive") and a qualitative dimension ("compulsive"). Concerning quantitative dimensions, exercise becomes excessive when its duration, frequency, or intensity exceeds what is required for physical health and increases the risk of physical injury (Davis & Fox, 1993). Excessive quantities of exercise have been associated with disturbed eating attitudes and weight preoccupation (Vansteelandt et al., 2007). According to qualitative dimension, exercise becomes compulsive when it is characterized "by maintenance of a rigid exercise schedule, increasing priority over other activities to maintain the pattern of exercise, detailed record keeping, and feelings of guilt and anxiety over missed exercise sessions" (Johnston, 2011). In other words, the compulsive quality of exercise has been associated with an increased drive for thinness, and increased disordered eating attitudes and behaviors.

If the studies about physical activity in AN and BN are mostly based on retrospective design, self-report questionnaires, and/or interviews, one can notice that limitations of retrospective design with self-report measures include (a) the possibility of socially desirable responses which can lead to an underreporting of physical activities, (b) the limited access of clinicians to behavior occurring in secret, (c) the complexity of accurately recalling physical activity and (d) retrospective bias and cognitive distortions linked to memory (Fazio et al., 1981). In order to remediate these limitations, few studies have attempted to use objective assessment like accelerometers quantifying physical activity (Klein et al., 2007; Probst et al., submitted) Furthermore, it is useful to study the inter-individual and intra-individual variability in physical activity in AN patients and BN patients (Probst et al., submitted).

Another theoretical and practical question arises analyzing the behavior of over-exercise. Many clinicians struggle with the question: "How much exercise is too much, and when does exercise become unhealthy?" Different important factors like the nutritional state, age, and previous experience with physical activity will influence the assessment as to whether the level of activity is excessive. It is arbitrary and personally

Excessive exercise

In a majority of cases, physical activity (here excessive exercise) starts in an innocent way. A person wants to lose weight, and in desperation to be thin and lean, may resort to many ways of burning or "getting rid of" calories they have consumed. Unhealthy over-exercise is one of many forms of purging food and calories. Therefore the person achieves fitness goals to excel in his or her[1] sport, but then loses control. What may have begun as a solution to problems of low self-esteem has now become an even bigger problem in its own right. The need to exercise or to control weight is often tied to an irrational fear of fat and weight gain (see diagnostic features). Physical activity is used to legitimize low weight and sport is used as an excuse not to eat, or to burn calories. This ends up with body and spirit ravaged by starvation, binge eating, purging, and frantic compulsive exercise and can lead to eating disorder pathology. Care givers have to keep in mind that during recovery persons suffering from anorexia or bulimia may increase exercise purging as they reduce vomiting or laxative use. This is a form of symptom substitution.

---

[1] Since the vast majority of eating disordered patients are women, we will speak only about "she" and "her."

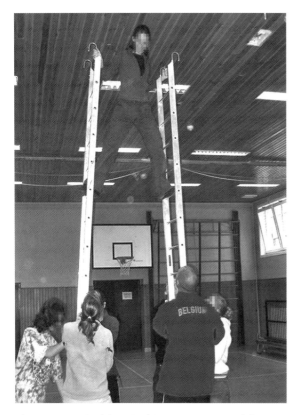

Figure 10.2 - Ladders. In this situation one of the participants has to climb the ladder supported by the others. It requires bravery, and trust in their abilities, and the capacity to control emotions like fear and fatigue. It is a very exciting activity for the climber as well as for people that have to support the ladders.

related; but for non-athletes, more than an hour of vigorous exercise more than 5 times per week can be dangerous, and could be an indication for the development of an eating disorder (see Chapter 11). Depending on the individual, the urge to move can take many forms, and periods of increased and reduced activity levels can alternate.

10.1.3 Prevalence and comprehensive functioning of excessive exercise

Concerning the prevalence of high level physical activity, rates ranged from 37% to 81% for patients with AN and from 20% to 57% for patients with BN (Davis et al., 1994, 1998, 2006; Hebebrand et al., 2003; Holtkamp et al., 2004; Klein et al., 2007; Peñas-Lledó et al., 2004). According to Davis et al. (1994), 75% of anorexia and 54% of bulimia patients are characterized by excessive movement. Schroff et al. (2006) estimated the prevalence of excessive exercise for people with ED at 39%. Probst (2005) found that 60% of hospitalized patients with ED have taken part in competitive sport at some point in their lives. As mentioned above, these large ranges of prevalence can explain the variety in terminology beyond the methodological heterogeneity. Independently of different prevalent rates, Beumont et al. (1994) observed that excessive exercise is more common in patients who are overwhelmed by anorexic preoccupations about weight and shape than in those for whom the illness appears to relate to family problems and attempts to manipulate the environment.

Concerning the association between physical activity and psychopathological features, a theoretical model was proposed by Davis et al. (1995). In this analytical model, physical activity, obsessive-compulsiveness and starvation influence each other in reciprocal ways. Some authors confirmed partially this model in patients with ED and mainly in patients with AN (Shroff et al., 2006; Solenberger, 2001; Brewerton et al., 1995). These authors found significantly higher scores of weight preoccupation in excessive exercisers than in non-excessive exercisers. They concluded that physical activity was a form of coping with anxiety.

Authors who were focused on a separate AN sample highlighted that (a) depression and anxiety is more common in excessive exercisers than in non-excessive exercisers (Brewerton et al., 1995; Holtkamp et al., 2004; Klein et al., 2007; Peñas-Lledó et al., 2004), and (b) weight preoccupation was significantly related to the level of physical activity (Davis et al., 1995). However, other authors indicated contradictory results (Davis et al., 1998; Brewerton et al., 1995; Klein et al., 2007). Other authors (Solenberger, 2001; Murphy et al., 2004) who focused on path analysis have found that there may not be a direct association between exercise behavior and ED symptoms. Cook and Hausenblas (2011) found that exercise dependence served as a mediator (but not a moderator) for the relationship between exercise behavior and eating pathology. This unidirectional causal model suggests that an individual's pathological motivation to exercise (i.e. exercise dependence), and not exercise behavior per se, is the critical component that plays the mediation role in the context of ED.

10.1.4 What is the motivation to exercise?

Biopsychological approach clarifies the role of hyperactivity in ED, precisely. A first and obvious explanation is that physical activity is simply an effective method of caloric expenditure and appetite suppression fulfilling the desire to lose weight. The amount of physical activity increases voluntarily, not for fun but from a preoccupation with weight (burning calories, ignoring hunger) and body shape. Food intake is carefully weighed against physical activity. These patients present an inadequate sense of fatigue, a special alertness, and claim to know no fatigue. Where others sustained effort is tiring, they continue their physical activities regardless of their poor physical condition as usual without complaint. Is this a desensitization to fatigue, or is it a denial? Secondly, there is abundant evidence that obsessive-compulsive behavior plays an important role in hyperactivity and has become a ritualized stereotype. The movement behavior of these patients show compulsive characteristics. They handle tight schedules with repeated activities (e.g. cleaning) and in exercise or sports, resembling a compulsory ritual. An involuntary or irresistible urge to exercise: here they feel constantly obliged to be doing something. They cannot find peace. Some patients may feel guilty if they are not sufficiently physically active. A third explanation is that hyperactivity may play an important role in affect-regulation (Probst, 2003; Vansteelandt et al., 2007). Compulsion is also a way to escape feelings of vacuum or a manner of regulating emotion (for example reducing negative feelings). Physical activity is stress reducing.

10.1.5 Conceptual framework for physical activity treatment for eating disorders

The comprehension of the relationship between physical activity and ED can explain why physical activity is often contraindicated in patients with ED and why most therapists ban physical exercises from their ED therapy programs. Nevertheless, certain path analysis revealed that the caloric requirement for weight gain during refeeding is not predicted by the patient's exercise behavior (Birmingham et al., 2004). In other words, a high level of exercise is not necessarily an obstacle to weight recovery in patients with ED because satisfactory levels of weight gain are achieved despite moderate levels of exercise (Hausenblas et al., 2007). From this empirical example, there may be benefits to using physical activity, under medically approved conditions, as an ED intervention.

As mentioned above (see §10.1.1), regular physical activity is associated with improvement in several physiological, psychological, and social benefits that are risk factors, maintenance factors,

Osteoporosis in eating disorders

Osteoporosis in ED as a consequence of eating disorder behavior is a new research subject. From these studies, we learned that we have to be careful with proposing specific physical activities. On the other hand, in more non-physically active ED, the positive role of physical activity on an increased risk of osteoporosis is well known. Controlled exercises can have a positive impact on the bone density of adolescents without compromising weight increase.

outcomes, or diagnostic criteria for ED (Davis et al., 1993). For physiological benefits, regular physical activity results in reductions in chronic pain, substance abuse, obesity, osteoporosis, and insomnia (Stice, 2002; Stice & Shaw, 2004). Psychologically, physical activity results in improvements in the malleable ED risk and maintenance factors of self-esteem, anxiety, depression, negative mood, and body image (Hausenblas & Fallon, 2006; Landers & Arent, 2003).

Significantly, patients with ED often cite controlling negative mood as a main reason for exercising (Long et al., 1993). Finally, physical activity results in improved social bonds and relations (Carron et al., 1996). Because patients with ED may have disturbed social relations (e.g. isolated eating and reduced social contact (APA, 2000), physical activity may aid in improving social behaviors. In short, theoretical justification suggests that by improving physical fitness through regular healthy physical activity, patients with ED may experience improved self-esteem, body image, and reduced sensations of bloating and distension during eating (Fossati et al., 2004). Additionally, physical activity promotes self-regulation. Therefore, physical activity may reduce bodily tensions and negative mood and increase tolerance to everyday stress, which are all triggers for binging and purging (Alpers & Tuschen-Caiffier, 2001).

According to Hausenblas et al. (2008), a conceptual framework illustrates how regular physical activity results in improvements in several malleable physiological, psychological, and social risk and protective factors for ED (Figure 10.3). More specifically, this framework is based on the fundamental principle that a reciprocal relationship occurs whereby physical activity results in improvements in well-being, and improved well-being results in increased physical activity. Simi-

larly, a reciprocal relationship occurs whereby improved well-being results in decreased ED risk factors, maintenance factors, and outcomes, which ultimately results in decreased ED prevalence. Physical activity also has the benefit of being self-sustaining, socially acceptable, and highly accessible, as well as having low cost and minimal side effects compared with traditional treatments. Also of great importance, the physical activity environment can be tailored to maximize overall effectiveness and long-term adherence via cohesive group physical activity classes and can be fostered within a socially enriched leadership environment.

10.2 A CONCEPTUAL PROPOSAL

This therapeutic and preventive model of ED comes from the multidimensional conception of self-concept and ED (Shavelson et al., 1976; Fox & Corbin, 1989; Marsh, 1997; Probst, 2005). The objective of this model is to increase self-concept components by adapted physical activity in clinical and non-clinical populations in order to decrease ED symptoms. Based on *reciprocal* or *bidirectional* direction between self-concept components (Feist et al., 1995; Marsh & Yeung, 1998), this model supposes that focusing on self-concept domains and sub-domains more relevant to therapeutic and preventive interventions will increase global self-esteem, which is seen as more stable. In order to achieve this objective, four steps can be described.

Step 1. Group composition A first diagnostic evaluation allows the formation of intervention groups. Firstly, the Eating Disorders Inventory (EDI; Maïano et al., 2009) and Self-Description Questionnaire (SDQ; Guérin et al., 2003) assesses the symptomatic level of ED and the level of each

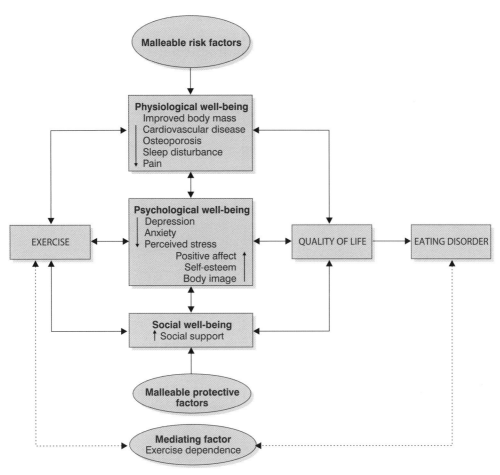

Figure 10.3 - Conceptual framework proposed by Hausenblas et al. (2008) for the effects of physical activity in eating disorders (reprinted with permission).

self-concept component for clinical ED (e.g. AN, BN, eating disorder not otherwise specified) and non-clinical ED (e.g. men and women from general population). From the global EDI score, one can identify the individual level of ED (for therapy) or individuals at risk of ED (for prevention), respectively. The scaled scores of SDQ – corresponding to emotional self-concept, physical self-concept and social self-concept – can discriminate individuals according to the lowest level among one of these components. Thus, from this diagnostic evaluation, three groups of clinical and subclinical individuals are constituted to propose three different therapeutic interventions according to specific need: (a) those whose emotional self-concept is the lowest, (b) those whose physical self-concept is the lowest, and (c) those whose social self-concept is the lowest. If SDQ and EDI are validated psychometrically (Stice &

Shaw, 2004), these self-reported questionnaires cannot avoid the denial demonstrated by individuals with ED (Kahn & Pike, 2001; Mathéron et al., 2002). In order to remediate it, clinical interviews can be conducted or other self-reported questionnaires can be included in diagnostic evaluation, such as the Toronto Alexithymia Scale (Loas et al., 1995), the Body Attitudes Test (Probst et al., 1995), etc.

Step 2. Objectives directly targeted by intervention
As regards Shavelson et al. (1976), objectives directly targeted by preventive interventions for each group are the increase in levels for (a) domains of self-concept, (b) sub-domains, (c) specific situations linked to self-concept. For instance, in the case of groups with lowest physical self-concept, their physical self-concept improves if the level of body attractiveness increases (Shav-

A case of a girl with anorectic behavior

For more than ten months, a twenty-year old girl came on a regular basis to the fitness club where she practiced at an intensive level. The girl applied 4 or 5 times a week and ran one hour at high intensity on the treadmill. She practiced individually, holding herself aloof. She had no contact with coaches or other practitioners.

After a time, the fitness coaches became concerned. Recently, they noticed that her weight had significantly decreased. She looked extremely lean and the coaches also received a number of concerned signals from her friends. Because of her intense exercise and her weight loss, fitness coaches suspected that her practice was possibly related to an eating disorder.

From their sense of responsibility, the coaches rightly asked how to deal with this behavior. The risk of letting her continue to play sports was too high. Moreover, there were many other users of the gym that were also worried about her behavior.

First, a soft approach was made with the question, "Do you practice with a kind of fitness plan," which resulted in a hostile response. She clearly did like that other people approached her.

What are possible guidelines in such extreme situations? Can such people be helped?

1. Don't hope it will go away if you ignore it. Don't try to keep the problem hidden by attempting to deal with it yourself when professional interventions are clearly appropriate.
2. Search for a professional who has experience with ED. The possibility exists, however well intended, that you will give the wrong message to the person.
3. Invite the person for a short meeting in which your concern about the degree of intensity and weight will be expressed. The coach who has the best rapport with the person should arrange this meeting privately. In an objective, non punitive way, list what you have seen and what you have heard that has led you to be concerned. Express support for the person and concern for their best interests. Be empathic and caring. Give a clear message that you believe there is a problem. Make clear that the manner in which they deal with their body is not adequate. It is not your job to refer to possible ED. Don't tell the person that you know they have a problem without giving your reasons and evidence.
4. If the center has devices for measuring body composition, you may ask them to submit to an examination of body composition. BMI lower than 16 and percent body fat below 15 are warning signs.
5. If they continue to deny the problem or are not open to a conversation you can refer them to the GP asking for a doctor's certificate of permission. If the doctor notes that there is a psychological problem, he will refer the person to a psychiatrist.
6. If they still refuse, you can ask them not to come to the gym because you don't bear the responsibility for any dangers. This gives a clear message that there is a problem. At that moment, it is their responsibility to seek help or not. The chance that they will visit another fitness center is great. It is clear that this step should not be taken lightly and preferably in consultation with a physician.

All these directives could possibly have no hold on the person. However, instructors cannot escape their responsibilities and have an obligation to express their concerns. To watch a person damage themself is not an option.

In the worst cases, this intervention will be a drop that could contribute to a later request for help. People who are not motivated cannot be helped. Denial is also a typical feature for this group. Dealing with people with such behavior, is sometimes an exercise in powerlessness.

elson et al., 1976). This increase of body appearance is dependent on perceptual, cognitive, subjective, and behavioral experiences lived positively (Probst, 2005). Among behavioral experiences, Probst (2005) lists avoidance behaviors and body checking.

The objectives are separately presented for each self-concept domain – corresponding to each group – but interrelation between self-concept component was empirically confirmed by some authors (Kowalski et al., 2003; Morin, 2011b). Consequently, even if the primary objective related to self-concept domain is to improve a specific self-concept domain, the improvement of the others constitutes secondary objectives. According to the aforementioned instance, the decrease of avoidance behavior or body checking involves positive changes in behavioral and cognitive experiences. These physical experiences increase the level of body attractiveness and the management of emotional state, and subsequently improve the physical and emotional self-concept.

Step 3. Interventional support This model proposes to use adapted physical activity in order to achieve the aforementioned preventive and therapeutic objectives. The use of adapted physical activity depends on the internal logic of physical activity and its adaptation related to dimension covered by its practice. Five types of physical activities are recognized here: (a) those in instable environments (e.g. climbing, canoeing), (b) those in stable environments (e.g. swimming, athletics), (c) those with an aesthetic and expressive target (e.g. dance, synchronized swimming), (d) those that are competitive (e.g. tennis, badminton), and (e) those that are cooperative (e.g. soft-ball, water-polo). These physical activities become adapted when applied in a preventive and therapeutic context. More precisely, adapted physical activities cover different dimensions (i.e. physiological/physical, sensory, cognitive, emotional, behavioral, communicative, relational, and symbolic) in order to improve self-concept domains. A comprehensive approach in the application of physical activities to self concept domains will show different improvements in overall self-concept. For example, gymnastics – physical activity in a stable environment – imposes on the individual (a) a management of emotion allowing improved emotional self-concept and (b) a specific cognitive processing which leads to the improvement of

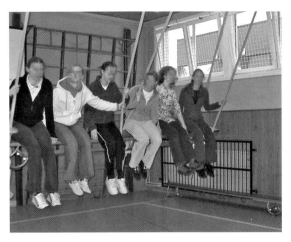

Figure 10.4 - Swing group. People are sat down on a bank suspended with ropes to the ceiling. They have to find a way to climb on the bank, permitting everybody to find a place. Then they all have to swing together. The aim of the situation is to collaborate, to help each other (e.g. when a member is afraid), and to deal with their own emotions.

physical self-concept. Furthermore, using adapted physical activity, this model allows the regulation of hyperactivity characterizing 50% to 70% of individuals with ED (Davis, 1994).

Step 4. Objective indirectly targeted by interventions Therapeutic and preventive interventions based in adapted physical activity which focus on direct improvement of self-concept domains and sub-domains also see an indirect increase of global self-esteem. According some studies in clinical and non-clinical populations, the directionality of the relationships between self-concept components called *causal flow* confirms the aforementioned *bi-directional* aspect (Monthuy-Blanc et al., 2010; Morin et al., 2011). Consequently, this model supposes that the increase of level of global self-esteem implies an increase of overall self-concept components.

10.3 A FLEMISH CLINICAL CONCEPT FOR PHYSICAL ACTIVITY AS AN INPATIENT TREATMENT APPROACH

The starting points for using physical activity within psychomotor therapy in the treatment of eating disorders are (a) the distorted body expe-

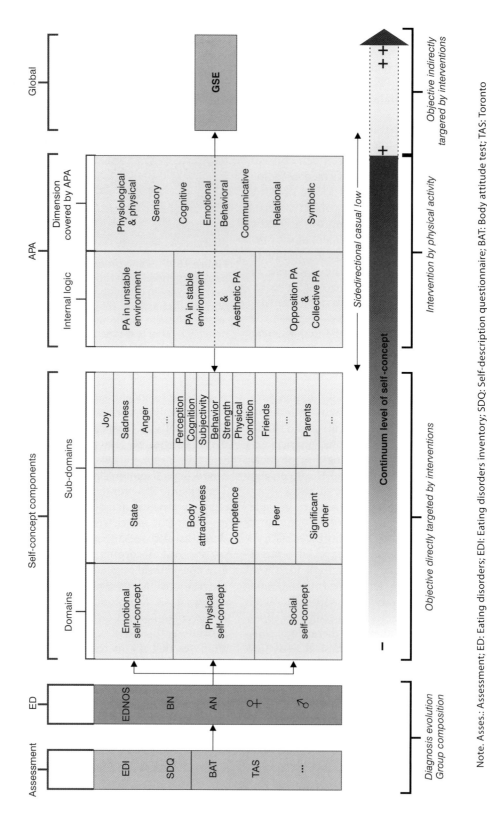

Figure 10.5 - ED: theoretical model for preventive and therapeutic interventions (Monthuy-Blanc & Probst, 2011).

Note. Asses.: Assessment; ED: Eating disorders; EDI: Eating disorders inventory; SDQ: Self-description questionnaire; BAT: Body attitude test; TAS: Toronto alexithymia scale; EDNOS: Eating disorders not otherwise specified; BN : Bulimia nervosa; AN: Anorexia nervosa; ♀: Women from general population; ♂: Men from general population; APA: Adapted physical activity; GSE: Global self-esteem.

PHYSICAL ACTIVITY AND MENTAL HEALTH − A Practice-Oriented Approach rience, (b) the observed hyperactivity, and (c) the fear of losing self-control. These points are deduced from the specific conduct pattern of ED (Vandereycken, Depreitere, & Probst 1987; Probst, 2005). The psychomotor approach focuses on the multidimensional aspect of the body experience (perception, cognition, attitude, behavior) with three specific objectives: (a) rebuilding a realistic self-image, (b) curbing hyperactivity, impulses, and tensions, and (c) developing social skills (Probst et al., 1995; Probst, 2006).

There are several ways to accomplish these objectives. From the wide array of possibilities (Vandereycken, Probst, & Van Bellinghen, 1992), one chooses the techniques which seem most effective in influencing the goals of ED patient. It is important to present the patient a safe and structured framework, where everyone knows the rules and where the therapist is sufficiently informative about the therapeutic setting. Care givers have to keep in mind that during recovery persons suffering from eating disorders may increase exercise purging as they reduce vomiting or laxative use. At that moment exercise is used as a form of symptom substitution.

The subject often experiences some measure of personal control and self-esteem by burning calories and losing weight. Even though it is a false sense of control, psychologically there is a brief, temporary sense of self-respect and anxiety reduction when "successfully" getting rid of calories by engaging in purging activity such as over-exercising.

It may sound contradictory that well-supervised and controlled progressive movement programs (fitness programs, aerobics, dance and creative movement [rhythmic exercises, free movement expressions], sports [swimming, volleyball and gymnastics], other physical activities) have been incorporated into our treatment. In our experience, it seems better to allow activity to a certain degree than to forbid patients to engage in controlled activities.

Today, these kind of activities have been commonly accepted in supportive surroundings (Beumont et al., 1994; Probst et al. 1999, Tokumura, Thien, 2003). This approach offers different thera-

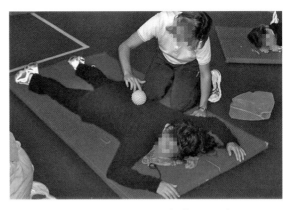

Figure 10.4 - Massage using a ball as mediator. Massage can be an important activity to facilitate communication and relationship with others, by reducing individual resistance.

peutic advantages: (a) the intensity of movement is controlled, (b) the opportunity for secret physical activities decreases, (c) the drive for movement is canalised, (d) the patients do not have the feeling that the only thing that matters is being fed, (e) the patients are given more responsibility, (f) it influence in a positive way physical and psychological well being, (g) it stimulate social contacts.

Of course some rules are taken into account. In our University Psychiatric Centre, campus Kortenberg (Belgium), physical activities may be restricted by the medical doctor until health and nutrition are sufficiently restored to support exercise. As a rule, reduction is temporarily imposed when patients' BMI is lower than 16. During therapy high-performance sport is discouraged, while recreational sport in groups encouraged. Even when partial recovery has occurred, advice of a physician and eventually a nutritionist will be necessary. Therapists have to monitor exercise closely, for instance using a physical activity monitor such as Sensewear or Actigraph.

Decisions about activity levels are also best made within the context of the therapeutic alliance and with concerns about weight being balanced against consideration of the person's physical and emotional need for exercises. Sometimes, it could be more helpful to encourage patients to experience what the absence of exercise means to them.

What can you do if a person is exercising beyond what is considered safe for his/her health?

1. REPORT OVER-EXERCISE TO THE PHYSICIAN AND TREATORS

    Because (young) people with ED, especially those with anorexia, may hide the purging aspect of their exercise from both themselves and those around them, watch for signs of too much exercise and report it to the (child's) physician and other professionals. They can assist in confronting unhealthy exercise practices and can set appropriate guidelines.

2. TALK TO ATHLETIC COACHES AND TEACHERS SUPERVISING THE TRAINING

    Upon talking to your child's physician, ask about the advisability of arranging contact between your child's physician and your child's school medical office and any sports coach your child may have.

    It is an important message to a recovering child that coaches, physical education teachers, and school medical staff are all willing to abide by physician recommendations for exercise when your child is in recovery. Information about your child's disordered eating and related health problems needs to be communicated to school personnel, coaches, and other athletic or dance teachers so that they can help enforce medical limits and guidelines for your child's safe participation in sports and athletics. For example, a child with anorexia who cannot retain body heat and is seriously underweight risks serious medical complications if allowed to swim in physical education or on a swim team.

3. ENCOURAGE TO TAKE TIME OUT FOR REST AND LEISURE

    Sometimes people with an over-exercise problem also have a compulsion to remain active.

    They are agitated with leisure or "down" time and manage to have little, if any, free time. Plan family time that includes rest and relaxation.

4. ENCOURAGE TO MAINTAIN A SOCIAL LIFE WITH PEERS (OUTSIDE OF SCHOOL)

    Ruminating about weight management and exercise rituals often causes social withdrawal and tense isolation from peers. You may notice that your child is disinvested in peer relationships when suffering from an eating disorder and/or over-exercising.

5. BE PATIENT WITH YOUR CHILD'S AGITATED "WITHDRAWAL SYMPTOMS" IF THEIR EXERCISE IS LIMITED BY TREATORS

    Your child with an eating disorder may become very anxious or tense if a care giver, coach, or dance teacher restricts exercise due to your child's poor health. Recall that over-exercise is a desperate attempt to maintain weight management. Any attempt to restrict it will likely be met with resistance.

6. IF YOUR CHILD OVER-EXERCISES AS A WAY OF PURGING FOOD, EXPECT SLOW, INCREMENTAL CHANGES IN THIS BEHAVIOR DURING RECOVERY

    Remember that a moderate amount of exercise, if sanctioned by your child's physician, is often health-building and increases appetite. During recovery, your child may experiment with decreasing over-exercise rituals, only to increase them again, hopefully temporarily, if he or she becomes scared of or actually experiences weight gain.

(continued)

7. HELP FIND OTHER WAYS OF FEELING IN CONTROL AND ORGANIZED

Over-exercise is often a way to feel in control and stable at times when life seems stressful, overwhelming or over-stimulating. You can help your child develop management techniques that will give them a sense of organization, efficacy, and being "on top of things." For example, talk about a time management schedule for school work. You can encourage your child to write out a schedule for homework and projects that are due.

Over-exercise is unhealthy. It is often ritualistic and compulsive in nature and is difficult to change. Young people with ED who use over-exercise as a means of purging food and burning calories are often resistant to giving up over-exercise. It is a coping mechanism from the perspective of the sufferer – one that offers a temporary sense of control and goal-achievement. While you can empathize with your child's motivation to "hang on" to over-exercise, you can also encourage your child to let go of distorted thoughts surrounding exercise. You can act as a role model and teach a healthy perspective on moderate exercise, and you can teach your children other ways, to feel good about themselves and their ability to manage their lives.

Adapted with permission from Haltom (2004).

Eating disorders in athletes **11**

Johana Monthuy-Blanc, Maud Bonanséa

As mentioned in the former chapter, patients with eating disorders (ED) frequently use physical activity for losing weight, compensating for binge eating, and regulating negative affects/emotions. If we accept the complicated relationship between ED and physical activity, we can consider the problem from the other side as well: ED in athletes. Two important questions arise: does sport participation represent a high risk factor for eating disorders, and do athletes represent a high risk population for eating disorders?

11.1 EATING DISORDERS SPECIFIC TO ATHLETES

Beyond the aforementioned diagnosis of clinical ED, two main subclinical ED specific to athletes can be identified: anorexia athletic and reverse anorexia (or muscle dysmorphia).

At the beginning, *anorexia athletica* characterized the female runner but now these terms refer to the *female athlete triad* (Figure 11.1). Anorexia athletica is characterized by the body image distortions, as is anorexia nervosa, wherein the body image desired is that of an excellent athlete (Vinci et al., 1999). As shown in Table 11.1, five diagnostic criteria have been defined by Sundgot-Borgen (1993).

Reverse anorexia (which usually concerns men) is characterized by muscle gain and obsessive preoccupation with physical appearance. Reverse anorexia is often associated with compulsive behaviors and anabolic steroid consummation (Pope et al., 1997). Numerous authors

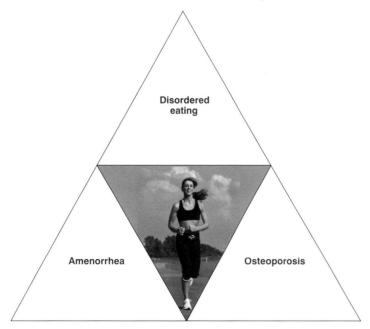

Figure 11.1 - Female athlete triad: characteristic disorders.

Table 11.1 - Diagnostics of anorexia athletica

Female athletes must exhibit the following five criteria for a positive diagnostic:

(1) Excessive fear of becoming obese

(2) Restriction of caloric intake

(3) Weight loss

(4) No medical disorder

(5) Gastrointestinal complaints

Additionally, one or more of the following criteria must be met:

(1) Disturbance in body image

(2) Compulsive exercising

(3) Binge eating

(4) Use of purging methods

(5) Delayed puberty

(6) Menstrual dysfunction

conceptualize ED in athletes along a continuum of eating behaviors. Koszewski et al. (1997) suggested that this continuum can range from anorexia nervosa to obesity (see Figure 11.2) or from dysfunctional eating behaviors to clinical eating disorders such as anorexia nervosa and bulimia

(Figure 11.3). Most researchers tend to agree with the second continuum (Torstveit & Sundgot-Borgen 2005).

11.2 PREVALENCE AND AETIOLOGY

Despite literature reporting a low prevalence in clinical ED (2% to 3%), 5% to 33% of male athletes and 15% to 65% of female athletes present sub-clinical ED (Beals & Manore, 2000; Bonci et al., 2008; Puper-Ouakil et al., 2002). Among these athletes, a history of ED was reported in 20% of female and 80% of male athletes. More precisely, menstrual dysfunction occurs in 3.4% to 66% of female athletes as compared with 2% to 5% in nonathletic women (Rumball & Lebrun, 2004). Concerning competition level, results from recent reviews have demonstrated that the women competing at an elite level exhibited significantly higher prevalence of ED symptoms as compared with nonathletes or athletes competing in lower levels (Beals & Manore, 1994; Byrne & McLean, 2001; Sundgot-Borgen, 1994). Only 18% of Black athletes reported the use of pathogenic weight control methods, as compared to 33% of their White counterparts, and less than 23% of Black athletes have ever dieted as compared to 69% of White athletes (Thompson & Sherman, 1993).

The biopsychosocial approach allows an understanding of the aetiology of ED in athletes (Figure

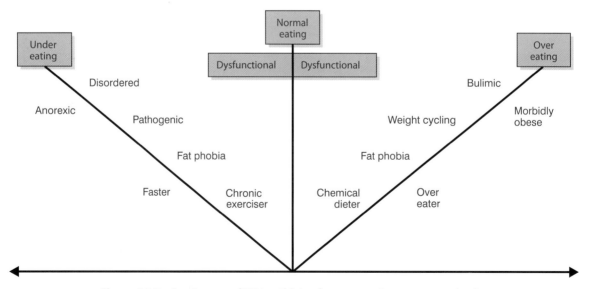

Figure 11.2 - Continuum of ED in athletes from anorexia nervosa to obesity.

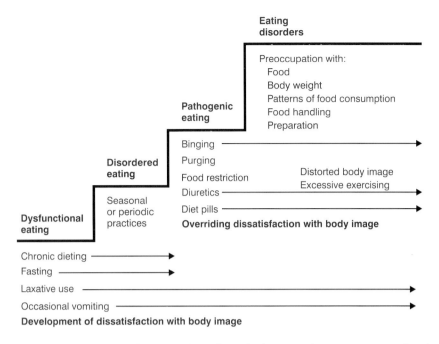

Figure 11.3 - Continuum of ED in athletes from dysfunctional eating to eating disoders.

11.4). Thus, biological (ethnic background, age, gender, loss/gain of weight, puberty, menstrual cycle and endorphin secretion), psychological (personality, perfectionism, self-esteem, body image and diet) and sociocultural factors (society, family, trainers, teammates, physical activity/ sport and life events) contribute to ED development (Puper-Ouakil et al., 2002; Sherman & Thompson, 1993). In other words, a female Caucasian elite gymnast with low weight and perfectionist tendencies presents a greater risk of developing ED than a male African basketball player in club context with high self-esteem and friendly relationships with teammates.

11.3 PHYSICAL ACTIVITY/SPORT: A SOCIAL RISK FACTOR

In regard to the biopsychosocial aetiology, physical activity (and more precisely sport participation), is one potential risk factor for developing ED. The sport environment demands that athletes are exposed to body shape and weight pressures unique to the sport. This can be ex-

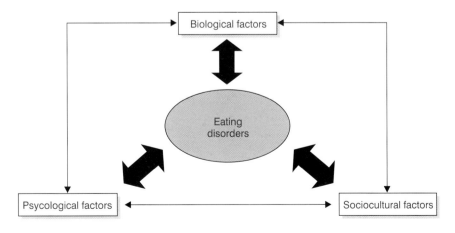

Figure 11.4 - Biopsychological approach of eating disorders in athletes.

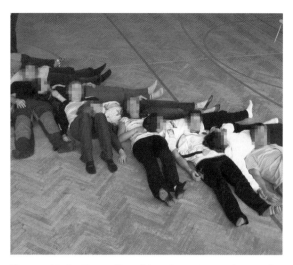

Figure 11.5 - Group Breathing. Participants lay on the ground, leaning their head on the belly of another participant. The task is to identify a univocal rhythm of breathing. It is necessary to come in contact with their personal capacity to listen to themselves and to perceive the breathing rhythm of the others.

plained by two main qualities. First, sport, with its emphasis on obtaining an optimal weight for athletic performance, represents a subculture that intensifies industrial societal pressures to be thin, thereby increasing the risk of developing an ED. Second, it has been shown that coaches, judges, and teammates can encourage unhealthy eating and weight management behaviors that escalate into dysfunctional disorders. Thus, researchers who focused on sport components leading to ED in athletes determined five sport classification systems:

- lean versus nonlean (Ashley et al., 1996; Petrie, 1996; Sundgot-Borgen & Corbin, 1987);
- thin body build versus normal build (Davis & Crowles, 1989);
- fostering the attainment of a thin physique versus low weight not being a central concern (Warren et al., 1990);
- endurance, aesthetic, weight-dependant, ball game and technical sports (Sundgot-Borgen, 1993);
- endurance, aesthetic, weight-class, anti-gravitation, technical, ball game sports and power (Torstveit & Sundgot-Borgen, 2005).

In summation, one can retain that overall sport classification systems depend on dichotomous classification: leanness sports where suc-

cess or performance requires that participants present a particular thin appearance, and non-leanness sports where a low body weight is not the fundamental nature of the sport. For example, Torstveit and Sundgot-Borgen (2005) encompassed endurance, aesthetic, weight class, and anti-gravitation in leanness sports, and technicality, ball game, and power in nonleanness sports. Empirically, numerous authors revealed that the women competing in sports which emphasize leanness and/or a low body weight (gymnastics, dancing, figure skating, judo, etc.) exhibited the highest prevalence of ED (Beals & Manore, 1994; Byrne & McLean, 2001; Hausenblas & Carron, 1999; Smolak et al., 2000; Sundgot-Borgen, 1994; Sundgot-Borgen & Torstveit, 2004). More precisely, a current review about sports and symptoms of ED in the greatest risk population – adolescent girl athletes – revealed: (a) a significantly higher frequency of overall ED symptoms in rhythmic gymnasts than in synchronized swimmers; (b) girls participating in power sports showed double risk for ED symptoms compared with their counterparts practicing other sports (endurance, aesthetic, weight class, anti-gravitation, technical and ball game); (c) a lack of significant differences in the frequency of ED symptoms among leanness and nonleanness sports (Monthuy-Blanc et al., 2010).

11.4 PREVENTION AND TREATMENT OF ED IN ATHLETES

At the Vancouver Winter Olympic Games in 2010, the International Olympic Committee asserted its responsibility to protect the health of the athlete and more precisely to prevent and treat ED in athletes. Since the nineties, some countries (e.g., Canada, France, USA, United Kingdom) underscore the need to lead a prevention policy upstream in directed institutions and downstream in professionals who have direct contact with athletes. In this way, the National Athletic Trainers' Association (NATA) and National Collegiate Athletic Association (NCAA) insist on performing a pre-participation examination (PPE) or periodic health evaluation (PHE) of all elite athletes (cf. Bonci et al., 2008; Ljungqvist et al., 2009). Nevertheless, it should be noted that prevention programs for ED in athletes mainly exist in the context of elite levels. As mentioned by Beals, Brey & Gonyou (1999), prevention and treatment of ED in all sport competition levels should be organized into three broad categories including primary, secondary, and tertiary prevention (Table 11.2).

Concerning primary and secondary preventions, any behaviorist would attest to the fact that increasing knowledge alone is not likely to change behavior. Education is certainly an important part of any eating disorder prevention program, but if it is to be effective it must be accompanied by a change of beliefs and behaviors of athletes and athletic staff. Thus, the prevention strategies employed should focus on de-emphasizing body weight and body composition, promoting healthy eating behaviors, destigmatizing disordered eating, and recognizing and encouraging the athlete's individuality while fostering a team environment (Beals, 2004).

Concerning tertiary prevention, if the athletic staff are not already directly involved in ED treatment, support and cooperation are necessary to the successful treatment (Beals, 2004). Furthermore, NATA specified some therapeutic guidelines to treat ED in athletes (Bonci et al., 2008). These mainly focus on optimization of caloric intake and in more serious cases, pharmacologic treatment in comorbid cases, the role of the athletic trainer and parents in a therapeutic team, and the importance of communication between athletic staff and therapeutic team within each organization.

Table 11.2 - Definition of prevention of ED in athletes

Primary prevention	Educational programs designed to prevent development of an ED
Secondary prevention	Identification and subsequent intervention
Tertiary prevention	Treatment of athletes who developed an ED

11.4.1 General guidelines

Overall, experts within the field of ED prevention agree that an efficient baseline for prevention programs can be summarized in three words: *identification* (screening), *prevention* (education), and *treatment* (intervention). NATA defines precisely seven general recommendations of ED prevention for athletes (Bonci et al., 2008). These recommendations focus on the need to educate the main actors of sport (athletes, coaches, certified athletic trainers, administrators, and other sport personnel) in ED prevention and to constitute a competent multidisciplinary team of caregivers with athletics administrators in order to implement a comprehensive management protocol from detection to treatment of ED in athletes (Table 11.3).

From scientific review of literature, Beals (2004) identifies four steps leading to efficient ED programs. First, it is essential to gain the support of the athletic administration to allay their fear of losing

Table 11.3 - ED prevention for athletes: general recommendations of NATA

1. Constitute a health care team of qualified caregivers who should represent multiple disciplines, including medicine, nutrition, mental health, and athletic training

2. Identify an athletics administrator who has the authority to take action when unexpected events and worst-case scenarios challenge the scope of existing resources and expertise

3. Implement a comprehensive management protocol from detection to treatment of of ED in athletes

4. Enlist the support and input of risk-management personnel and legal counsel in planning, developing, and implementing the management protocol

5. Establish a screening approach along a continuum of eating behaviors during the PPE

6. Develop policies that clearly define the appropriate responses of coaches when dealing with athletes regarding body weight issues and performance

7. Design mandatory structured educational and behavioral programs for all athletes, coaches, certified athletic trainers, administrators, and other support personnel to prevent ED

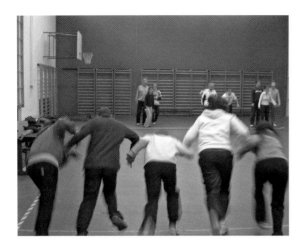

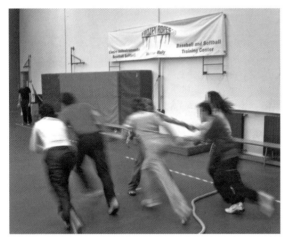

Figure 11.6 - The adding relay. Groups are in competition, they have to run back and forth across the room adding a person at each cycle.

control of athletes. This can best be accomplished by providing the administration with evidence of the ED team's expertise (statement of credentials, letters of recommendation, curriculum vitae) and involving the administration in the development and implementation of the ED program (program component, program protocols, assembling team members, etc). The next step in successful programs implementation is to get the athletic staff on board. If the athletic trainer exhibits resistance, one must (a) convince them of the ED team's expertise, (b) involve them in program development and implementation, and (c) maintain open lines of communication. It is imperative to make every effort to openly demonstrate the expertise of the ED team, because the athletic trainer is "on the front line," so to speak (Beals, 2004).

Third, the ED program cannot be effective if the athlete does not trust the ED team. The athletic trainer acts in a mediation role, because if they endorse the program, chances are the athlete will follow suit. Most ED prevention experts use team educational sessions and focused discussion groups in order to share perceptions of ED. And last, no efficient ED program exists without a committed and cohesive ED team. As shown in Figure 11.7, the patient with ED is in a central position and is the focus of treatment by the surrounding ED team, constituted by a physical nutritional, and mental health provider. The link between the different actors in the ED program must be made in order to improve communication and make decisions together.

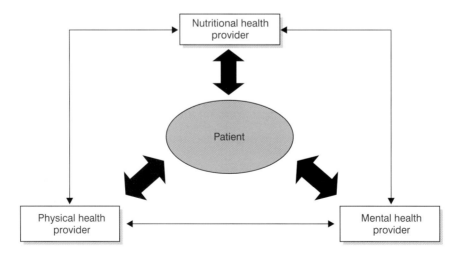

Figure 11.7 - Representation of relationship between ED team and patient with ED.

Guidelines for appropriate weight loss in sport leanness based on the recommendations of Rhea et al. (1996)

1. A health care professional experienced in working with ED should assess the athletes to determine that they are at minimal risk for developing an eating disorder as a result of a weight loss plan.
2. The athlete's weight should be higher than the medically recommended body weight
3. The athlete should agree with the decision to lose weight.
4. A dietician should be responsible for determining the target weight range, designing an eating plan and monitoring the program.
5. The weight loss program should be discontinued if any weight-related or psychological difficulties emerge.
6. Athletic performance is actually increasing as weight decreases.
7. If performance is not enhanced, the weight loss program should be discontinued.
8. If performance is enhanced, the weight loss regimen should not be continued beyond the target weight range.

11.4.2 Specific guidelines

Beyond the general guidelines, it is possible to specify prevention programs according to characteristics of the athlete such as their competition level, age, sport category, etc. In this section, we focus on the three significant environments of the athlete: *sport environment* (athletic trainer), *family environment* (parents) and *elite environment* (need for weight loss). Concerning athletic environment, an athletic trainer's primary responsibility is to assist athletes in maintaining optimal health (Vaughan et al., 2004). The athletic trainer's guidelines should be limited to six main recommendations (Rhea, 1996; Thompson & Sherman, 1993; Vaughan et al., 2004): (a) focus on genetic distinction and individual limitations to avoid setting weight goals based on appearance, generic standards or tables; (b) initiate progressive weight control programs to control pathogenic weight techniques; (c) eliminate groups weigh-ins to prohibit negative comments and pressure surrounding body weight; (d) participate in the health of athletes by detecting signs of ED; (e) initiate dietary intervention with a dietitian by focusing on caloric and nutritional needs based on sport category, duration, gender, and food preference; and (f) base training on positive input in order to im-

Table 11.4 - Athletic environment of the athlete: trainer's guidelines

1. Recognize individual body composition differences
2. Discourage rapid weight loss methods
3. Respect confidentiality concerning body composition and weight assessment
4. Detect signs and symptoms of ED
5. Work on weight loss and gain with a nutritional health provider
6. Give positive feedback

prove protective factors such as self-esteem (Table 11.4).

The parents of the athlete have a similar role to fill in the protection of their child's health. Powers (2000) proposes splitting the guidelines for parents into 12 recommendations linked to weight loss, resetting of weight goals, amenorrhea, excessive exercise, inappropriate dieting behavior, negative trainers, use of exercise to purge, use of exercise to cope, avoidance of tasks of adolescence, athletic performance and weight loss, participation in high-risk sports, and unrealistic sport achievement expectations.

Obesity and exercise in psychiatric patients

12

Jannis Alexandridis

Obesity is one of the most serious public health challenges of the 21st century (WHO, 2007). Obesity is an exceptionally heterogeneous disorder in terms of its aetiology, physical and behavioral presentation, and association with adverse health problems. Fortunately, there exists a very broad range of interventions and treatments. From this plethora of themes, this chapter gives emphasis to physical activities which are most relevant to a movement therapist from a holistic approach including psychotherapeutic methods. It will focus on physical activity as a therapeutic treatment for obesity in a clinical population of obese adults.

12.1 WHAT OVERWEIGHT AND OBESITY ARE

Overweight and obesity are defined as abnormal or excessive fat accumulation that may impair health.

Body mass index (BMI) is a simple ratio of weight to height that is commonly used in classifying overweight and obesity in adult populations and individuals. It is defined as the weight in kilograms divided by the height in meters squared (kg/m^2).

BMI provides the most useful population-level measure of overweight and obesity, as it is the same for both sexes and for all ages of adults. Although BMI is highly correlated with percent body fat, it does not provide information about body composition. Table 12.1 shows the World Health Organization (WHO) classification of weight and obesity levels by body mass index (WHO, 1998). However, it should be considered a rough guide because it may not correspond to the same degree of fatness in different individuals.

Excess weight does not always reflect excess fat. For example, some muscular athletes may be overweight but not necessarily obese. BMI may overestimate obesity in muscular or athletic persons and may underestimate obesity in older persons who have lost lean tissue with age and decreased exercise. In addition to BMI, it is particularly important to assess the body composition e.g., proportion of lean body mass, fat mass and distribution of fat (Grilo, 2006).

12.2 THE AETIOLOGY OF OVERWEIGHT AND OBESITY

The fundamental cause of obesity and overweight is an energy imbalance between calories consumed and calories expended. However, this is an oversimplification; obesity is a markedly heterogeneous condition and multifactorial in its aetiology. That basic energy imbalance can occur by a variety of complex genetic, biological, environmental, psychological, social, and behavioral factors that can differ across individuals and groups and even within individuals across their own lifespan. Levels of physical activity, inactivity, and

Table 12.1 - The International Classification of adult overweight and obesity according to BMI (WHO, 1998)

Classification	BMI (kg/m^2)
Overweight	≥25.00
Obese	≥30.00
class I	30.00 - 34.9
class II	35.00 - 39.9
class III	≥40.00

sedentary behavior are such factors. There is a clear, inverse relationship between physical activity and weight gain. The modern environment is currently obesogenic and toxic, showing a trend towards decreased physical activity. This is evident in the increasingly sedentary nature of many forms of work, changing modes of transportation, and changing lifestyles.

12.3 CONSEQUENCES OF OVERWEIGHT AND OBESITY

Overweight and obesity are associated with medical complications that lead to increased mortality and morbidity. Although the psychosocial consequences are the primary focus of this section, one must not forget the highly preventable physiological consequences associated with overweight and obesity.

12.3.1 Physiological consequences of overweight and obesity

Generally, mortality and health risk factors increase progressively as waist circumference (and thus BMI) increases. Common medical problems include: insulin resistance, type 2 diabetes, hypertension, dyslipidemia, cardiovascular disease (primarily heart disease and stroke), gallbladder disease, respiratory disease (obstructive sleep, apnea, asthma), musculoskeletal disorders (especially osteoarthritis, gout, and lower back pain), and some forms of cancer (endometrial, breast, colon).

12.3.2 Psychosocial consequences of overweight and obesity

In addition to the medical problems and mortality, obesity is associated with several psychosocial consequences and mental illnesses.

Overweight and obese individuals are often targets of bias and stigma, and suffer from psychological distress and consequent symptoms of low self-esteem, low self-worth, and guilt. "They are often subjected to prejudice and discrimination in a society that glorifies thinness" (Wadden, Womble, Stunkard, & Anderson, 2004). These social consequences are serious and pervasive. They are vulnerable to negative attitudes in multiple facets of living including places of employ-ment, medical facilities, mass media, interpersonal relationships, educational institutions and physical activities.

Obese persons suffer from greater body image dissatisfaction. When such concerns with appearance exist, they tend to seek treatment (Grilo, 2006; Sarwer & Thompson, 2006).

In addition to body image problems, obesity has a negative impact on health-related quality of life (HRQOL). This concept has been explored since the 1970s and refers to a person or group's perceived physical and mental health over time. Obesity affects important aspects of HRQOL, including physical health, emotional well-being, and psychosocial function. Both cross-sectional and longitudinal studies have shown HRQOL to diminish as BMI increases from normal to obese. Furthermore, HRQOL is used to measure the efficacy of treatment for obesity (Seidell & Tijhuis 2002; Bish et al., 2006).

Obesity is often accompanied by mental illnesses such as depression and binge eating disorder (BED). There is a reciprocal association over time between depression and obesity. Luppino (2010) reports, in his systematic review and meta-analysis, that obesity increases the risk of depression in initially non-depressed individuals by 55 percent and depression increases the risk of obesity in initially normal-weight individuals by 58 percent. The link between obesity and later depression is more pronounced among Americans than among Europeans (Luppino et al., 2010). On the other hand, BED expresses a much different relationship with obesity. Binge eating disorder was included in 1994 in the *Diagnostic and Statistical Manual of Mental Disorders-IV* (DSM-IV) as a provisional diagnostic category requiring further study. The prevalence in the general population is 2%; BED is 1.5 times more common in women than men. Up to 30% of participants in weight loss programs meet criteria for BED (de Zwaan & Friederich, 2006). Binge eating is characterized by consumption of an objectively large amount of food in a brief period during which the individual experiences a subjective loss of control. With BED, overeating is not followed by purging or other compensatory behavior, which distinguishes this condition from bulimia nervosa. In obese individuals with BED, psychopathology such as depression, greater symptoms of borderline personality disorder, lower self-esteem, and Axis I disorders including substance abuse or dependence is significantly more common compared to obese persons without BED (Wadden et al., 2004). Therefore it is important to differentiate between obese individuals who do and do not have an eating disorder in addition to their weight problem.

Despite these psychosocial consequences and mental illnesses, the heterogeneity of obesity must be considered in reference to the psychological status of the individual. One must also consider that obese individuals in clinical populations are different than obese individuals in non-clinical populations. "Among persons encountered in clinical settings and actively seeking treatment, approximately 10-20% are likely to suffer from clinically significant symptoms of depression, negative body image, or impaired health–related quality of life. Such problems are most likely to occur in women (particularly from higher socioeconomic status levels) in those with BED, and in those with extreme obesity (i.e, BMI$\geq$ 40 kg/m^2) and its attendant health complications" (Wadden et al., 2004; Luppino, 2010). The great majority, in spite of their hostile environment and psychological distress, appear to have essentially normal psychological functioning (Wadden et al., 2004).

12.4 THE TREATMENT OF OBESITY

For effective management of overweight and obesity, multiple treatments can be taken: a multi-disciplinary approach, pharmacotherapy, or bariatric surgery.

The multidisciplinary approach, recommended by virtually all countries with public health agencies, consists of a standard combination of diet, exercise, and behavioral modification. It incorporates a dietary-nutritional component (which for this text's purpose is irrelevant and therefore not discussed), physical activity and exercise interventions (which will be discussed in further detail below), and behavioral treatment, which refers to a set of principles and techniques designed to help overweight individuals reverse maladaptive eating and activity habits.

Pharmacotherapy should be used as an additional tool only by patients who are at increased medical risk. Medication should be used alongside diet, exercise, and behavior changes, not as a substitute. Without lifestyle changes, medication is unlikely to be effective.

Bariatric surgery offers the best chance of losing the most weight quickly, but can pose serious risks. It is recommended for individuals who are severely obese (BMI >40 kg/m^2), who have serious weight-related health problems, or a combination of the two.

12.4.1 Role of physical activity in preventing and treating obesity

Physical activity and sedentary lifestyle can be seen not only as causes for the pathogenesis of obesity, but also as an effect (i.e, physical inactivity caused by weight gain and obesity). Analyses from several (cross-sectional as well as longitudinal) studies indicate a reciprocal relationship between physical activity and obesity. However, the direction of the association is still unclear (Hu, 2008). Therefore, there is a great need for prospective randomized trials that show clear cause and effect.

On the other hand, physical activity and exercise as an approach to obesity is established as a basic treatment module in addition to diet therapy and behavioral treatment. The establishment of this treatment is obvious because physical activity is the most easily controllable way to increase caloric consumption.

12.4.2 Role of physical activity in weight management

The impact of physical activity on weight management has been the main subject of virtually all obesity studies for the last several years; in particular, the effect of physical activity on the prevention of weight gain, on weight loss, and on the prevention of weight regain after weight loss. In a position stand from the American College of Sports Medicine (ACSM), currently-available data on the role of physical activity in weight management was reviewed. Appropriate Physical Activity Intervention Strategies for the previously listed three categories were recommended (Donnelly et al., 2009).

The data on the role of physical activity in the prevention of weight gain over time is not clear, but most studies have found that increasing physical activity attenuates gain in weight or waist circumference during midlife. Physical activity of 150 to 250 min/wk with an energy expendature equivalent to 1200 to 2000 kcal/wk will prevent

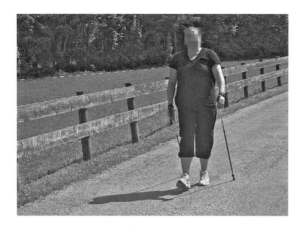

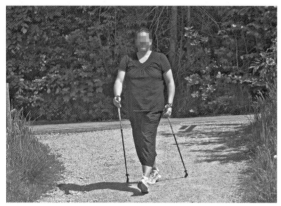

Figure 12.1 - Nordic Walking. This is an aerobic activity adapted to stimulate people to move in natural environments, which activates the aerobic metabolism and tones up several muscles. Walking can prevent skeletal diseases and can be used to cope with stress, depression and anxiety.

weight gain greater than 3% in most adults (Evidence Category A) (Donnelly et al., 2009).

The amount of weight loss through physical activity without diet restriction is generally modest; however, laboratory studies that provide supervision and greater doses of physical activity compared to outpatient studies tend to show weight loss at or above 3% of initial weight. Physical activity <150 min/wk promotes minimal weight loss, physical activity >150 min/wk results in modest weight loss of approximately 2–3 kg, physical activity >225–420 min/wk results in 5 to 7.5 kg weight loss, and a dose–response exists (Evidence Category B). Physical activity combined with diet restriction provides a modest additional-weight loss compared to diet alone, and this additive effect diminishes as the level of diet restriction increases (Donnelly et al., 2009).

The role of physical activity for weight maintenance after weight loss is essential. In several studies, high levels of physical activity have been found to predict success in long-term weight loss maintenance (Hill & Wyatt, 2005). According to the National Weight Control Registry in the US, the primary key strategy for long-term successful weight loss is to engage in high levels of physical activity (Wing & Phelan, 2005). Some studies suggest 200 to 300 minutes of physical activity per week during weight maintenance to reduce weight regain after weight loss, and it seems that "more is better." However, there are no correctly designed, adequately powered, energy balance studies to provide evidence for the amount of physical activity to prevent weight regain after weight loss (Evidence Category B) (Donnelly et al., 2009).

In addition to weight control, increased physical activity is consistently associated with other health benefits. There is a clinical significance to physical activity treatment, even when the criterion of successful weight loss of 5% to 10% is not achieved. Significant reductions in total body fat, abdominal obesity, or both, and significant improvements in cardiometabolic risk factors can be achieved with or without weight loss (Ross, 2010).

Furthermore, mortality risks associated with excess weight may be offset among those who are physically active. There is a dose–response association in that higher levels of physical activity produce a greater reduction in mortality risk among overweight and obese adults. Regardless of body weight, adults who are physically active have more health benefits and a reduced risk of mortality compared to those adults who are unfit and sedentary (Fontaine, 2010; LaMonte & Blair, 2006).

12.4.3 How does physical activity work?

The importance of physical activity for weight management and control can be shown Figure 12.2 from Baker and Brownell (2000). These are potential pathways through which physical activity can influence weight management. Although there is cumulative evidence about the physiological pathways, less attention has been given to these.

There is consistent evidence that physical activity increases psychosocial well-being and thus compliance to physical activity regimens (Hu, 2008).

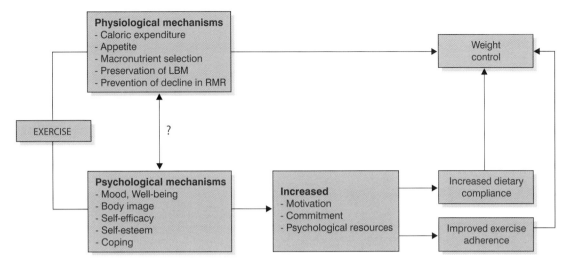

Figure 12.2 - Proposed mechanisms and potential pathways linking exercise and weight control (From Baker & Brownell 2000. Physical activity and maintenance of weight loss: physiological and psychological mechanisms. In C. Bouchard [Ed.], *Physical Activity and Obesity* pp. 311-28, with permission). LBM, lean body mass; RMR, resting metabolic rate.

Mannix et al. (2005) see all psychological effects of exercise (see Figure 12.1) as extremely beneficial and useful for obese people wanting to lose weight. Research resulting from a range of dietary measures confirms the commonly-known experience that restrictive eating behavior leads to depression, anxiety, fatigue, and irritability. This was evident in half of all dieters studied (Mannix et al., 2005).

Physical exercise can help people with obesity who want to lose weight through stress reduction. It improves self-assessment and self-concept, two areas that often are highly reduced after many years of living with obesity.

The growing sense of personal control and efficacy obtained by exercise may indirectly influence eating habits and, due to small success experiences, other positive lifestyle changes.

Movement therapists should elucidate the importance of physical activity for improved mental functioning and well-being to patients.

The fact that physical activity and training triggers immediate feelings of well-being should neither be underestimated nor overlooked (Mannix et al., 2005).

Physical activity and weight control are in part related to psychological mechanisms; however, these relationships are largely hypothetical. Research in the field of physical activity and weight maintenance has overlooked the potential role of psychological variables.

The inability to separate the psychological effects of physical activity from the physiological effects is a major obstacle in recognizing the causal role in obesity.

The psychological effects of physical activity result from either biological or cognitive factors, or they result from a complex interaction between the physiology and psychology.

Baker and Brownell (2000) emphasized the special importance of cognitive factors of self-esteem and self-efficacy in association with weight management.

12.5 THE REALIZATION OF PHYSICAL ACTIVITY ON OBESITY

The specific realization of physical activity on obesity is an adaption of general methodology of physical activity for a specific population. It takes into account the specific psychological, physiological, and social premises of the obese population.

12.5.1 Assessment of the obese adult patient

In addition to a medical evaluation, a complete medical history, including age of onset, family history, a behavioral assessment of eating and exercise behavior, smoking, alcohol use, and previous weight loss experience are crucial for a movement therapist.

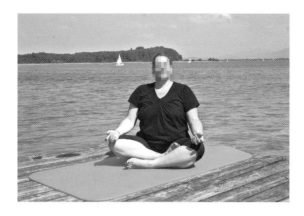

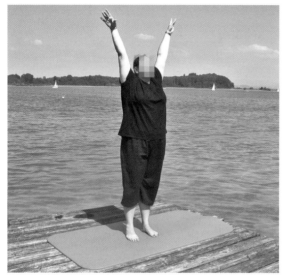

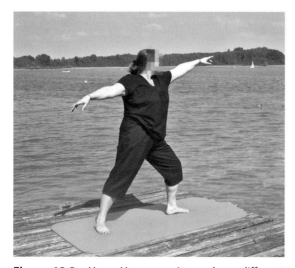

Figure 12.3 - Yoga. Yoga permits work on different levels of human functioning body awareness, physical and psychological sensations, relaxation, perception of limitations and a general flexibility which gives more agility in all kinds of movements.

Specific to physical activity and exercise behavior, the assessment of exercise history, current physical activity levels and fitness levels, and preference (i.e, type of activity) are very important. Assessment of attitudes toward the physical activity and exercise, and finally, the stage of readiness for exercise are very helpful for the followed prescription of physical activity.

12.5.2 Prescription of exercise - how much exercise is needed?

Determining the optimal duration, intensity and type of training needed in order to promote weight reduction remains a prominent question in research.

Current guidelines from the American College of Sports Medicine (ACSM) recommend "that adults participate in at least 150 min/wk of moderately-intense physical activity to prevent significant weight gain and reduce associated chronic disease risk factors.

Furthermore, there is likely a dose-effect of physical activity with greater weight loss and enhanced prevention of weight regained with doses of physical activity that approximate 250 to 300 min/week (approximately 2000 kcal/week) of moderately-intense physical activity" (Donnelly et al., 2009).

These recommendations are consistent with primary health-enhancing physical activity recommendations:

- 30 minutes of moderate intensity physical activity to be regularly performed five days per week,
- or 20 minutes of vigorous intensity activity at least three days per week,
- combinations of moderate- and vigorous-intensity activity are possible to meet this recommendation (Haskell et al., 2007).

These recommendations are general and widely accepted (WHO, 2010).

Through these recommendations, the risk of cardiovascular factors will decrease and mortality rate will minimize, though weight will not necessarily be lost (see §12.4.3).

However, individual circumstances such as new evidence on the dose-response relationship between physical activity and obesity should be taken into account. These recommendations should be accordingly modified (Sjöström, Hagströmer, & Ruiz, 2008).

In the American guidelines, moderate-intensity is defined as 3.0 to 5.9 Metabolic Equivalent (METs). While performing moderate-intensity physical activity, breathing and heart rate are noticeably faster, but one can still carry on conversation. The term includes all forms of everyday activities which lead to a medically effective increase in energy consumption.

This new thinking about physical activity and exercise led to the concept of lifestyle physical activity, which particularly encourages non-active people to integrate moderate physical activities into their daily life.

Lifestyle physical activity examples include walking briskly (1 km/9-12 min; 3.2 km in 30-40 min), light raking leaves or gardening, light snow shoveling, actively playing with children, biking at a casual pace, etc.

Such activities may take place during occupational duties, household work, or even as a means of transportation. For an activity to be effective, it must not be of high intensity, take place in a special place like the gym or tennis court, or be completed temporally contiguous to a single training session.

The advantage of the guidelines regarding the concept of moderate physical activity is that they expand the view of sports and exercises. The most important benefits of regular, moderate intensity physical activity compared to high intensity include:

- easy implementation in practice for severely obese patients (especially at the beginning of weight loss);
- daily performance possible;
- better tolerated with more compliance from patients;
- significantly lower risk of injury;
- eliminates the need for major medical preliminary examinations;
- relatively equal and favorable changes in BMI and body composition.

Hopefully, by incorporating such activities into daily life, adherence to exercise can be more easily maintained.

12.5.3 Types of physical activity - what types of exercise are appropriate?

In addition to lifestyle physical activity, two other types of physical activity are predominantly discussed in current literature: aerobic exercise and resistance exercise. Flexibility training is mentioned as a valuable component to both exercise regimens.

Aerobic activities or endurance training are highly recommended because of the health enhancing effects (cardiorespiratory fitness, energy expenditure and fat loss). For the treatment of obesity, they require moderate or vigorous-intensity efforts. Different types of aerobic activities include walking, water aerobics, bicycling, aerobic dancing, hiking uphill, jogging, etc. The moderate intensity aerobic activities also enable untrained people to achieve these effects and raise calorie consumption. Endurance sports can also be easily performed by obese people while for the most part protecting their joints. Studies from the United States show that walking has become the most popular form of aerobic exercise for the obese (Jakicic, 2003).

The number of studies concerning resistance training as an exercise intervention is significantly less than the number concerning aerobic training, due to the fact that resistance training is not as effective for weight loss. Resistance training consumes lower levels of energy and fat during sessions of equal duration. "Resistance training increases fat-free mass when used alone or in combination with weight loss from diet restriction" (Donnelly et al., 2009). A greater benefit can be achieved when resistance training and diet restriction are combined with aerobic exercise. Although it should be combined with aerobic exercise, the inclusion of resistance training can help obese individuals build strength and preserve lean body tissue. No evidence is currently available regarding "prevention of weight regain after weight loss or for a dose effect for resistance training and weight loss" (Donnelly et al., 2009 p. 466).

While aerobic type activities and resistance training are vital components of maintaining or increasing overall fitness, an exercise program should also incorporate flexibility training. These exercises focus on enhancing posture and flexibility and minimizing stiffness, as well as helping gain confidence in balance and mobility. The addition of these activities will create a well-rounded program for overall physical function.

Furthermore, as with any exercise program, the sport history and the current needs and interests of the patient should always be considered. For optimal adherence, the following topics should be considered: *suitable versus unsuitable, intermit-*

Methodological principles
in the treatment of obesity

External Differentiation. The movement therapists should be sensitive to physical restraints of the patient and offer an exercise program with a variety of different physical activities and sport types (aerobic activities through walking, cycling, or, aqua jogging; or resistance training through weight training or use of other exercise equipment such as medicine balls, bands, and dumbbells).

Internal Differentiation. The patient needs to have different training options within his or her own physical activity performance capabilities. For example, if a patient is unable to stand for long periods of time, activities like badminton should be performed in a sitting position using a stool or chair. Use of exercise bands with differing levels of resistance is also recommended.

Individualization. Although useful guidelines and recommendations from the health organizations exist, *one-size-fits-all intervention* is not practical for everyone within a given population. Exercise programs which are tailored to the individual's needs seem to be more effective, and therefore accordingly advised. The consideration of the current health status, fitness level, performance, needs, preferences, interests and sport history serve as the best, individualized exercise program prescription for the patient. He or she should have the freedom to choose a pleasurable activity, and even be able to vary the regularity of his or her activities. Consider starting the exercise program at a level suited to the patient's capabilities.

Equilibrium. Sometimes it is important to de-emphasize exercise intensity and emphasize staying active, rather focusing on "effort" or minor issues e.g. is it better to exercise before or after a meal, mornings or evenings. The key is to encourage performance and achievement without pressuring and overwhelming the patient. The ideal dose of physical activity must also not underwhelm.

Holism. The consideration of the complete person, physically and psychologically, in the exercise program emphasizes the need for sensitivity, particularly to the psychological barriers of the obese person.

Heterogeneity. Although obese people generally have low fitness levels and poor physical performance, there is a great heterogeneity in levels and rates of changes in occurrence within and between populations. Individuals' sex, age, culture and ethnicity must be taken into consideration.

Transparency. "Why we are doing what we are doing?." It is the therapist's responsibility to make the exercise program and different therapeutic steps clear and understandable to the patient. Trust, safety and empowerment can all be attributed to transparency.

Reinforcement. Experiencing positive reinforcement and performance praise from the movement therapist are crucial elements in improving exercise compliance.

Modeling. Obese persons should model their physical activities and exercises on those of other individuals, like their therapists.

tent *versus traditional continuous exercise, home versus in-group exercise, and lifestyle versus structured exercise.* Current research has neither provided a clear and concrete answer to, nor favoritism for or against these questions. Therefore, more research regarding these topics is needed.

12.5.4 **Methodology**

The three basic didactic principles of physical activity are:
- easy to difficult;
- familiar to unknown;
- simple to complex.

They should be also considered in the prescription and the realization of the exercise treatment.

In addition, further methodological principles should be taken into account by a movement therapist: external differentiation, internal differentiation, individualization, equilibrium, holism, heterogeneity, transparency, reinforcement, and modeling (Textbox 12.1).

12.5.5 Aims of the exercise program

People with obesity often have high expectations and set unrealistic goals such as rapid weight reduction. In regards to their sports and physical activity, they are uncertain about and underestimate their physical performance. Their exercise program goals should be measured regularly with even small successes reinforced. For example, regular participation in an exercise program, regardless of whether or not weight reduction is achieved, is an important goal (Vögele, 2003).

Generally, developing an exercise program consists of well-designed goals. Although found more commonly in other applications, SMART: Specific, Measurable, Achievable, Realistic and Tangible is a dynamic and multifunctional concept that can also be applied to exercise programs. Furthermore, the designed exercise program must be safe, effective and pleasant to prevent patients from quitting or becoming prematurely unmotivated (Mannix et al., 2005; Munsch & Margraf, 2003).

More important than the goal of weight loss is the stabilization of the reduced body weight. In addition, the risk of diseases associated with obesity should be minimized, health behavior improved, and the quality of life must also be a primary goal. The following list presents additional goals of an exercise program.

Functional level
- improvement of body functions and physical performance;
- renewed ability to perform physical activities.

Relationship level
- group cohesion in a protected environment of equals; obese experience with other obese people;
- gain of confidence in the body's abilities;
- improved body image through self-acceptance;
- overcome fears and shame about body image;
- increase self-esteem;

- renewed pleasure in physical activity.

Metalevel
- relationships between physical activity and psychological well-being recognized;
- mediation of motivational strategies to change the old, reduced physical activity levels into integrated lifestyle physical activity.

12.5.6 Behavioral techniques to increase and maintain physical activity

The routine use of behavior therapy strategies to promote physical activity are helpful to weight loss, and therefore recommended. Implementation of such strategies, based on learning principles, provide tools for overcoming barriers to compliance with physical activity changes.

The following strategies can be used by the movement therapist to modify patient's movement behavior.

Self-monitoring of physical activity. Self-monitoring, observation, and record-keeping of physical activity through direct observation methods such pedometers, accelerometers, heart rate monitors or self-reported methods such as records, diaries, logs, and recalls increase awareness of behavior patterns and *are essential to objectifying movement behavior.* Additionally, patients record feelings, reactions, thoughts, events, and reviews, as well as the time and place associated with physical activity events.

Goal setting. Setting behavioral (e.g., exercising 4 days weekly, each for 30 min.) and outcome (e.g., walking 400 m further each exercise session) goals regarding exercise and physical activity can be motivating for obese people (see also section 12.5.5).

Stress management. Stress is a large contributor to obesity. By incorporating stress management techniques such as relaxation, meditation and autogenic training, situations leading to overeating can be alleviated.

Stimulus control. By prompting the occurrence of target behaviors as well as the identification of stimuli, physical activity may be encouraged. Examples: keep the Nordic Walking Poles in sight,

Table 12.2 - Unrealistic and realistic exercise goals for obese people

Unrealistic goals and inaccurate beliefs	Realistic goals and beliefs
I will exercise every day for one hour	I will exercise three times per week for one hour
Exercising and sports are only for skinny people	Everything is for everybody. There are no requirements to starting your individual exercise program
Physical activity and exercise are always competitive	I am doing this for myself. I don't need to compete with others. My focus is on paying attention to my own needs
I am always compared to other people	Remember for whom you are doing this: yourself. Don't worry about competing with others, but instead concentrate on your goals
Sport (Exercise) is associated with grades and athletic performance pressure	Define your personal goals and see them as your grades. Compare your perceived level of performance with the level on which you have started
Walking means to go 10 min per km	I am proud to go my own pace. Moderate intensity exercise can yield positive health results. It doesn't have to hurt to be effective
When I play badminton, I sweat and smell unpleasantly	I can play badminton. It is normal to sweat while exercising

color dots to prompt exercise initiation or leave sport bag in the car to go directly to the exercise venue after work.

Problem-solving. During the initiation and maintenance of an exercise program, the participating obese individual may encounter a number of problems with time and setting (also §12.5.7).

Problem-solving, in the context of physical activity, is the correction of problem areas. Some of the methods that can be used are:
- identification and detailed definition of a specific problem (e.g., time management, employment, transportation issues, adverse weather, injuries, holidays, mood, negative self -talk etc.);
- brainstorming potential solutions;
- weighing the benefits and the disadvantages of each solution;
- selecting, planning, and implementing the solution with the highest potential for ratification;
- evaluating outcomes.

Contingency management. Contingency management can be used to rectify behavior through a reward system. Patients can either be rewarded from an external source such as the movement therapist, or from an internal source, themselves.

For example, a proper reward for training is not a sumptuous meal, but rather the purchase of a CD. The movement therapist could reward the patient with verbal encouragement, compliments, or by offering an exercise chosen by the client.

Cognitive restructuring. Cognitive restructuring requires people to modify unrealistic goals and inaccurate beliefs about weight loss, body image, and physical activity to help change self-defeating thoughts and feelings that undermine weight loss efforts and other physical activities.

This can be accomplished through replacement of negative, dysfunctional, and unrealistic thoughts with more rational thinking (Table 12.2).

Social support. As with ethnicity, sex, and age, a person's social support network must be examined. With a strong support network, weight reduction and physical activity are more easily promoted and maintained. Such a network may include family, friends, work colleagues or online contacts. This group provides crucial motivation and positive reinforcement.

Psychoeducation. This is a method to help patients and their families understand and learn about obesity and its impact on their lives. Psychoeduca-

Barriers to physical activity for obese people

Physiological barriers:
- the wearing of personal body weight
- orthopedic problems – osteoarthritis, other degenerative changes in the lower extremities, lower back pain
- reduced motor skills through the body abundance – soft tissue barrier
- coordination difficulties or balance uncertainty
- declining performance
- possibly a consequent increased risk of injury (Mannix et al., 2005; Wirth, 2003; Vögele, 2003)

Psychological barriers:
- belief that exercise is inconvenient
- low self-confidence in sports and exercise
- lack of knowledge gained from experience
- embarrassment or shame about attending a gym or walking in the street
- past negative experiences
- teasing by peers
- being picked last for teams
- lack of social support
- poor physical performance
- burden of excess weight
- low fitness level

Other barriers:
- lack of time
- lack of interest
- inappropriate facilities and equipment
- lack of tailored exercises programs
- associated costs (e.g., membership, trainer, home equipment)

tional group sessions serve here to specify the development of physical activity issues associated with obesity. Addressed topics are: the role of physical activity and exercise as a therapeutic agent against obesity, management of self-organized physical activities, information about a physical activity plan including type, frequency, intensity, duration etc. In a discussion forum, participants also can share their thoughts, feelings and experiences about physical activities with the group.

Prevention of relapses. Relapse in obesity treatment appears in many forms. Two such relapses are weight regain and failure to adhere to an exercise program (§12.5.7). Therefore, relapse prevention training should help obese persons persist in their exercise adherence.

For optimal relapse prevention, the patient needs to identify a high-risk situation (e.g., change in work schedule; therefore, I can no longer participate in my walking group) and apply an adequate coping response (I will go walking by myself, or go to the gym). By removing self-deprecating feelings, setbacks can be either addressed or completely avoided.

12.5.7 Exercise adherence and barriers to physical activity

Exercise adherence, getting started and continuing with an exercise program are challenges. High dropouts rates, nearly 50% within the first six months of an exercise program, are very common (Dishman, Washburn, & Heath, 2004). Maintenance of exercise participation is a predictive factor for successful weight management;

however, obese persons have a number of physical, psychological, psychosociological and economic barriers to exercise. Some of them are very common, like lack of time, and some are obesity related like the physical burden of excess weight. Barriers include both physiological and psychological aspects (Textbox 12.2) and should be taken into consideration and addressed by the movement therapist in correlation with the patient's circumstances not only for the selection of an initial exercise program, but also as an intervention component used in the therapeutic setting.

12.6 CONCLUSIONS

Obesity is a chronic disease which needs life-long treatment, long-term management, and continuous care. Physical activity and exercise are important components in both prevention and treatment of obesity. In addition to weight management, physical activity has beneficial physical and mental health effects and improves quality of life. Movement therapists must consider not only physiological, but also psychological and clinical issues regarding the use of physical activity as part of obesity therapy. The most prevalent problem is adherence to an exercise program. Behavioral techniques such as psycho-education help increase physical activity and should be used more often and strongly by the movement therapist as a part of the movement treatment. The ultimate goal is incorporating physical activity as a permanent part of one's lifestyle.

The role of **physical activity** in the treatment of **attention deficit hyperactivity disorder** 13

Marika Berchicci & Maurizio Bertollo

13.1 INTRODUCTION

"The Story of Fidgety Philip" is a book of children's poems, published in 1845 and written by a German psychiatrist, Heinrich Hoffman. He described a child called Philip that "[…] won't sit still; he wriggles and giggles, […] swings backwards and forwards, and tilts up his chair […]." Hoffman provided a perfect description of what we know as Attention Deficit Hyperactivity Disorder (ADHD), predominantly hyperactive-impulsive type. Half a century later, in 1902, Sir George F. Still published three lectures to the Royal Academy of Physicians in London in which he described a group of 43 children with behavioral problems. He suggested that the cause was genetic, not poor child rearing. The complex symptomatology of ADHD has not changed since the first descriptions. However, the historical evolution of the ADHD concept firstly emphasized the hyperactivity and poor impulse control (American Psychological Association [APA], 1968); subsequently, neuropsychological methods and techniques evidenced behavioral inattention and performance deficits of attention (APA, 1980). Overall, ADHD is currently described as a neurobiological disorder characterized by chronic and developmentally age-inappropriate symptoms of inattention, hyperactivity, and/or impulsivity, which occur for at least six months in at least two domains of life, beginning prior to the age of 7 years (APA, 2000). Nowadays, ADHD is the most prevalent childhood psychiatric disorder (Nair et al., 2006). The symptoms, usually associated with a variety of psychiatric comorbidities, are related to a catecholaminergic dysfunction in the prefrontal cortex and striate areas, as shown by neuroimaging and neurobiological studies. Children with ADHD exhibit also a peripheral catecholamine (CA) deficiency, which can be detected during biochemical, physical, and cognitive tests (Medina et al., 2010). The Fourth Edition of the Diagnostic and Statistical Manual of Mental Disorder (APA [DSM-IV-TR], 2000) differentiates three subtypes of ADHD: predominantly inattentive (ADHD-I), predominantly hyperactive-impulsive (ADHD-H), and combined (ADHD-C). ADHD affects 5% to 10% of school-aged children; boys are six to ten times more likely to be referred for the disorder, and three to four times more likely to be diagnosed when compared to girls (Willcutt & Pennington, 2000). Ethnic group, family, and socio-environmental factors influence the recognition of ADHD through the degree of acceptance of externalizing behavioral traits and informant agreement (Stefanatos & Baron, 2007). An alternative diagnostic criteria used in the diagnosis of ADHD is the ICD-10 Clinical description (WHO, 1992), which refers to ADHD as *hyperkinesia*. Current research suggests that neurobiological factors play an important role in the development of ADHD. More specifically, the cerebellum (see Cherkasova & Hechtman, 2009 for a review), the frontal regions, the cingulate cortex and associated striate regions, as well as the basal ganglia and the parietal cortices, are frequently cited as neural correlates of ADHD (Dickstein, Bannon, Xavier, Castellanos, & Milham, 2006; Sowell, Peterson, Thompson et al., 2003). An additional hypoactivity has been found in the dorsal anterior cingulate cortex that facilitates complex and effortful cognitive processing and modulates reward-based decision-making, as documented by two more recent meta-analyses (Dickstein et al., 2006; Valera, Faraone, Murray, & Seidman, 2007).

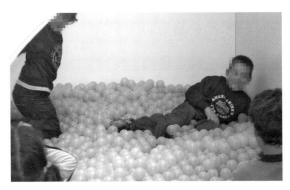

Figure 13.1 - Pool of balls. Children having fun time in a pool of balls. Free play could have positive impact on emotion management and imagination.

Moreover, MRI studies comparing children with ADHD to controls found that children with ADHD had all four lobe volumes smaller than the controls (see Krain & Castellanos, 2006 for a review). However, the most structural differences are in the prefrontal cortex. The dorsolateral prefrontal cortex (DLPFC) which is the region that affects vigilance, attention shifting, planning, executive control, selective and divided attention, and working memory (Duncan & Owen, 2000), in conjunction with the ventrolateral prefrontal cortex (VLPFC), which is linked with behavioral inhibition and has documented involvement in stop-signal task (Aron, Fletcher, Bullmore, Sahakian, & Robbins, 2003), represent a core deficit in frontal lobe function that underlies its various cognitive and behavioral manifestations in ADHD (see Bush, Valera, & Siedman, 2005 for a review). These structural and functional dysfunc-

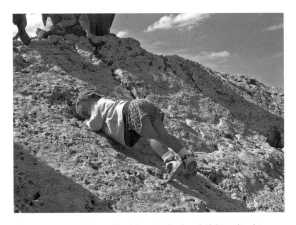

Figure 13.2 - Free climbing. A little child is climbing a rock. Free climbing helps children to consolidate basic skills and to cope with risk situations.

tions may reflect the poor executive function in children with ADHD. The role of executive function involves central control processes, such as planning, organizing, shifting and sustained attention, regulating alertness, modulating emotion, facilitating working memory, and having the ability to self-regulate actions. One comprehensive theory well accounted for in literature is the *Barkley's hybrid model* (Barkley, 1997) of ADHD that identifies behavioral inhibition as the core executive function affected in ADHD. More specifically, he refers to the difficulty of stopping a habitual and dominant response, and to alert their response following corrective feedback and goal-directed motor behavior (Dawson & Guare, 2004), as well as diminished self-control, timing, flexibility, and novelty (Barkley, 1997). Evidence supports that these executive function deficiencies involve numerous impairments in social life, such as disruptive behavior, cognitive deficits, higher frequency of risk taking behavior, difficulties in family and peer relationships, and also an increased risk of obesity. Moreover, there is a characteristically higher incidence of anxiety and depressive symptoms, stemming from low self-esteem (Barkley, 1990; Weiss & Hechtman, 1993). Executive function deficits are also associated with poor academic performance, which places a heavy load on the school system (Altemeir & Horwitz, 1997). ADHD has long-term negative outcomes for many children, including decreased educational attainment, work performance, and occupational stability (Barkley, 2002; Barkley, Fischer, Smallish, & Fletcher, 2006). Learning problems are an especially common comorbid diagnosis in ADHD among school-aged children (Pliszka, 2007), which contribute to academic performance and productivity. In addition, writing deficits (Marcotte & Stern, 1997), central auditory processing problems (Breier, Gray, Klaas, Fletcher, & Foorman, 2002), and speech and language disorders often co-occur with ADHD (Bruce, Thernlund, & Nettelbladt, 2006). Further, motor coordination signs were found in 60% of children with ADHD when compared to controls, with excessive mirror movements, difficulties in the execution of complex motor sequences and slower reaction time (Stefanatos & Baron, 2007). A considerable number of children with ADHD may have difficulties when performing locomotor and object control skills (Harvey & Reid, 2005), as well as in timing. Furthermore, in a recent study Barry et al. confirmed the existence of hypoarousal in ADHD (Barry et al., 2012).

13.2 PHYSICAL ACTIVITY AND ADHD: THEORETICAL OVERVIEW

Multidisciplinary literature has documented the beneficial effect of physical exercise on brain functions and cognition (Hillman, Erickson, & Kramer, 2008). Exercise not only improves physical health, but exerts its positive effects on the cognition at the molecular, cellular, behavioral and systemic levels. Further evidence indicates that participation in sports activity has been associated with the reduction of mental disorders (e.g., anxiety and depression) and physical disorders (e.g., cardiovascular disease, obesity, breast and colon cancer) across the lifespan.

There is evidence that aerobic physical activities, which improve cardio-respiratory fitness, are beneficial to cognitive function and selectively improve executive function performance in the general population (Etnier, Nowell, Landers, & Sibley, 2006), in healthy older adults (Angevaren, Aufdemkampe, Verhaar, Aleman, & Vanhees, 2008; Colcombe & Kramer, 2003), and in children (Sibley & Etnier, 2003). However, physical activity has been relatively unexplored as a behavior that could benefit children with ADHD.

An overview of current literature on the relationship between physical activity and cognition will be provided as a rationale for approaching an understanding of the affect on children. For example, older adults tend to experience declines in executive processes coupled with selective increased brain tissue density and loss of frontal, parietal, and temporal cortices, which were found reduced as a function of cardiovascular fitness (Colcombe et al., 2003). In adjunction, higher levels of aerobic fitness were found associated with increased hippocampal volume and better memory function in older humans (Erickson et al., 2009). Exercise also enhances neurogenesis; a positive correlation was found between physical exercise and hippocampal neurogenesis (Winter et al., 2007), raising the hypothesis that exercise improves learning through its effect on the hippocampus (Fabel & Kempermann, 2008), changing the function of neurotransmitter systems.

Animal studies and studies with older adults demonstrate that the deficiencies of central cate-

cholamines in cognitive (Anderson et al., 2000), biochemical (Girardi et al., 1995), and physical (Wigal et al., 2003) tests are decreased after physical activity (Hillman, Castelli, & Buck, 2005). Upregulation of dopamine and norepinephrine were found in animal studies. In addition to catecholamines, the release of neurotrophic factors, like brain-derived neurotrophic factor (BDNF), nerve-growth factor (NGF), or insulin-like growth factor (IGF-1) is increased in the brain after daily physical exercise.

In particular, serotonin receptors activated by physical activity enhances BDNF expression in hippocampal cells (Vaidya et al., 1997) and BDNF treatment increases tryptophan hydroxylase expression in raphe nucleus neurons (Siuciak et al., 1998). This complex neurobiological mechanism plays a key role in the learning process (Cotman & Berchtold, 2007). A similar picture has emerged in human studies indicating that physically active behaviors influence cognitive functions and the supporting brain structures.

In humans, the P300 component of event-related potential (ERP) had larger amplitude and a shortened latency in attentional challenging tasks. It seems that in humans, physical exercise affects executive functions more than other cognitive processes (Colcombe & Kramer, 2003). Lambourne (2006) found that the working memory capacity of young adults with a high level of fitness differed from those who did not practice exercise.

This is one of the few studies investigating the relationship between cognition and physical activity in adolescents. Overall these findings suggest that the exercise-induced increase of catecholamines and neurotrophic factors might improve learning and induces changes in activity of frontal lobes, which facilitate mental concentration, decision making, memory, planning, and creativity (Caterino & Polak, 1999; Winter et al., 2007).

There is considerable support for the view that regular physical exercise is associated with elevation in mood states (Tomporowski, 2003) and modulates stress and anxiety, which have detrimental effects on memory and learning, contributing to behavioral problems (Adlar & Cotman, 2004; Howells, Russell, Mabandla, & Kellaway, 2005).

Physical activity has been found to positively impact many of the same neurobiological and cognitive factors that are implicated in ADHD. Intense exercise increases blood flow and heightens levels of endorphin and acetylcholine in the brain. The increase in endorphin levels promotes a feeling of wellbeing and reduces the effects of certain secondary symptoms such as depression. Exercise is also effective at reducing hyperactivity and restlessness by making it easier to sit still for a longer period of time.

Physical activity as an intervention in the classroom has been found to impact some of the difficulties that students with ADHD may present, such as the target child's ability to focus, and contributes to improved achievements in math class. For example Azrin, Vinas, and Ehle (2007) suggest that for children with hyperactivity, vigorous scheduled physical activity might be effective to reinforce calmness and increase academic performance.

Another benefit of exercise is that it may discourage children from other endeavors that may make ADHD symptoms worse. The best examples of these wrong behaviors are television, video, and computer games. Television, video, and computer games take up a lot of time that could be used for activities such as interacting with others and involvement in physical activity programs. These sedentary activities promote passivity, give immediate gratification, and promote solitary behavior.

A considerable number of children with ADHD may have difficulties when performing locomotor and object control skills (Harvey & Reid, 2005). Most children with ADHD seem to be novice in movement skill performance and even though they know different action terms, they are not able to refer to the terms with their peers in an appropriate manner, as if they have only a superficial understanding of both movement skills and the purpose of the actions. Such differences in skill confirm a substantial atypical development of procedural and declarative knowledge in children with ADHD (Harvey et al., 2009), as already reported for adults with physical disabilities (Williams & Davids, 1995).

Medina et al. (2010) found better reaction times and lower impulsivity after exercise than that observed among normal individuals immediately. Their results also confirm the assumption that the child's attention deficit can be minimized through physical activity independently from pharmacological medication.

13.3 TREATMENTS

ADHD treatment is based on a multimodal approach that combines psychosocial intervention and medical therapy (Kutcher et al., 2004), even though for many years, particularly in the United States, *pharmacotherapy* has been the most applied intervention in ADHD treatment. The stimulants represent the class of psychotropic medication most commonly prescribed for children with ADHD, which are considered to be catecholamine agonists. It is important to note that while stimulants are effective in the management of the behavioral and cognitive symptoms associated with ADHD, such as inattention, over-activity and impulsivity, there is little known about the long-term changes in academic achievement, the wide individual variation in therapeutic effectiveness, and the optimal dosage level. Another criticism of stimulant drug therapy is represented by the side effects, such as sleep disturbance, appetite suppression, headaches and stomachaches, irritability, motor tics, and social withdrawal (Pliszka, 2000). Moreover, medication does nothing to promote healthy lifestyle behaviors.

Since it is well recognized that children with ADHD devote little time to play or be active with other children, *play therapy* should be a good additional treatment (Davenport & Bourgeois, 2008; Johnson, Rasbury, & Siegel, 1997). Psychologists have determined that a child expresses a great deal through play, which is the idea behind play therapy. It allows children to play in a controlled environment, leaving the adults to observe their behavior. For example sensorimotor play involves the different senses (e.g., tactile, acoustic, and visual experiences, kinaesthetic and proprioceptive stimuli). Practice play contributes to the development of coordinated motor skills needed for later structured game playing and sport. In symbolic play, also called make-believe play, a child transforms an object into other objects and acts toward them. The social play revolves around social interaction with peers. Constructive play occurs when a child uses their imagination and skills to create a product. The play therapy develops problem solving skills, imagination, fine motor skills, and self-esteem, selectively impaired in ADHD, thus can be beneficial in achieving a good outcome.

Recently, some authors and clinicians have introduced *neurofeedback*, or EEG biofeedback in the therapy setting (Arns, De Ritter, Strehl, Bre-

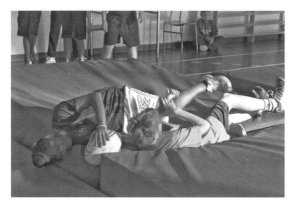

Figure 13.3 - Tumble play. Children involved in tumble play have valuable opportunities to build social and emotional bonds.

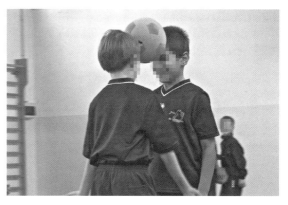

Figure 13.4 - In pair transport. Children have to organize their action with those of a partner to realize the transportation of the ball. This activity requires coordination, precision and couple communication.

teler, Coenen, 2009; Leins, Goth, Hinterberger, Klinger, Rumpf, & Strehl, 2007), even though it was first applied in 1976 by Lubar and Shouse. EEG activity from ADHD children presents different waveforms when compared to control children. Specifically, the EEG brain waves tend to be of larger amplitude and show excess theta activity along with lower amounts of beta activity (Lubar, 1991). This pattern of brain wave activity usually indicates a sleep or day dreaming state, rather than an alert and focused state. The goal of EEG biofeedback training is to alter these abnormal brain waves by decreasing theta waves, while simultaneously increasing beta waves. In EEG biofeedback training, the therapist explains to the child the connection between what is happening in their cortex and what is recorded on the EEG. Using an electroencephalograph to monitor the brain waves and a system of positive reinforcement, the children learn how to make their brains become more attentive. The result is that there is a significant reduction in ADHD symptoms and improvements in behavior, relative to how well the children learn to control their own brain function. When an ADHD child is given a task requiring attention, instead of increasing beta waves, sometimes he increases theta waves, the day dreaming brain wave. These children have what is known as a high theta/beta ratio and neurofeedback technique could normalize this ratio (Fox, Tharp, & Fox, 2005; Fuchs, Birbaumer, Lutzenberg, Gruzelier, & Kaiser, 2003; Gevensleben et al., 2009).

Behavioral management, which includes cogni-

tive behavioral therapy, parent-training, classroom, academic and peer-related interventions, has also been widely studied for children with ADHD.

Despite the strength of evidence for behavioral interventions, it may be unsuccessful due to the need for continued intervention, the complexity of the therapy, dependence on cooperation between parents and teachers, and the relatively high cost of implementing behavioral interventions (Barabasz & Barabasz, 2000).

Thus, behavioral therapies are typically not adequate for bringing children into normal ranges of functioning (Antshel & Remer, 2003; Fiore, Becker, & Nero, 1993; Hinshaw, 1992); additionally, stimulant medications do not show improvement in basic physical skills and involve numerous side effects (Rowland, Lesesne, & Abramowitz, 2002).

Despite combined treatment necessitating the involvement of multiple professionals in the care of children with ADHD and their families, it represents the gold standard in ADHD treatment and is often recommended as the first-line treatment option due to the many problems faced by children with ADHD. The desirable treatment should be socially valid, functionally based, should be specifically tailored to the identified disorder subtype and suited to the child, family and socio-environmental context. Physical activity reflects these features, and it may represent an additional treatment intervention and can prove helpful in minimizing a number of primary and secondary symptoms.

13.4 SUGGESTIONS FOR PHYSICAL ACTIVITY INTERVENTION

Exercise works in a positive way to regulate behavior, improve mood, develop coordination, improve self-esteem, focus attention, and regulate activation. In particular, a specific type of physical activity is *movement therapy*, which is based on sensorimotor activity, like many pedagogical interventions. The latest treatment of ADHD espouses sport as an alternative to prescription drugs. This approach advocates body training and daily walks in natural surroundings such as gardens or woods. It is claimed that the above-mentioned approach can enhance cognitive processes and free tensions in feelings. Indeed, psychomotor education encourages the use of all senses and promotes movement, emphasizing the link between physical and emotional behavior. Physical activity also induces healthy habits. Disorganization, stress, and poor sleeping are all symptoms of ADHD that make it hard to be active and healthy. Exercise reduces anxiety, impulsiveness and hyperactivity associated with ADHD, improves sleep quality and contributes to weight management. Working out empowers persons to release pent-up energy. Post-exercise elevation of brain chemicals improves concentration and may make it easier for people to make lifestyle choices after a workout. Scheduling workouts and adhering to that schedule creates order and establishes a routine, both of which benefit someone suffering with ADHD.

The literature agrees with suggesting at least 30 to 60 minutes per day of moderate to vigorous physical activity for ADHD children, in order to regulate adrenergic system and to use physical activity as catecolaminergic agonist, in favor of a reduction of pharmacological prescriptions.

The lack of clinical randomized control study, which uses the psychomotor intervention, along with structured adapted physical activity and/or exercise, is a limitation in this area. There is also a need for shared procedures in physical activity settings. In this paragraph we would like to advise and propose a first step toward the understanding of procedures and activities that may attenuate ADHD symptoms, stemming from the six characteristics most frequently seen in children with ADHD. These are hyperactivity, perceptual motor impairment, emotional instability, general coordination deficit, disorders of attention, and executive function impairments.

Recently, Verret, Guay, Berthiaume, Gardiner, & Béliveau (2010) tried to prove the effect of a structured physical activity program, which may have clinical relevance to the functional adaptation of children with ADHD. In particular, Tantillo and colleagues (2002) developed physical exercise and sport activity programs specifically designed to improve psychomotor ability, cognitive processes or biochemical level.

A successful approach to adapted physical activity programs with children needs to start with skill development. Different programs have been used to improve psychomotor abilities and skills development. For instance, the psychomotor tradition refers to Le Boulch (1979), Vayer (1982) and Aucouturier (2005) programs, whereas in a school educational context there are the physical education activities suggested by Pangrazi (2004), and in sport education programs the proposal of Siedentop and Tannehill (2000).

In relation to the definition of a structured program of physical activity for ADHD children, the problems lie not only in the exercises or its contents, but also to the procedure and the teaching strategies. For instance, Hallowell and Ratey published an interesting brochure titled "50 Tips on the Classroom Management of Attention Deficit Disorder."

Based on our experience, we believe that a good theoretical framework and applied setting for defining a structured physical activity program is the Five Step Strategy (FSS). The FSS is a metastrategy that has been developed specifically for enhancing the learning of self-paced motor skills (Singer, 1988). The FSS emphasizes the appropriate use of cognitive processes before, during, and after a skill performance. It is a sequential organization of five stages (Textbox 13.1). The FSS should help individuals who are learning a new motor skill to increase their self-confidence, to concentrate on the task at hand, and to create a self-monitoring system. The adaptation of this strategy to children affected by ADHD is very useful, because it follows the same metacognitive strategies used in cognitive behavioral therapy, extended to motor and physical activity.

FSS theoretical framework application could represent a useful structure for ADHD children, implementing specific exercise, mainly derived from the psychomotor and movement therapy tradition, as described in Table 13.1.

The five stages of Five Step Strategy
to enhance the learning of self-paced motor skills

1. *Readying*: helps individuals to create an optimal arousal state before performance by identifying and controlling emotions that may be disruptive to performance itself. ADHD children need higher levels of arousal than others because they are hypoactivated (Douglas, 1988). Readying can help improve their arousal levels to more appropriate and controllable levels, prior to cognitive and behavioral performance as well.

2. *Imaging*: involves visualizing the desired outcome of the intended act (i.e, the correct execution of the task). Imaging has been shown to facilitate motor-skill acquisition, and it may be particularly important for ADHD children, because they tend to have problems with self-regulation mechanisms (Schunk & Zimmerman, 2003).

3. *Focusing*: involves orienting one's attention to a relevant cue. This type of attentional focus should help individuals to block out internal and external distractions that impede learning (Broadbent, 1982). Since ADHD children have a more difficult time attending to important stimuli relevant to the task and blocking out external distractors, this sub-strategy should help them focus better on the task at hand.

4. *Executing*: involves performing the task with a clear mind (i.e, without focusing on the mechanics of the skill).

5. *Evaluating*: involves the learner in analyzing the quality of performance. Analyzing what was done right and what was done wrong is essential to learning a skill. This sub-strategy promotes a self-monitoring system and the adjustment of future performances based upon the assessment of previous performance outcomes.

13.5 SUMMARY

Hoffman, as early as 1845, provided a perfect description of what we know as Attentional Deficit and Hyperactivity Disorder (ADHD), currently described as a neurobiological disorder characterized by chronic and developmentally age-inappropriate symptoms of inattention, hyperactivity, and/or impulsivity, which occur for at least six months in at least two domains of life, beginning prior to the age of 7 years. Nowadays, ADHD is the most referred childhood psychiatric disorder, affecting 5% to 10% of school-aged children. The symptoms, usually associated with a variety of psychiatric comorbidities, are related to a catecholaminergic dysfunction in the prefrontal cortex and striate areas, as shown by neuroimaging and neurobiological studies, as well as in the cerebellum. The structural and functional dysfunction, especially in the prefrontal brain, may reflect the poor executive function in children with ADHD. The role of the executive function impaired in ADHD involves central control processes, such as planning, organizing, shifting and sustained attention, regulating alertness, modulating emotion, facilitating working memory, and having the ability to self-regulate actions. Evidence supports that these executive function deficiencies involving numerous impairments in social life, such as disruptive behavior, cognitive deficits, higher frequency of risk taking behavior, difficulties in family and peer relationships, and an increased risk of obesity. Executive function deficits are also associated with low self-esteem and a consequent higher incidence of anxiety and depressive symptoms, and with poor academic performance, which places a heavy load on the school system. ADHD has long-term negative outcomes for many children, including decreased educational attainment, work performance, and occupational stability. Further, motor coordination signs were found in 60% of children with ADHD when compared to controls, with excessive mirror movements, difficulties in the execution of complex motor sequences and slower reaction time, difficulties when performing locomotor and object control skills, and difficulties in timing. Combined treatments represent the gold standard in

Table 13.1 - ADHD: physical activity intervention

Area of intervention	Rationale	References or theoretical framework	Program focus	Suggested exercises
Behavior and cognitive functions	Exercise improves cognitive ability and regulates behavior	Verret, Guay, Berthiaume, Gardiner, & Béliveau (2010)	Aerobic activity, strength training, and motor skills training	To perform at least a 45-min exercise routine 3 times per week supervised by a PE teacher maintaining moderate to vigorous intensity in each session, possibly using heart rate monitor.
Calming hyperactivity	Physical activity to reinforce calmness	Azrin, Vinas, Ehle (2007); Lapierre and Aucouturier (1978)	Locomotor skills Movement	Run and stop on signal; change direction on signal; run with different steps; run at different speed.
Arousal, activation focusing and emotion regulation	Modulate the arousal level: high activation can be lowered, high and low arousal level can be reinterpreted, low activation felt as unpleasant can be increased	Bertollo and Carraro (2003), based on IZOF model (Hanin, 2000) and Reversal Theory (Kerr, 1987)	Relaxation Muscle to mind Mind to muscle	Laying into ball-pond. Breathing exercises or progressive relaxing (Jacobson). Meditation, visualization, passive relaxing (A.T.).
	Develop the ability to concentrate and be aware of feelings in a controlled, coordinated, and skilful manner, promoting psychosocial development	Therapeutic Eurhythmy (TE) (Majorek, Tüchelmann, & Heusser, 2004)	Coordination and skills Rhythms Sounds and speech	Throw a ball or a rod to each other to a rhythmically spoken poem; move a copper ball with the fingers of one or two hands; carry out different patterns of jumping over rods; walk the rhythm, and the meter of a poem; clap and/or walk different types of rhythms; make specific patterns of movements with arms, hands, fingers, and legs to spoken letters in a sequence, e.g., BMDNRL; jump or execute specific arm movements for the five vowels.
Perceptual motor skill, general motor development	Enhance the ability to receive, interpret and respond successfully to sensory information, throughout movement activity	Frostig (1975); Le Boulch (1979); Vayer (1982); Pangrazi (2004)	Gross motor activities	Rolling, crawling, walking, running, jumping and landing, hopping, skipping, galloping, leaping.
			Vestibular activities	Roll over balls, forward and backward rolls, spinning, balance, scooter boards, skipping with and without ropes, jumping activities.
			Visual motor activities	Manipulation, such as eye-hand co-ordination (e.g., striking), eye-foot coordination activities (e.g., kicking), ball activities (e.g., throwing and catching).
			Auditory motor activities	Temporal awareness. Singing, rhymes and chants. Responding to auditory cues/commands.
			Tactile activities Lateralization activities	Massage, direct touch, and rolling. Bilateral movements, either simultaneous or parallel. Unilateral movements (i.e, one side of the body). Cross lateral movements, such as simultaneous movement of different limbs on opposite sides of the body (e.g., crawling).

(continued)

			Awareness	Body awareness, such as that of one's hands, feet, arms, elbows, stomach, back, etc. Spatial awareness, such as the use of topological and Euclidean concept wherein the child explores the space using different types of locomotion.
General coordination	Coordination improvement for the awareness of physical self, emotional and physical security, increase in confidence, and awareness of environment	Rintala, Pienimaki, Ahonen, Cantell, & Kooistra (1998); Gross motor training (Kiphard, 1994); Developmental Movement Method (Sherborne, 1990)	Gross motor training	Walk and run, climb a ladder, jump on a trampoline, rhythmic jump on the floor, skip with a rope, dynamic balance walking tasks, throw at a target, kick and strike a ball, jump over and crawl under a bar, static balancing tasks, rolling tasks; to be completed 2-3 times per session. Awareness of the body (using one's hands, feet, arms, elbows, back, etc.) and space (crawling, walking, running in the room, etc.), work in pairs (rolling, swinging, pulling, etc.) and as a group (making a circle/tunnel and moving, etc.).
	Enhance motor learning in general, in particular the transfer of skills to activities of daily living for DCD children. Also useful for ADHD children	Neuromotor Task Training (Schoemaker & Smits-Engelsman, 2005)	Body awareness training	The tasks are different for each child, depending on its individual needs as well as the expectations, capabilities, and motivation of both the child and its parents/guardians. The focus of exercise is on the interactions between the child and its environment that will result in acquiring new or improved motor functions, and special attention is paid to how therapists teach the children.
Attention, memory and cognitive process	The concentration required during physical activity to one's bodily movement increases post-exercise focus, attention and memory	Berchicci & Bertollo (2009)	Sports	Taekwondo, martial arts, ballet, yoga, dance, or any physical activity that requires deep mental concentration.
			Other physical activities	Catch just the blue ball, or the all the balls except the red one. Inverse repetition of hand's movements.
Executive functions and learning	Physical activity to improve brain chemicals	Gapin & Etnier (2009)	Aerobic exercise	Acute bouts of moderate aerobic exercise (i.e, 20 min).
	Complex program of integrated sensory stimulation incorporating visuomotor and vestibular therapy. It is created specifically to stimulate and improve the efficiency of the cerebellum	Dyslexia, dyspraxia and attention disorder treatment (DDAT) (Mackie et al., 2007)	Visuomotor and vestibular therapy	Balance board; throw and catch of bean bags (including throwing from hand to hand with careful tracking by eye); practice of dual tasking; stretching and coordination exercises.

ADHD treatment and are often recommended as the first-line treatment option due to the many problems faced by children with ADHD. Behavioral therapies are typically not adequate in bringing children into normal ranges of functioning, and stimulant medications do not show improvement in the basic physical skills and involve numerous side effects. The desirable treatment should be socially valid, functionally based, should be specifically tailored to the identified disorder subtype and suited to the child in a family and socio-environmental context. Physical activity reflects these features, and it may represent an additional treatment intervention and can be proven helpful in minimizing a number of primary and secondary symptoms. Exercise works in a positive way to improve mood, develop coordination, improve self-esteem, and release the excess energy that is so common in hyperactive children; all beneficial in managing attention deficit disorder with hyperactivity.

Physical activity has been found to positively impact many of the same neurobiological and cognitive factors that are implicated in ADHD. Intense exercise increases blood flow and heightens levels of endorphin and acetylcholine in the brain. The increase in endorphin levels promotes a feeling of wellbeing and reduces the effects of certain secondary symptoms such as depression. Exercise is also effective at reducing hyperactivity and restlessness by making it easier to sit still for a longer period of time. Physical activity as an intervention in the classroom has been found to impact some of the difficulties that students with ADHD may present, such as the ability to focus, and contributes to improved achievements in math class.

The *Five Step Strategy* (FSS), which is a Cognitive Behavioral Educational Intervention, is a meta-strategy that has been developed specifically for the enhanced learning of self-paced motor skills (Singer, 1988). It is a sequential organization of five processes: *readying, imaging, focusing, executing,* and *evaluating.* The FSS should help individuals who are learning a new motor skill to increase their self-confidence, to concentrate on the task at hand, and to create a self-monitoring system. FSS theoretical framework application could represent a useful program for ADHD children, implementing specific exercise, mainly derived from the psychomotor and movement therapy tradition.

Sport and adolescents with severe conduct disorders 14

Christophe Maïano

14.1 INTRODUCTION

Conduct disorders, "*that is to say, of persistent disruptive and aggressive behaviors, are the most common form of childhood psychiatric problem in the community and in referrals to child mental health facilities in the West*" (Hill, 2002). Indeed, across the majority of the epidemiological studies performed in the industrialized western world at any one time, between 5% and 10% of eight- to 16-year-olds have conduct problems (i.e., oppositional, disruptive or aggressive behavior problems), and the ratio of boys to girls is 4 or 5:1 (for a review see Angold and Costello, 2001). Historically, these problems of conduct have been identified as a constellation of behaviors that can be characterized as: (i) a disorder; (ii) groups of behaviors; or (iii) specific behaviors or subtypes of behaviors (Hill, 2002). Conduct disorders are defined in the Diagnostic and Statistical Manual of Mental Disorders (DSM-IV; American Psychiatric Association, 1994) as: "*A repetitive and persistent pattern of behavior in which the basic rights of others or major age-appropriate societal norms or rules are violated, as manifested by the presence of three (or more) of the following criteria in the past twelve months, with at least one criterion present in the past six months: (i) aggression toward people or animals, (ii) destruction of property, (iii) deceitfulness or theft, and (iv) serious rule violations*". In addition to meeting the above criterion the disturbance in behavior must cause significant impairment in social, academic, or occupational functioning (American Psychiatric Association, 1994). In the DSM-IV system two subtypes of conduct disorders are described: childhood-onset type has its onset prior to age ten and adolescent-onset type involves the first appearance of symptoms at age ten or older (American Psychiatric Association, 1994).

Clinically, adolescents with conduct disorders can be characterized by chronic patterns of aggressive and antisocial behavior (i.e., actions contrary to the rights of others and rules of society), such as yelling, insulting, throwing or breaking of objects, bullying, fighting, material deterioration, stealing and various misdemeanors (Bassarath, 2001; Frick, 2001; Hill, 2002; Waddell, Lipman, & Offord, 1999). According to Hill (2002), these antisocial behaviors are either "reactive" (i.e., occur in response to actual or perceived threat) or "proactive" (i.e, initiated by the individual), and may follow three different pathway patterns: (i) "overt" (i.e, characterized by bullying followed by early fighting and proceeding to more serious violence); (ii) "covert" (i.e., starting with lying and stealing and going on to more serious damage to property); and (iii) "authority conflict" (i.e., in which oppositional and deviant behaviors are prominent). Additionally, "*adolescent antisocial behavior that breaks the law (and gets caught) may result in contact with police and the courts; the terms delinquent and young offender would then apply*" (Bassarath, 2001). Consequently, conduct disorders represent a constellation of antisocial behaviors, in which a subgroup of youths with severe conduct disorders will be labeled as "delinquents" or "offenders" (Bassarath, 2001; Waddell et al., 1999).

Analysis of the psychosocial characteristics of adolescents with conduct disorders reveal that they exhibited a low self-concept, a high activity level, risk taking, attentional problems and impulsiveness (Bassarath, 2001; Hill, 2002). Then, their relationships with peers and non-peers are mostly unstable and marked by conflict (for a review see Vitaro, Tremblay, & Bukowski, 2001). Additionally, the adolescents with conduct disorders generally lack interest in social activities, and their few centers of interest tend to be quite limited (Frick, 1998). Therefore, their investment in leisure or extracurricular activities is inclined to remain superficial and temporary, and these activities must represent constant sources of immediate satisfaction to be maintained (Hill, 2002). Finally, the assessment of their intellectual abilities usually reveals an intellectual quotient (IQ) over 85, with higher performance IQ than verbal IQ (Teichner & Golden, 2000). Yet, despite their "average" intellectual abilities, these adolescents often have learning disabilities in reading, spelling, writing and math, as well as deficit in executive functions (i.e., abilities implicated in successfully achieving goals through appropriate, effective actions). These executive deficits concern abstract reasoning, language comprehension, problem solving, mental planning, anticipation, concept development, space-time orientation, self-control and the sensorimotor and oculomotor systems (for a review see Lynam & Henry, 2001).

Etiologically, a number of authors have identified multiple risk factors over the past 20 years (Bassarath, 2001; Hill, 2002; Waddell et al., 1999). These researchers have explained conduct disorders in adolescents by referring to internal and external factors. At an external level, the literature has identified (i) emotional deprivation (for a review see DeKlyen & Speltz, 2001); (ii) family influences, such as frequent shifting of parental figures, large family size, inconsistent management with harsh discipline, and so on (for a review see Maughan, 2001); and (iii) community and societal contributions, such as high unemployment rates, social disorganization, and subcultural deviance, among other contributors (for a review see Maughan, 2001). At an internal level, the literature has identified (i) neurophysiologic disturbances, such as low resting pulse rate or low electrodermal response (for a review see Hill, 2001); (ii) biochemical disturbances, such as low blood plasma level of g-amino-butyric acid (GABA), dopamine β-hydroxalase or central serotonin (5-hydroxyindoleacetic acid) (for a review see Herbert & Martinez, 2001); and (iii) genetic influences (for a review see Simonoff, 2001).

In sum, conduct disorders are serious and complex conditions, both for the affected youths and society. These disorders are further complicated by a plethora of biopsychosocial risk and protective factors that are implicated in its aetiology (Bassarath, 2001; DeKlyen & Speltz, 2001; Herbert & Martinez, 2001; Hill, 2001, 2002; Maughan, 2001; Simonoff, 2001).

14.2 SPORT AND SEVERE CONDUCT DISORDERS: THEORETICAL OVERVIEW

Since the end of the 1970s, sport[1] has been widely used as either "prevention" or "rehabilitation" means for adolescents with conduct disorders. The prevention hypothesis posits that sport participation is likely to prevent the onset of conduct disorders; whereas the rehabilitation hypothesis supposes that sport participation may help the adolescents with conduct disorders "readjust to, or cope with, their environment in a more socially desirable manner" (Segrave & Hastad, 1984). Historically, the psychological and sociological perspectives that are frequently proposed in support of these hypotheses have exclusively focused on a specific subgroup of youths with severe conduct disorders: those labeled as "delinquents" or "offenders." Consequently, this theoretical overview, based on the substantial literature review of Segrave (1983), will exclusively focus on severe conduct disorders.

14.2.1 Psychological perspectives

Recapitulation theory. This theory, popularized by Hall (1902), "*maintained that all individuals were born with certain predispositions for inappropriate and disruptive behavior which could only be weakened or modified through*" sport (Segrave, 1983). For the advocates of this theory antisocial behaviors occur when the opportunity, for individuals to discharge their aggressive impulse through sport were restricted or not possible (Andrews & Andrews, 2003). Consequently, sport provided a "*splendid*" motive against vices that could weaken and corrupt the body (Mason & Wilson, 1988).

Surplus energy theory. This theory initiated by Spencer (1873) proposed that sport may induce a

---

[1]   In this paper, the term "sport" will be used to refer to physical activity, exercise and athletic involvement. This reflects the ways those terms are used in the scientific literature on adolescents with conduct disorders. Although fine distinctions can be made between those concepts, they are beyond the scope of this chapter.

tension-reduction, *"whereby energy not expended through work builds up in the individual until it reaches a bursting point. This surplus energy can be expended eufunctionally, in the form of wholesome activity, or dysfunctionally, in the form of delinquent behavior"* (Segrave, 1983). Therefore, sport has often been supported on the basis that it allows individuals to *"blow off steam"* in a positive rather than a destructive way (Segrave, 1983).

Personality theory. For Segrave (1983), *"several theoretical positions have maintained that participation in sport enhances the development of certain personality traits that mitigate against delinquency; the rationale being (...) that by developing wholesome personalities and social human being, it helps assure a situation in which antisocial attitudes do not flourish"*. One of the various aspects of personality that has received particular attention in the relationship between sport and severe conduct disorders is the general self-concept. Indeed, several studies conducted in either the general education system (i.e., regular education classes and resource rooms) or the segregated education system (i.e., segregated classes in a specialized establishment) have demonstrated that adolescents with conduct disorders frequently present a low level of global self-concept in comparison with their non-conduct disorder counterparts (Al-Talib & Griffin, 1994; Barry, Frick, & Killian, 2003; Evans, Levy, Sullenberger, & Vyas, 1991; Harter, Whitesell, & Junkin, 1998; Levy 1997; Maïano, Ninot, Bilard, & Albernhe, 2002; Sprott & Doob, 2000; Sweitzer, 2005). For most of these authors, the antisocial behaviors of these adolescents often represent a response to a lack of global self-concept (Segrave, 1983). Consequently, sport participation may be used as a significant means to enhance individuals' global self-concept and thus precludes involvement in antisocial behaviors.

Stimulus-seeking behavior. This theory initiated by Donnelly (1981) and Sales (1971) proposes that individuals with severe conduct disorders *"actively seek stimulation from the environment once their primary drives are satisfied, or even before they are satisfied. Delinquency is viewed as the product of (...) a high need for stimulation"* (Segrave, 1983). Therefore, advocates of this model argue that all forms of sport offering a highly challenging and demanding environment that channel energy and appetite for excitement or danger will offer a viable substitute for offending or delinquency (Andrews & Andrews, 2003; Segrave, 1983).

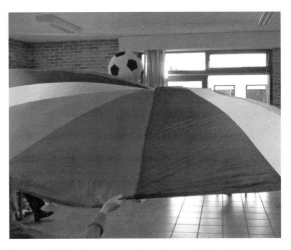

Figure 14.1 - Parachute. Keeping a ball aloft by moving a parachute or a big sheet could be an enjoyable play that requires collaboration and coordination among participants.

14.2.2 Sociological perspectives

Boredom theory. Scholars from this theory (Bordua, 1960; Briar & Piliavin, 1965) have posited that antisocial behaviors developed because adolescents have nothing better to do with their time (Segrave, 1983). Therefore, *"for many years participation in sport has been advocated on the grounds that it occupies the spare time of youthtime that could otherwise be used in deviant behavior"* (Segrave, 1983).

Subculture theory. This theory developed by Sutherland and Cressey (1966) argued that the antisocial behavior of these adolescents is *"learned within peer groups through the communication of both the techniques for committing the criminal act, and the motivations, drives, and rationalizations to justify these actions"* (Mason & Wilson, 1988). Thus, to offer alternatives to these antisocial behaviors it is hypothesized *"that one must not seek to displace the delinquent sub-culture, rather to reproduce the experiential elements of such sub-cultures"* (Andrews & Andrews, 2003). As a solution, scholars suggest the importance of "natural sport" containing variables which closely resemble those of delinquent sub-cultures: (i) de-emphasis on competition; (ii) focus on personality constructed goals; (iii) minimal regulations; and (iv) individual or small group in nature (Andrews & Andrews, 2003).

Strain theory. Advocates of this theory (Merton, 1938; Cohen, 1955) argue that *"certain members of* society, largely as a result of their relative class position, are driven to delinquency in order to achieve goals they are denied through legitimate channels" (Segrave, 1983). Thus, these individuals may use illegitimate channels of goal achievement. The advocates of this theory argue that antisocial behavior is often the expression of a frustration felt toward achievement criteria that they cannot attain (Segrave, 1983). Consequently, sport may function as an alternative means to achieving these goals (Purdy & Richard, 1983).

Social control theory. This theory, formalized by Hirschi (1969), supposes that individuals who have developed a strong social bond with various components of conventional society (e.g., attachment, commitment, involvement, belief, etc.) are more likely to conform. Accordingly, advocates of this theory posit that participation in structured sports should serve as a *"prophylactic against delinquency by encouraging youths to develop a commitment to conformity"* and thus discouraging delinquency (Guest & McRee, 2009).

14.3 RECOMMENDATIONS

The purpose of this third section is to provide key elements that should be taken into consideration when designing a sport program or curriculum that may be theory-driven and adapted to the characteristics and needs of adolescents with conduct disorders.

a. *Characteristics of the participants.* As already mentioned in the introduction, adolescents with conduct disorders represent a constellation of aggressive and antisocial behaviors (e.g., yelling, insulting, bullying, fighting, material deterioration). Consequently, the selection and the profile of youths who will participate is one of the essential decisions to be made, because it plays a fundamental role in designing the most effective program.

b. *Setting.* In order to effectively deal with the full complexity of conduct disorders in adolescents and their social consequences, the policies of many western countries orientate these adolescents toward either segregated classes (i.e., resource rooms or self-contained classes in the general education system) providing an adapted educational support, or specialized establishments, security units, and detention centers. Therefore, the specificities of these various settings (e.g., functioning, professionals, rules)

should be taking into consideration when designing the sport program or curriculum.

c. *Conditions of inclusion in the program.* Regarding the characteristics of adolescents with conduct disorders, it is preferable that programs include only voluntary participants who have volunteered and are motivated. Indeed, as already mentioned in the introduction, these adolescents generally lack interest in social activities, and their investment in leisure or extracurricular activities is inclined to remain superficial and temporary. However, if the program is to take place in a specialized establishment, security unit, or detention center, or as an alternative to institutionalization it may be essential that their participation is obligatory.

d. *Size of the group.* A group comprising six to ten participants may represent an optimal choice (Mason & Wilson, 1988). However, this number may be adjusted to the characteristics of the adolescents with conduct disorders (i.e., severity of the antisocial behaviors) and the rules of the setting (i.e., limited numbers of adolescents in a group).

e. *Supervision.* The staff-participant ratio should be 1:3 or 1:4 (Mason & Wilson, 1988). Nevertheless, this ratio should be adjusted to the characteristics of: (i) the adolescents with conduct disorders, (ii) the setting, and (iii) the type of sport program.

f. *Objective(s) of the program.* Based on the aforementioned theoretical models on the relationship between sport and conduct disorders, several objectives could be offered when designing the program or curriculum: (i) to develop personality characteristics (e.g., self-concept, confidence, motivation); (ii) to develop social skills and commitment to conformity (e.g., respect of others, communication); (iii) to discharge aggressive impulse; (iv) to induce a tension-reduction; (v) to offer a high level of stimulation; (vi) to develop sport skills and physical fitness; or (vii) to relieve the boredom of these adolescents with nothing better to do with their time.

g. *Categories of programs.* According to the literature (e.g., Mason & Wilson, 1988; Segrave, 1983), three categories of programs could be proposed to adolescents with conduct disorders: (i) interscholastic athletics; (ii) sport; or (iii) outward bound (i.e., high risk activity program). The decision to follow one or more of these programs should be related to the objective(s) of the program or curriculum.

h. *Mode of competition*. Although there are differing opinions on the place of sport competition in the prevention or rehabilitation of adolescents with conduct disorders (Segrave, 1983; Mason & Wilson, 1988), five approaches could be proposed: (i) competing against peers with conduct disorders; (ii) competing against the self; (iii) competing against the environment; (iv) competing against adolescents without conduct disorders; and (v) competing in a group mixing youths with conducts disorders and those without.

i. *Type of sport activities*. A wide range of sport activities could be offered to adolescents with conduct disorders. However, their inclusion in a program or curriculum should be theory-driven and related to the purpose of the program or curriculum. For example, the *stimulus-seeking behavior* theory hypothesized offering challenging and demanding sport activities which channel energy and appetite for excitement or danger to deal with the high need for stimulation in these adolescents. Inversely, advocates of the *subculture theory* propose to offer "natural sport," containing variables which closely resemble the culture (e.g., de-emphasis on competition, minimal regulation) of adolescents with conduct disorders.

j. *Dose of sport*. The dose of sport is comprised of three components: the frequency (i.e., amount of time per week), the bout duration (minutes), and the intensity (i.e., moderate to vigorous). Based on the aforementioned theoretical models on the relationship between sport and conduct disorders, it is possible to act on one or several of these parameters. For example, if the objective of the program is to discharge the aggressive impulse of these adolescents (as suggested by the recapitulation theory), it is advised to propose a vigorous intensity. Inversely, if the purpose of the program is to occupy the spare time of these adolescents (as suggested by the boredom theory), it is preferable to both increase the frequency and the bout duration.

k. *Length of the program*. According to the literature (Mason & Wilson, 1988), the length of the program may range from one week to six months. For example, Mason and Wilson (1988) argued that outward bound programs are usually three to four weeks long. However, this parameter should be adjusted to the specificities of the program (e.g., objective, category) and to the time of institutionalization.

Conduct disorders: summary/guidelines

- Conduct disorders are defined as a repetitive and persistent pattern of behavior in which the basic rights of others or major age-appropriate societal norms or rules are violated
- Clinically, adolescents with conduct disorders are characterized by chronic patterns of aggressive and antisocial behaviors (such as yelling, insulting, throwing or breaking of objects, bullying, fighting, material deterioration, stealing, etc.)
- Adolescents' antisocial behaviors are either "reactive" (i.e., occur in response to actual or perceived threat) or "proactive" (i.e., initiated by the individual), and may follow three different pathway patterns: (i) overt, (ii) covert, and (iii) authority conflict
- Conduct disorders represent a constellation of antisocial behaviors, in which a subgroup of youths with severe conduct disorders are labeled as "delinquents" or "offenders"
- Psychosocial characteristics reveal that adolescents with conduct disorders exhibit: (i) a low self-concept, (ii) a high activity level, (iii) risk taking, (iv) attentional problems, and (v) impulsiveness
- Peer and non-peer relationships, in adolescents with conduct disorders, are mostly unstable and marked by conflict
- Adolescents with conduct disorders generally lack interest in social activities, and their few centers of interest tend to be quite limited
- Despite their "average" intellectual abilities, adolescents with conduct disorders often have learning disabilities (i.e., reading, spelling, writing and math) and deficit in executive functions (e.g., abstract reasoning, language comprehension, problem solving, mental planning, anticipation, concept development, space-time orientation)
- Etiologically, several internal (i.e., neurophysiologic disturbances, biochemical disturbances, and genetic influences) and external factors (i.e., emotional deprivation, family influences, and community and societal contributions) may explain the development of conduct disorders in adolescents
- Historically, sport has been widely used as either "prevention" (i.e., prevent the onset of conduct disorders) or "rehabilitation" (i.e, readjust to, or cope with, their environment in a more socially desirable manner) means for adolescents with conduct disorders
- The theoretical models that are frequently proposed in support of these hypothesis (i.e., prevention or rehabilitation) have drawn their rationale from several psychological and sociological perspectives
- Four psychological theories on the relationship between sport and conduct disorders are available in the literature: (i) recapitulation, (ii) surplus energy, (iii) personality theory, and (iv) stimulus-seeking behavior
- Four sociological theories are proposed in support of the relationship between sport and conduct disorders: (i) boredom, (ii) subculture, (iii) strain, and (iv) social control
- Eleven key elements should be followed to design a sport program or curriculum that may be theory-driven and adapted to the characteristics and needs of adolescents with conduct disorders: (i) characteristics of the participants; (ii) setting; (iii) conditions of inclusion in the program; (iv) size of the group; (v) supervision; (vi) objective(s) of the program; (vii) categories of programs; (viii) mode of competition; (ix) type of sports activities; (x) dose of sport; and (xi) length of the program

Physical activity and people with intellectual disability (mental retardation) 15

Erica Gobbi, Ilaria Ferri, Attilio Carraro

15.1 INTELLECTUAL DISABILITY

The term "Mental Retardation" (MR) is going to be replaced as it has been judged to have gained a prejudicial meaning and it will likely be changed to "Intellectual Disabilities" in the near future. Mental retardation is perhaps the best known form of disability but its definition is still in progress. The Diagnostic Statistical Manual-IV (DSM-IV) diagnostic features (American Psychiatric Association, 2000) single out three criteria characterizing a person with mental retardation, these being a *"significantly subaverage general intellectual functioning (Criterion A) that is accompanied by significant limitation in adaptive functioning in at least two of the following skill areas: communication, self-care, home living, social/interpersonal skills, use of community resources, self-direction, functional academic skills, work, leisure, health, and safety (Criterion B). The onset must occur before age 18 years (Criterion C)"* (p. 42). In this definition "general intellectual functioning" refers to intelligence quotient (IQ) obtained by specific assessment instruments (individually administered intelligence tests generally used are the Standford-Binet IV and the Wechsler Intelligence Scale for Children III), and current cutoff point for mental retardation is IQ of about 70 (considering a measurement error of 5 points in assessing IQ).

"Adaptive functioning" refers to how effectively persons cope with common life demands and how well they meet the standards of personal independence expected of someone of their particular age, group, sociocultural background, and community setting.

To provide input into the DSM-5, the AAIDD (American Association on Intellectual and Developmental Disabilities - formerly the American Association on Mental Retardation) recommends the following three edits/changes (AAIDD 11th Edition Implementation Committee, 2010):

1. To use as the criterion for significant limitations/deficits in adaptive behavior, "performance that is approximately two standard deviations below the mean of either (a) one of the following three types of adaptive behavior: conceptual, social, and practical, or (b) an overall score on a standardized measure of conceptual, social, and practical skills.
2. To insert the word "approximately" before the words "two or more standard deviations" for both criterion A (IQ) and B (adaptive behavior).
3. Insert a statement indicating that a change in terminology (from mental retardation to intellectual disability) does not result in a change in one's eligibility for services and supports.

So, although mental retardation remains the formal and proper diagnostic term defined in the DSM (currently in the 4th text-revised edition), our intention is to use the term intellectual disability (ID) in coordination with the term adjustment in the publication of the DSM-5.

Individuals with ID are typically classified into four different categories based on their level of functioning or severity as measured as reflected by the ratio of mental age to chronological age, or intelligence quotient (IQ). Subaverage intellectual functioning is defined as an IQ score of at least two standard deviations below the mean, or approximately 70 to 75 or below, the classification based on Diagnostic and Statistical Manual of Mental Disorders-IV-TR, and the International Classification of Diseases-10 presented in Table 15.1, however these features hide the wide variety among persons with ID.

Table 15.1 - Classification of ID based on DSM-IV-R and ICD-10

Class	IQ
Profound mental retardation	Below 20-25
Severe mental retardation	20-25 to 35-40
Moderate mental retardation	35-40 to 50-55
Mild mental retardation	50-55 to 70-75

15.1.1 Prevalence and aetiology

Prevalence of ID is generally estimated by a normal curve theory. Mild, moderate, severe, and profound degrees of intellectual disability refer to two, three, four, or five standard deviations below the normal IQ for the general population, so about 2.3 percent of the entire population fit into this group.

The largest group of persons with ID, about 90% of cases, fall into the "mild" category (Handapp & Dykens, 2003). This group appears similar to the general population; persons can be educated and may function quite well in society. Some are able to live independently, hold jobs, marry, raise a family, and may simply appear slow or in need of extra help. More persons with mild ID come from minority and low-SES backgrounds (Strømme & Magnus, 2000), and their disease is generally not associated with substantial behavioral problems.

Persons with "moderate" ID are the second most commonly diffused and are considered trainable, but almost all require lifelong support in navigating everyday life. They learn best through repetition and some are included in supervised workshop programs.

Cases classified as "severe" and those classified as "profound" are people that show concurrent physical or ambulatory problems, or other concurrent diseases (e.g., heart or respiratory impaired conditions). These persons tend to display more behavioral problems, require special lifelong assistance and generally learn only basic eating, toileting, grooming and dressing behaviors.

Aetiology of MR can generally be split into organic (known medical cause) and non organic (unknown or familial/environmental causes).

Medical etiologies identified of ID can be classified as (i) prenatal, (ii) perinatal, or (iii) postnatal by time of onset (Grossman, 1983). Prenatal causes refers to genetic disorders or alcohol exposure in utero; perinatal causes to premature birth and includes the period extending from the 28th week of pregnancy to the 28th day following birth; and postnatal causes involve head trauma and exposure to lead. However, in about 40% of ID cases the causes cannot be found, and also involve environmental factors in the development of this impairment.

15.2 RATIONALE FOR PHYSICAL ACTIVITY IN INTELLECTUAL DISABILITY

Although there is scant information on health behaviors of individuals with ID, there is substantial evidence that fitness levels are low (Graham & Reid, 2000; Fernhall & Pitetti, 2001) and that people with ID experience high rates of morbidity associated with hypoactive disease (Sutherland, Couch, & Iacono, 2002). Persons with an intellectual disability comprise a subgroup that is considered at elevated risk for health problems associated with inactivity (Rimmer & Braddock, 2002) and have high obesity rates (Rimmer, Braddock, & Fujiura, 1993), higher rates of diabetes and high blood pressure (Rimmer, Braddock, & Marks, 1995; Draheim, McCubbin, & Williams, 2002; Janicki, et al., 2002).

In the population with ID it is more likely that physical activity patterns go unnoticed or unstudied because these people are generally not included in large-scale population studies (Temple, Frey, & Stanish, 2006).

However, studies concerning this population report that only about 20-30% of adults with ID meet the current health promotion recommendation (Stanish & Draheim, 2004), and that youth with ID demonstrate lower levels of cardiovascular fitness, muscular strength, and higher levels of obesity than peers without ID (MacDonncha, Watson, McSweeney, & O'Donovan, 1999).

There is a critical need to establish stronger evidence that examines the effects of various doses and modalities of exercise on key health outcomes (i.e, mental health, physical functioning). It's difficult to make comparisons between studies when there isn't a rigorous design (e.g., randomized controlled trial); different instruments are used and no two persons with ID are the same. In the next paragraphs we intend to summarize the most relevant results obtained in research with ID persons, pointing out physical and mental health benefits that reported statistical significance, is to support the concept that persons with ID can achieve the same physical activity levels as the general population, and that beneficial effects can establish the use of exercise in clinical and community practices for various subgroups of people with ID.

15.2.1 Physical and mental health benefits

Given the risk for obesity and chronic disease in people with ID, research focused primarily on fitness level, body composition, muscular strength, and endurance and flexibility. Sedentary behaviors are exhibited in most people with ID, and researchers progressively gave attention to enhancing physical activity participation. To investigate sources of reinforcement and predictors of PA participation, studies on exercise effects were conducted examining more areas of the persons involved (e.g., depression, quality of life).

Based on the review published by Rimmer et al. (2010), we report a selection of studies showing significant improvement and excluding the study specifically referring to people with Down Syndrome (Table 15.2).

There are two non-randomized controlled trials (Carmeli, Zinger-Vaknin, Morad, & Merrick, 2005; Ewing, McDermott, Thomas-Kroger, Whitner, & Pierce, 2004), three pre versus posttrial (Elliot, Dobbin, Rose, & Soper, 1994; Mann, Zhou, McDermott, & Poston, 2006; Pommering et al., 1994), and one randomized controlled trial (Seagraves, Horvat, Franklin, & Jones, 2004). Two of these studies involved participants in educational intervention (Ewing et. al, 2004; Mann et al., 2006), two proposed aerobic exercise (Elliot et al., 1994; Pommering et al., 1994), one study combined modality of exercise (Carmeli et al., 2005), and another examined strengthening exercise (Seagraves et al., 2004). The majority of studies report outcomes referring to functional, musculoskeletal, cardiorespiratory and metabolic health, so there are especially variables related to physical health. However, some studies do investigate mental health, so well being, maladaptive behaviors and cognitive aspects were examined.

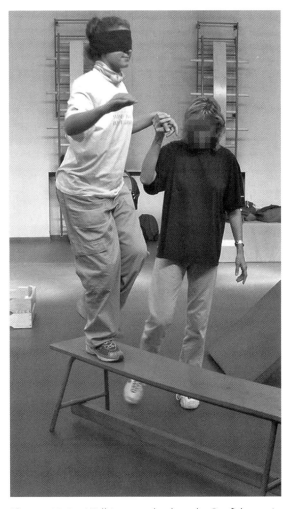

Figure 15.1 - Walking on the bench. Confidence in the other is a central objective. A variety of movement situations can be created to stimulate cooperation and contact.

15.3 PRACTICAL IMPLICATIONS FOR PA-INTERVENTIONS IN PEOPLE WITH INTELLECTUAL DISABILITY

Individuals with ID adapt to increased levels of physical activity in much the same way as individuals without disabilities. A direct relationship exists between fitness levels and engagement in physical activity, which is why health agencies worldwide continue to promote importance of sustained activity over attaining a state of fitness for the general public (Stanish & Frey, 2008). An adequate amount of PA must be assessed accord-

Table 15.2 - Characteristics and results of exercise intervention research on persons with ID

Study	Experimental design	Participants	Setting	Type of intervention	Frequency description	Length of treatment	Outcomes
Carmeli et al. (2005)	non-RCT	group A: 10 group B: 12	Foster home residential	Combined exercise	3 days/wk A: balance and strength B: general exercise	6 months	↑ well being ↑ strength ↑ Functional Reach Test ↑ balance (TUGT)
Ewing et al. (2004)	non-RCT	ID = 92 non ID = 97	Group teaching	Education	Knowledge of healthy eating, self-report of fruit and vegetable intake, exercise	8 weeks	↓ BMI
Elliot et al. (1994)	pre vs. post	n = 6	Residential	Aerobic exercise	General motor activities: bike, stepper, weight lifting. Vigorous aerobic exercise: treadmill 20 minutes	5 sessions	↓ maladaptive and stereotypic behaviors (vigorous ex)
Mann et al. (2006)	pre vs. post	n = 192	Residential	Education	Steps to Your Health Program 90 minutes. Optional brisk walk	8 classes	↓ BMI ↑ exercise frequency ↑ knowledge on diet/ nutrition/exercise/stress
Pommering et al. (1994)	pre vs. post	n = 14	Community-based	Aerobic exercise	Supervised optional training sessions 4 days/wk	10 weeks	↑ VO$_2$max ↑ O$_2$ pulse ↑ maximum ventilation ↑ exercise stress test duration ↑ flexibility
Seagraves et al. (2004)	RCT	Ex: 7 C: 7	High school	Strengthening	2 days/wk 3-4 sets of each exercise 8-12 rep.	10 weeks	↑ isometric strength

Note: non-RCT = non randomized controlled trial; pre vs. post = pre-post design; RCT = randomized controlled trial; ID = Intellectual Disability; Ex = Exercise Group; C = Control group; BMI = Body Mass Index; VO$_2$max = Maximal Oxygen Uptake.

ing to the general activity guidelines of the WHO (2003): 30 minutes of moderate to vigorous intensity physical activity on all or most days of the week, or 10,000 steps per day. Therefore, the greater need for researchers is to develop and test interventions that encourage individuals with ID to initiate and maintain physical activity (Rimmer & Braddock, 2002; Rimmer, Braddock, & Pitetti, 1996). Lavay and McKenzie (1991) reported significantly increased aerobic fitness levels in adults with ID after participation in short-term activity programs like walking or jogging (3 days per week for 12 weeks) with some supervision and encouragement.

Other researchers investigated the effectiveness of a 12-week (3 days/week) low-impact aerobic dance program for improving cardiovascular endurance in adults with ID and trying to determine whether aerobic dance is motivating to individuals with ID (Cluphf, O'Connor, et al., 2001): they assess that adults with ID will be active if provided enjoyable opportunities like aerobics, but the direct involvement of others (i.e, staff, families) is needed to facilitate participation and promote adherence. The findings of these studies further indicate that individuals with ID increase levels of engagement with positive extrinsic reinforcement. Based on the literature reviewed, there is evidence that people with ID will engage in meaningful physical activity if they have the opportunity to do so. It is a common opinion that individuals with ID are not motivated to seek out opportunities to be physically active, therefore reinforcement strategies and high supervision have to be used in efforts to promote activity. Moreover it is known that family members, residential care providers, employers, and/or other individuals that support people with ID play a role in identifying opportunities to engage in activity and assist with partici-

pation. Therefore, an important step toward improving health behaviors is ensuring that care providers have the knowledge, skills, and resources to facilitate healthy living, and it is critical that people with ID perceive the benefits of physical activity (Mann, Zhou, McDermott, & Poston, 2006).

Functional health is the most commonly targeted health outcome, which included walking capacity, functional independence, balance, quality of life, motor function, and pain reduction. This was followed by musculoskeletal health, which includes muscle strength, muscular endurance, flexibility, bone mineral density, and cardio-respiratory health (Rimmer, et al., 2010). Furthermore, PA propositions for people with ID can aim to ameliorate and reinforce work-related tasks, and enjoy but also profit from participation in recreational and leisure activities (Guidetti et al., 2010). Therefore, it is important to knock down barriers and segregated environments that can inhibit successful promotion of skills development and programming (Whorton, Morgan, & Nisbet, 1994). A number of studies have investigated the important relationship between PA and autonomy in connection to health. Autonomy refers to self-determination, independence, and self-care, but is also strictly related to controlling actions, decision-making, wishes and desires, and making decisions about one's own life and health. This suggests the awkwardness of the argument and underlines the need for a general reflection about all that characterizes the environment and the context in which activities are proposed: safety/contents, inclusion, frequency and intensity, activity modification, instructional strategies, group dimensions, competition, enjoyment, and co-morbidity are all elements that the PA instructor has to combine in the activity programs.

Physical activity-interventions in people with intellectual disability: summary/guidelines

There are many suggestions for strategies that could be considered when implementing programs for people with ID. Encouraging people with ID to engage in physical activity is one of the most important proposals suggested by researchers.

An ideal program centered around encouragement, must include:
- settings that provide interaction between people with ID and the general population (inclusion);
- low to moderate intensity activities like warm ups and walking;
- strategies and positive reinforcement that build personal motivation and self-esteem;
- social interaction between individuals and participants;
- involvement of participants in activity selection and decision making;
- age-appropriate activities and repetition of common actions;
- programs based on community environments;
- participants, needs and preferences with a deep focus/attention on their abilities;
- quick program changes to satisfy participants, abilities;
- progress supervision, participants, goal tending and final recognition of improvements.

In accordance with these suggestions based in the scientific literature, it is important to note some other aspects when setting an intervention to enhance PA participation:
- the accessibility of the propositions in terms of barriers and task difficulty: these have to be adapted to people's abilities;
- the meeting structure: repetitiveness gives a sense of safety and allows the reinforcement of skill acquisition. New requests or tasks have to be entered respecting didactic progressions and particularly subjects responses;
- contents: each group session is planned around some macro-objective established from people's needs and wishes; physical abilities like coordination, muscle strength, muscular endurance, or flexibility;
- group composition: it is important to guarantee an adequate level of attention and support to each participant of the group, to facilitate cooperation and socialization, to raise consciousness of their own limits and abilities;
- rules: a suitable behavior foreseeing the respect of shared rules and recognition of roles;
- climate: competition and comparison have to be moderated and used in order to ameliorate communicational and relational competences (e.g., collaboration, tolerance, challenge, attention to team-mates) and not only physical abilities;
- intensity: frequency and duration of the activities have to be modulated according to people's capabilities; pauses and recovery are important moments for promoting self-consciousness.

Physical activity – psychomotor therapy and elderly with **psychiatric disorders** 16

Seppe Deckx

16.1 BRIEF DESCRIPTION OF THE CHARACTERISTICS OF THE DISORDER

In this chapter we discuss the elderly that are included in a unit for older people with psychiatric disorders and the place that psychomotor therapy (PMT) and physical activity (PA) can have in the treatment of this elderly.

When we consider that our society will face an increasingly aging population in the next years, we understand that this will undoubtedly lead to an increased demand for attention and care for the elderly, with or without psychiatric problems. Moreover, one can expect the number of older people with psychiatric problems to increase in the coming years. Dilip & Jeste (2000) provide some explanations for this increase: better and earlier diagnosis, reduced social stigma for psychiatric disorders, and overall improved healthcare.

Before moving on to PA & PMT it is important to know which elderly are included on a psychiatric ward. When we consider the profiles of older psychiatric patients, we can distinguish between two major groups. The first group is those who suffer from dementia, mainly due to a neurodegenerative disease. The other group we can describe as patients with functional psychiatric disorders. Obviously, the approach of the psychomotor therapist or physiotherapist will differ between the two groups.

16.1.1 Dementia

The descriptive term dementia refers to the cognitive problems in patients, usually because of

a neurodegenerative disorder. Neurodegenerative disorders are brain diseases that gradually become worse (Deelman 2004). Examples are Alzheimer's disease, dementia in Parkinson's disease, and frontotemporal lobar degeneration. Neurodegenerative diseases always have a major impact on patients because cognitive, emotional, and motor functions are affected, individually or in combination with each other. The ability to function independently is lost. Yet there are some kinds of dementia that are not gradually evolving (vascular dementia). We must also make it clear that dementia is not always the result of a neurodegenerative disorder. It can also be caused by a tumor or AIDS. Not all forms of dementia affect the same brain functions and consequently they have different courses.

Older people with dementia will not necessarily be referred to a psychogeriatric unit. This happens only when a diagnostic clarification is needed, or when the elderly states problems due to dementia resulting in the situation at home or in the rest home no longer being tenable. These are problems of various kinds: behavioral problems, mood-related problems, psychosis-related problems, etc. Examples include agitation, aggression, depression, apathy, delusions, hallucinations, false recognitions, etc. The reason for an inclusion in a psychiatric hospital is to get these problems under control by a multidisciplinary approach followed by referral to a rest home.

16.1.2 Functional psychiatric disorders

Among the functional psychiatric disorders we understand a broad spectrum of disorders. Some of the most common are mood disorders, schizophrenia, anxiety disorders, personality disorders and substance dependence. This can include disorders that start later in life (late onset) but also chronic disorders that have been present for a long time (early onset).

For an extensive discussion of both the neurodegenerative and functional disorders we refer to the DSM-IV classification (American Psychiatric Association 2001).

16.2 THEORETICAL SCIENTIFIC VIEW WHY PA MAY BE IMPORTANT FOR THIS DISORDER

Why do we need PMT & PA on a psychogeriatric ward? Why do we try to motivate patients to participate in the therapy? Why should older people have to be physically active? Why not leave an elderly patient in his or her seat?

16.2.1 Quality of life

To answer these questions, we introduce the term "quality of life." This refers to a person's perception of their position in life in the context of culture and value systems in which they live, in relation to their goals, expectations, standards and concerns. It is a broad concept that brings together physical health, psychological state, level of independence, social relationships, personal beliefs, and relationship to salient properties of the environment in a complex manner.

International authors often stress the absence of a generally accepted definition of quality of life in dementia. To fill this gap, Ettema et al. (2005) defined quality of life in dementia through a multi-dimensional assessment of the person in their environment in terms of adaptation to the observed effects of dementia. They also developed a promising new tool (QUALIDEM) for measuring this.

The more active elderly, the longer their quality of life remains at a satisfactory level. PA promotes endurance, balance, muscle strength, flexibility, agility and coordination, reduces the risk of chronic health problems and fall incidents, and promotes overall well-being. In other words, PA in later life is an important resource for an active and independent functioning and thus increased quality of life (Figure 16.1). Indeed, being physically active also effects the ability to take advantage of public services, visit friends or acquaintances, participate in activities or take part in social life.

16.2.2 The adaptation process

Elderly hospitalized in a psychogeriatric ward have to face many disruptions in their psychological functioning and behavior (Dröes 2001, Bron 1994). This is not only caused by organic factors (e.g., in dementia) but also by psychological and social factors.

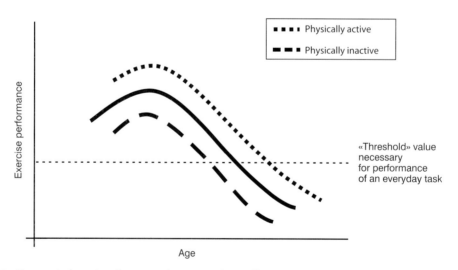

Figure 16.1 - Change in functional capacity between physically active and physically inactive persons in relation to age.

The acceptance process usually plays an important role. A patient with (devoloping) cognitive problems often notices their own degradation and must cope with it. Moreover, there is an increasing dependence on others. Also, growing somatic problems may entail dependence. Patients hospitalized for the first time in a psychiatric hospital often fear (rightly) stigma or the loss of friends. Older people who have lost a partner may still have to go through a long process and are at risk to end up in social isolation. The self image of older persons included in a psychiatric unit often suffers from this confrontational experience.

It is a challenge to help the elderly adapt to and cope with the changing circumstances in their situation. Hence, we talk about adaptive tasks. These can be displayed in the adaptation-coping model (Dröes 2001, Figure 16.2):

Some adaptive tasks are:
- coping with disability;
- maintaining an emotional balance;
- maintaining a positive self-image;
- preparing for an uncertain future;
- develop an appropriate relationship with the care staff;
- maintain social relationships;
- dealing with the hospital environment.

The above stated adaptive tasks are not exhaustive and there can be described many different adaptive tasks. The stress and emotional response that such tasks entail, and the associated coping mechanisms, are determined by the meaning patients give to the changes made. This process is called cognitive assessment and the process is influenced by personal, illness-related, material, and social environment factors. This adaptation-coping model is psychodynamically oriented and is used because more and more attention has been focused on an experience oriented approach. Psychodynamic therapy offers specific movement activities in which participants experience success and confidence in themselves and others to make contact again with the environment.

16.2.3 Other models

Beside the adaptation-coping model, there are many other models that can be used as a basis for providing an appropriate PMT.

Therapy programs based on a cognitive or neurophysiologic perspective (functional training)

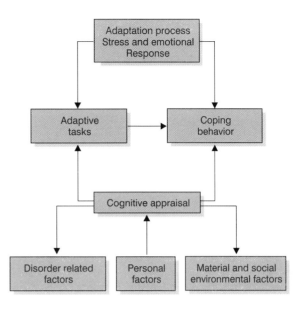

Figure 16.2 - Adaptation-coping model (Dröes, 2001).

use movement activities from the world of physical education, sports, and games. Through activation of PA one seeks to stimulate patients as an information processing system or to influence the underlying disturbing neurophysiologic processes.

Therapies based on a holistic perspective try to restore the bio-psycho-social system and use movement exercises (to promote self-image, self-expression and self-esteem), music, breathing exercises, and informal conversation as therapeutic agents.

Behavior therapy programs are based on behavioral principles and use verbal rewards, intrinsic rewards in games, or progressive relaxation exercises.

Often a psychomotor therapist works rather eclecticly and uses elements from different approaches. It is up to the reader to be critical and to assess the advantages and disadvantages of the use of certain models in practice. Often this will also depend on the population. A session with demented people obviously requires a different approach than a session with a patient with a psychosis.

16.2.4 Scientific evidence for the use of PA in older psychiatric patients

In recent scientific literature we can find a lot of arguments for the contributions PA can offer in the treatment of elderly with psychiatric disor-

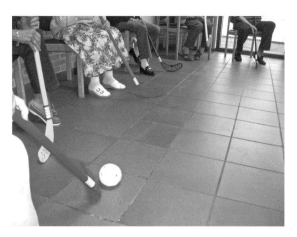

Figure 16.3 - Sitting game. Elderly can play hockey sitting in a circle and hitting a ball with a stick. Balance is not compromised and it does not need strength because of the close proximity of the chairs.

ders. Unfortunately this evidence is situated mainly on the somatic and motor levels. However, the search for arguments on the socio-affective and cognitive levels is much harder. Nevertheless, we will now try to give an overview addressing the somatic, motor, cognitive, and socio-affective levels, as well as some specific evidence for PA in dementia.

Scientific evidence on the somatic level

In general, the effect of PA on physical health is positive (Huijsman et al 1996). Moderate but regular PA is linked to a reduction in overall mortality in the elderly, has a positive contribution in the primary prevention of coronary heart disease, and has a positive effect on fat profile. PA also shows an improvement in body composition by reducing body fat, lowering blood pressure and preventing stroke and type 2 diabetes. Additionally, PA plays a known role in preventing some forms of cancer (especially breast and colon cancer), in increasing bone mass and in the prevention of fall incidents.

PA is inversely associated with insulin resistance and various related risk factors. Moreover, a low leisure activity is an independent predictor for the presence of the metabolic syndrome in older people. The metabolic syndrome is defined as a cluster of obesity, dyslipedemia, glucose intolerance, insulin resistance and hypertension. Performing regular PA, preferably recreational, may

simultaneously influence several predisposing factors with beneficial effects, even at an advanced age (Bianchi et al., 2008).

Caregivers should encourage their patients to perform aerobic PA as well as resistance training, not only in favor of physical health but also for the almost certain advantages in terms of brain health. Resistance training can prevent cognitive decline in the elderly through mechanisms in which IGF-1 (insulin-like growth factor that plays a role in cell growth) and homocysteine are involved. The latter is a sulfur-containing amino acid that is formed in the body. When its concentration is too high, the risk of heart attack, stroke, and peripheral arterial disease substantially grows.

An important positive side effect of resistance training is the proven role in reducing morbidity in the elderly. More specifically, resistance training moderates the development of sarcopenia. This is the loss of muscle mass and muscular strength in aging humans. The multifactor consequences include an increased fall and fracture risk and occurrence of physical limitations (Liu-Ambrose & Donaldson 2009).

There is some evidence for the effectiveness of progressive muscle relaxation plus guided imagery on osteoarthritis pain. There is limited evidence for the effects of meditation and tai chi for improving function or coping in older adults with lower back pain or osteoarthritis. Tai chi, yoga, hypnosis and progressive muscle relaxation are associated with pain reduction. All these methods are safe but more research is needed to determine their effect on chronic pain (Morone and Greco, 2007).

Relaxation may also play a role in the treatment of so-called irritable bowel syndrome (IBS), which occurs in approximately 20% of patients with schizophrenia and 25% of patients with depression (Blanchard et al., 1993). IBS is the collective name for a group of disorders that have in common the abnormal contractions of the bowel. IBS is one of the most common causes of abdominal pain and poor bowel movement.

For a broader overview of the various relaxation methods, we refer to Kerr (2000).

Scientific evidence on the motor level

According to Rolland et al. (2007), two occurences of one hour of walking, strength exercises, balance training, and agility exercises provide a slower decline in ADL (activities of daily living). Also, a high-intensity functional weight–bearing exercise program seems to reduce ADL decline related to indoor mobility for older people living in residential care facilities (Littbrand et al., 2009), however this program does not appear to have an overall effect on ADL outside of this specific population. In people with dementia, the exercise program may prevent decline in overall ADL performance, but continuous training may be needed to maintain that effect.

Overall, literature focusing on key variables such as intensity, type, and volume suggests that the best amount of activity is one which provides an improved cardiorespiratory fitness, strength, and (indirectly) balance. Fitness is associated with functional capacity and independence. Strength is linked to performance and ADL. Balance and mobility combined with strength are important components in preventing fall incidents. In this way morbidity and mortality also decrease. A recommendation for the elderly is as follows: use moderately intense cardio respiratory activities (e.g., brisk walking), perform strength training to maintain muscle mass, train specific muscle groups and perform balance exercises, mobility exercises and flexibility exercises (stretching) as much as necessary (Paterson et al., 2007).

PA is an important predictor of functional status. Sedentary older people can improve their functional status by reaching the recommended level of PA. Conversely, falling below the recommended level has an adverse effect on functional status. Given the importance of PA in maintaining independence and quality of life in older adults, it must be encouraged to meet the recommended guidelines (Morey et al., 2008).

Unfortunately, patients often do not see the full potential of these benefits because they are given vague or wrong instructions. Effective exercise prescriptions include recommendations on frequency, intensity, duration, and progression of the efforts following disease-specific guidelines. Changes in PA require multiple motivational strategies together with education about setting goals, self-monitoring and problem solving (McDermott & Mernitz, 2006).

Scientific evidence on the cognitive level

Some studies suggest that PA is associated with a reduced risk for developing dementia and Alzheimer's disease (Vogel et al., 2009).

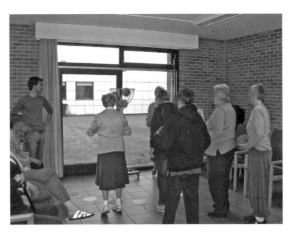

Figure 16.4 - Basketball. It is possible to recreate a sport action like the basketball throw for the elderly. Some cautions are necessary: the distance of the basket, weight and feature of the ball, and the use of a closed basket could help to maintain a secure environment which avoids failure.

In one study concerning adults with subjective memory problems, a six-month program of PA led to a modest improvement in cognition during a follow up period of 18 months (Lautenschlager et al., 2008). Objective measurements of total daily PA were associated with a wide range of cognitive abilities in the elderly. These findings support the link between PA and cognition in the elderly (Buchman et al., 2008).

There is, however, some evidence that a small but significant improvement in cognitive performance occurs in elderly who experience an increasing aerobic fitness (Boutcher, 2000). Even fitness at an age of 96 leads to improved strength and mobility (Leloup, 2007). It was also recently shown that strength training is relatively safe in the elderly (Sagiv, 2009).

Scientific evidence on the socio-affective level

PA is generally perceived positively by older people, due to experiences of improved functioning and social benefits (Fox et al., 2007).

Despite the problems commonly experienced by the elderly, there are often areas where they are still functioning. Examples are procedural learning, somatosensory perception, body schema, (understanding of) physical expression, movement (both motor and procedural), imitating motor action, and social skills (Dröes, 1994). Because

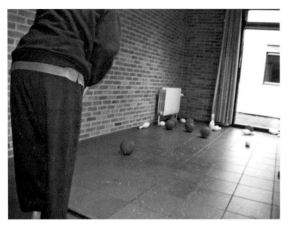

Figure 16.5 - Bowling. Elderly can safely participate in a bowling game. Bowling requires limited speed and strength, putting more emphasis on movement precision.

these residual possibilities are encouraged, these older people experience positive experiences which in turn could have a beneficial effect on body image. As (revised) self-image is important for continuity between past, present and future, it is clear that PA and PMT, through their effect on this self-image, can help in accepting the present and can aid in addressing the uncertain future (Dröes, 2001).

If we consider PA from a relational view, we can say that people not only enter into contact with the environment by observing, thinking, and speaking, but certainly also by moving. This body language has several components: facial expression, gestures, posture, vocal tone, physical proximity to others, and physical contact, to name a few. Movement is an alternative form of communication to maintain relationships with their environment (Dröes, 2001).

PA also has a beneficial effect on emotional balance and self-image. Despite problems in terms of memory, perception, or action, older people can usually still can take part in group movement activities. This often leads to success and a pleasurable experience which can compensate for present limitations, and thus has a positive effect on self-image (Dröes, 2001). Emotional stability and high self-esteem often go together in the elderly (Sonstroem, 1982).

Depressive symptoms in the elderly also result in an increase in abdominal obesity independent of overall obesity, suggesting that specific pathophysiological mechanisms link depression with

visceral accumulation of lipids. These results also help to explain why depression increases the risk of diabetes and cardiovascular disease and thus give a reason for introducing PA to fight this accumulation of lipids (Vogelzangs et al., 2008).

PA ensures a reduction of depressive symptoms. Moreover, the relationship between depressive symptoms and limitations in older people is moderated by PA. Caregivers should promote a moderate amount of PA as a possible means of intervention given this link between depression and limitations in later life, especially in those who have many physical and mental limitations (Lee & Park, 2007).

An exercise program can even be considered as an alternative to antidepressants for the treatment of depression in older people. Although antidepressants can induce a faster initial therapeutic response than exercise, the latter was equally effective in reducing depression in older patients with major depressive disorder after 16 weeks (Blumenthal et al., 1999). According to Blake et al. (2009), physical exercise programs seem to produce clinically relevant outcomes in the treatment of depressive symptoms in depressed older people. Exercise, though not appropriate for everyone in this population, may improve mood.

Relaxation can work on several areas: it could play a role in reducing anxiety, (chronic) pain, (tension) headaches, hypertension, depression and insomnia (Broota, 1990; Carroll, 1998; Eppley, 1989; Jacob, 1991; Jacobs, 1993; Mandl, 1996; NIH, 1996; Ost, 2000; Rankin, 1993; Seers, 1998). It is also a safe treatment.

Specific to the psychiatric field, Damen & Ouwens (2008) stated that anxiety and stress symptoms, which are often present in psychiatric disorders, are treatable via relaxation with one domain specific approach. Therefore, applied relaxation as a physical response can give answers to disturbing concerns because there is a connection between the personal influence on relaxation and the personal influence on churning thoughts. This can lead to an improvement in daily functioning. One disadvantage is that it can be threatening for patients with a psychotic disorder.

The better older people move, the less the costs for nursing and care in rest homes. A combination of aerobic activity, strength training, and flexibility exercises, plus increased general daily activity can reduce dependency on medication and a decline in the cost of health care, and simultane-

PHYSICAL ACTIVITY AND MENTAL HEALTH – A Practice-Oriented Approach

ously maintain functional independence and quality of life in elderly people (McDermott & Mernitz, 2006). The more elderly move, the higher their level of independent functioning and the better their self-esteem. By continuing to move, the age-related decline of physiological reserve slows. Even light exercise seems beneficial both for improving quality of life and to decrease the risk of falling, which in turn will lower the mortality rate (Ekwall et al., 2009).

Older persons reporting dizziness should be encouraged and perhaps helped to exercise. If one could increase PA among the elderly, it would reduce the number of falls, diminish medical costs, suffering for the individual, and be of paramount medicosocial importance to society.

Scientific evidence for PA in dementia

Without discussing the nature of the activity, Volicer (2006) has stated that the more hours patients are engaged in activities, the less they need to use psychotropic medication, the better their food intake is, and the more the patient's family is satisfied.

Friedman and Tappen (1991) specifically showed that walking for half an hour three times a week has a beneficial effect on the communication skills of patients with Alzheimer's Disease. When starting to use a wandering garden, the most significant changes in the fixed schedule of psychiatric medication in Alzheimer patients were reductions in antipsychotic medication and an increase in the number of residents who needed no antipsychotic medication (Detweiler et al., 2009).

Regular participation in PA can delay or prevent the emergence of behavioral problems in demented elderly living in a nursing home (Landi et al., 2004). Even aggressive behavior decreased (Holmberg, 1997). Mechling (2008) found that 20 minutes daily walking, later increased to 60 minutes twice a week, could lead to a reduction in restlessness, behavioral problems and fall incidents, and an improvement in balance and sleep.

Physical and mental activation, along with encouraging social interaction, lead, to slower cognitive, physical, social, emotional and functional decline. Also, Heyn et al. (2004) indicated that PA increases fitness, physical functioning, cognitive functioning, and positive behavior in people with dementia and related cognitive impairments. Teri et al. (2003) indicated that a combination of exercise and education for caregivers, related to behavioral problems in patients with Alzheimer's disease, improves patient's physical health and reduces their depressive symptoms.

Aerobic activities can improve cognitive and functional abilities in people with Alzheimer's disease by modifying neuropathological changes in the brain. Specific cognitive domains such as executive functioning (planning to perform motor tasks) are important for understanding the functioning of people with Alzheimer's disease (Yu et al., 2006). Group-based exercises can be especially effective in improving cognitive performances (Brown et al., 2009).

Moderately intense (mainly conducted in a chair) exercises seem to be associated with a decrease in depressive and anxiety symptoms in patients with Alzheimer's disease in both the short and long term (Edwards et al., 2008).

In the Netherlands, a Movement Activation Program was introduced in several rest homes. This had positive effects on behavior and cognition of demented elderly (Hopman-Rock et al., 2000).

Welden and Yesavage (1982) studied the effect of intensive relaxation training on behavioral problems.

The training consisted of exercises of progressive muscle relaxation, body-focused attention, imagination and self-hypnosis. It could be shown that relaxation training had a positive effect on all assessed behavioral aspects (psychiatric symptoms, eating, bathing, dressing and toilet problems, responsibility, communication, social interaction, and independence). Also, 42% of the participants no longer showed the need for sleep medication after the training.

16.3 TRANSLATING THEORY INTO PRACTICAL APPLICATIONS

Although PMT mainly is offered as a group therapy, there are still individual goals for each patient on the ward. This is something we try keep in mind throughout the whole therapeutic process. This is shown in figure 16.6.

16.3.1 Preparation

A good PMT requires good preparation. At the department level it must be determined how often

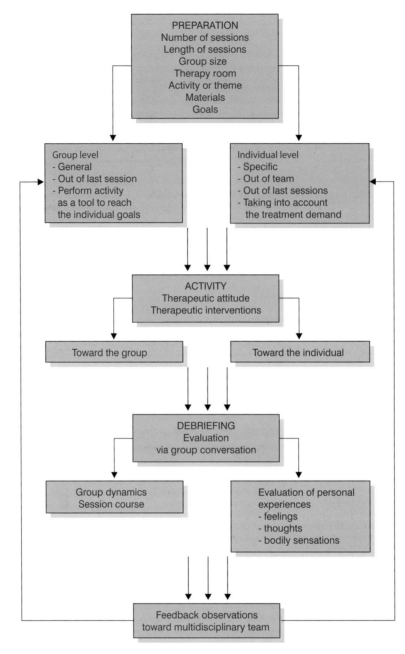

Figure 16.6 - Psychomotor therapy (PMT) in the elderly.

the elderly receive a PMT session per week. We can catalog this under the heading of policy issues (Probst & Simons, 2008). The needs of patients should be taken into account, as well as available hours of the therapist, and one has to achieve a balanced treatment program in which different therapies have their place (occupational therapy, music therapy, psycho-education, etc.). In this way there will be similar therapy programs every week. This structure is very important for psychiatric patients. The duration of a session is also established at this level.

When the therapist will provide therapy, they must take into account the group size. Especially with dementia, the group should not be too big because the therapist often must guide and give individual attention to patients within the group.

There should also be attention paid to a suitable

PHYSICAL ACTIVITY AND MENTAL HEALTH – A Practice-Oriented Approach

therapy room. Preferably, this is a separate room (sports hall, gym, pool, relaxation room), but a separate place on the ward can also be appropriate. This is of particular advantage to those elderly who are less mobile and might quit because of the distance to the therapy room. The elderly who suffer from incontinence symptoms (often triggered by exercise) can still participate in this way: their familiar toilet is nearby.

Still in preparation, the therapist must choose an activity or a theme to work with. As an example, the theme can involve confidence and the session can consist of various assignments on confidence and trust. An activity may be performing movement tasks blindfolded.

More specifically, the therapist chooses the materials. For example, patients can play basketball in a circle with one ball, or exercises can be chosen where each patient has a ball. These are but two examples and for most themes the only limit is the imagination of the therapist. Creativity is a must!

An important part of the preparation is setting goals. Here we distinguish between individual goals and group goals. At the group level, the goals are more general and one of them is often carrying out the activity as a means for reaching individual goals. Although group dynamics play an important role for each patient, the group goals and activities are still subordinate to the individual goals. This does not mean that there should be no attention paid to group dynamics. In a positive atmosphere the elderly feel better and are more motivated to continue participating in the PMT. Sometimes it can even happen that something happens in one session and that the therapist works with this the next session. Yet again a group dynamic is created by the behavior of the individual patient. Hence group goals are almost always also individual goals.

The individual goals are more specific. They can be drawn from the multidisciplinary team or may be made based on events in an earlier session. The preparation of these goals is preferably in consultation with the patient, taking into account the individual request for help. We must realize that it will not always be possible to do this: an elderly person with advanced dementia will usually fail to achieve a good discussion with the therapist. Yet here it is also important to consider whether that person has a specific request for help.

Finally, a good preparation includes a welcome and introduction. Some therapists do this by the

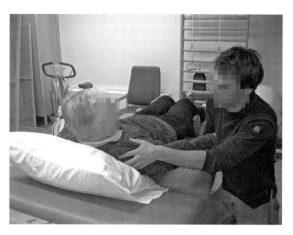

Figure 16.7 - Passive movement. The therapist can help elderly in improving the joint range of movement. Slow and sweeping movements, wherein secure assistance is required, are preferred.

personal greeting of each patient with a handshake but it can also be achieved by asking a short (personal) question that expresses your commitment as a therapist. Then the therapist explains what the program is and the purpose of the session.

16.3.2 Activity

During the activity the therapist has access to a whole arsenal of therapeutic techniques, and through their career this arsenal will only increase. We make a distinction between the attitude of the therapist and the interventions of the therapist.

The attitude can and should vary depending on the target group, but also from session to session or from person to person. When we talk about the target group it is clear that a demented elderly is more in need of an attitude that creates security than a 60-year old who has no cognitive problems but is included because of a personality disorder. If we consider the session, the therapist can sometimes steer the action to see how a patient deals with stricter rules, and then relaxing these rules in the next session to observe how a patient deals with less structure and guidance. Finally, if we consider the person, it is clear that one may benefit more from a motivational attitude (e.g., a depressed woman) and another from an approach with more boundaries (e.g., a hypomanic man).

There may also be a certain attitude toward the group (e.g., challenge to be creative in problem

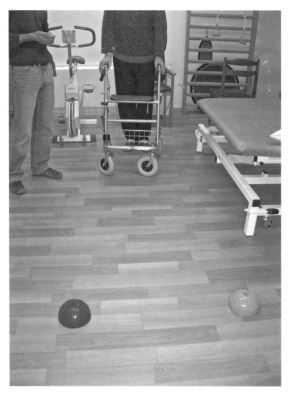

Figure 16.8 - Assisted walking. For elderly it is important to improve their walking abilities in order to maintain autonomy and independence. Walking supports can be useful.

solving) while the therapist guides within that group some people more than others (e.g., providing a psychotic patient structure within this challenge). There are of course different attitudes. Some examples: motivating, supportive, encouraging, creating security, humorous, respectful, guiding, challenging, structuring, ... It is also obvious that, for example, a provocative attitude is not always necessary but that another attitude is always needed (e.g., being respectful). It is important that older people are respected in their need for distance and in the correct use of their names. All too often diminutive words are used. A good rule might be: speak to the patient as you would like to be addressed.

A second aspect is the therapeutic interventions. Here we can distinguish between interventions in the activity (distribution of teams, assigning a particular role, time limits, rules, etc.) and materials (e.g., adjusting difficulty by using a smaller ball). In addition, there are interventions that focus more on the individual patient (e.g.,

insightful, confrontational or behavioral therapy techniques). Here it is clear again that the boundaries are individually based. The interventions take place during the activity but also – and especially – during the debriefing.

16.3.3 Debriefing

A group discussion almost always follows the activity. Although patients – especially at the beginning of their inclusion – don't always appreciate this, it is perhaps the most important part of the session. Here again we can distinguish between the group and individual level. At the group level there can be attention paid to the course of the session: "Was is possible for everyone to participate?" and "Was it a pleasant activity?" are two possible questions. Although they are important, these questions serve as a starting point for the individual level. Whether the activity was enjoyable can, for example, result in a negative answer and then it can be explored as to whether it was perceived like this by everyone and why this was so. In this way there can be found numerous entrance gates to address each patient. It can be a guide for the therapist to keep in mind three questions: "What were your feelings," "What were your thoughts," and "What were your physical sensations?" Again the experience of the therapist grows with each session. It is a common misconception in novice therapists that a failed activity is also a failed session. This is not so. On the contrary, sometimes sessions where patients do not come to a solution to a problem are the most interesting during the debriefing. The activity is secondary to the therapeutic process!

Finally, the therapist's observations have to be used in the regular assessment of the progress of the individual patient. This can be done by reporting on (weekly) multidisciplinary team meetings, but nowadays also increasingly by communication via electronic files or e-mail. Based on the combined observations of all disciplines, the evolution of the patient can be identified and new or modified goals can be made which are then retranslated into specific goals for the PMT.

The schedule that was outlined above can be used for older people with dementia and for other elderly but will obviously be filled in very different ways in the two groups.

16.3.4 **Challenges for the future**

The future of PMT in the elderly seems to promise some new options. Nevertheless, psychomotor therapy in the future will have a partly different view. As previously stated, the world of mental health will need to find answers to the problems that aging brings. This implies more work in the field of psychogeriatrics. If psychomotor therapy as a discipline is able to profile enough (Probst & Simons 2008), there will also be a lot of job opportunities for the psychomotor therapist.

There will probably be an increasing tendency to work with modules in the near future. This means that a series of sessions on a particular theme is offered for which patients can register themselves. We can imagine number of modules. Some examples:
- start to walk;
- yoga;
- relaxation;
- mindfulness;
- dealing with physical deterioration;
- aquagym;
- body oriented work.

It is up to the therapist to find their own modules and content. These modules can be offered in a ward, but most likely working with out patients will see greater development. This is possible in group sessions but individual sessions are also a possibility.

Other new ideas for psychomotor therapy will have to arise from the creativity of the therapist or the demand for care from the elderly population. It is a challenge for the therapist to reinvent psychomotor therapy in older people again and again and thus achieve a position within health care that makes PMT a vital part in the treatment of older people with psychiatric problems.

It will also be important for the psychomotor therapist to be informed of the latest developments or scientific insights. In this way the therapist can respond quickly to new trends within PMT to continue to offer the best care in his therapy. An example is the recent introduction of yoga as a form of PMT in people with schizophrenia (Vancampfort et al., 2009).

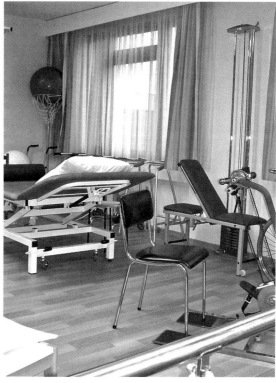

Figure 16.9 - Gym room. A typical room in which elderly can practice a variety of movement situations with the support and supervision of an exercise specialist. Several facilities and equipments could be effective with elderly in order to adapt physical activity.

The scientific research deserves more attention in the future. In writing this contribution we had to establish that there is very little scientific literature of a sufficient level on this subject available.

These findings convince us, as Probst and Simons (2008), that PMT in general but specifically with elderly needs to prove itself more. Otherwise there is a risk that other disciplines will increasingly invade the domain-specific medium of the PMT or that PMT will merge into a weakened form (adapted physical activity).

16.4 SUMMARY AND GUIDELINES

An overview of the similarities and differences of PMT in patients with dementia and patients with functional psychiatric disorders is shown in Table 16.1.

Table 16.1 - PMT: similarities and differences in patients with dementia and patients with functional psychiatric disorders

	Dementia	*Functional psychiatric disorders*
Number of sessions	– preferably 5 sessions per week (in practice not always feasible) – in the morning at the same time of day (afternoon often more sleepy or family visits)	– preferably 5 to 8 sessions per week (in practice not always feasible) – more activity options: aqua therapy, relaxation oriented – preferably at the same time of day (fixed structure)
Duration of the session	– 30 to 45 min – part of the time is spent collecting the patients	– 30 to 45 min – more abilities (e.g., being in time as part of the therapy: orientation in time and space)
Group size	– involve as many patients as possible – ideally up to 10 persons: possibility for individual support within the group	– often 8 to 14: more opportunities for "team-oriented" activities
Therapy room	– a separate therapy room close to the ward (recognisable + better orientation) vs. on the ward (less mobile patients can participate)	– ideally separate therapy room with attention to recognisability, fixed structure and therapy atmosphere
Activities	– aerobic activities – flexibility exercises/gymnastic forms – lifestyle body movement – perceptual locomotion/sensory-locomotion – functional training – relaxation training – dancing	– aerobic activities (e.g., swimming) – resistance exercises (e.g., fitness) – flexibility exercises/gymnastic forms – lifestyle body movement – more emphasis on relaxation training – dancing
Materials	– adapted recognisable, colored and light materials – easy to handle – provoke movement + stimulating contact	– all materials
Goals	– motor – cognitive – socio-affective	– motor – cognitive – socio-affective
Therapeutic attitude	– giving security – motivating – structuring – supportive	– giving security – motivating – structuring (or not for observational goals) – supportive
Interventions	– demonstrating – verbalizing – discuss psycho-social problems – attention to non-verbal communication – facilitate effective components	– demonstrating – verbalizing – discuss psycho-social problems – attention to non-verbal communication – facilitate effective components – more focus on reflection!
Evaluation and feedback	– LOFOPT – BPMT– demonstration – Others: gait, balance, endurance,…	– LOFOPT – Others: gait, balance, endurance,…

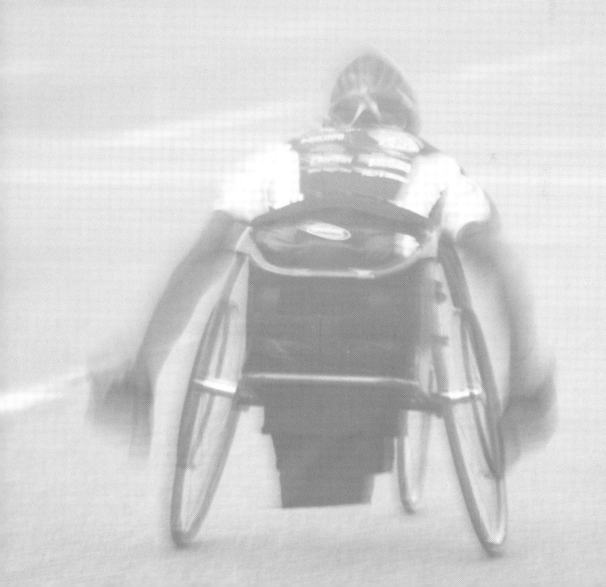

Section 3

Instruments

Assessment and evaluation **instruments** of **physical activity** to use in people with **mental health problems**

Attilio Carraro, Michel Probst

Parallel with the growing interest in physical activity, exercise, and mental health, the attention for research in this field is increasing.

Within the scope of this book it is not possible to give an overview of all physical activity assessment tools that can be used in the context of mental health; the authors refer to different valuable textbooks (Disch & Mood, 2010; Malina, Bouchard, & Bar-Or, 2004; Morrow et al., 2011; Welk, 2002) which give great attention to this topic.

Besides the use of instruments related to physical activity and exercise monitoring, psychological inventories are crucial in the field of mental health (Conti, 1999). Physical activity has been shown to have the capacity to increase the feeling of psychological well-being. Psychological tests help to evaluate the accuracy of different psychological theories and provide information on the mental health status of the participants.

The problem with these kinds of instruments is the inappropriate use and interpretation of results. To overcome these problems, the authors advise a search for specialists that are familiar with psychological testing and evaluation. The description of questionnaires is limited to international, well known and reliable valid instruments. Most of the questionnaires are translated in different languages.

The aim of this chapter is to provide the reader an overview of several selected instruments specifically related to physical activity and mental health that are frequently used in clinical practice.

An overview of different assessment methods in the field of physical activity and mental health is reported in Table 17.1.

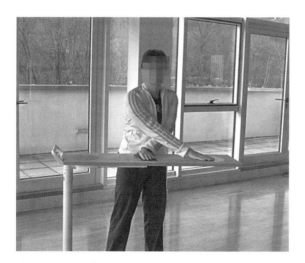

Figure 17.1 - Plate tapping. The test aims to measure the speed of repeated limb movement during a defined, semi-precise task.

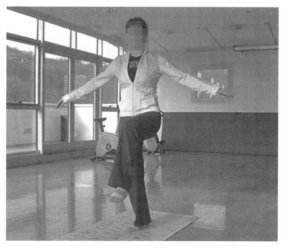

Figure 17.2 - Single leg balance test. The aim is to evaluate whole body balance.

Table 17.1 - Assessment methods in the field of physical activity and mental health

Measures of physical activity	Remarks
Self-report instruments	This technique is often used in mental health. In a short time and in an inexpensive way, the researcher captures a lot of qualitative and quantitative information. The disadvantage is the translation of the questionnaire, the standardization, the reliability, validity, interpretation of results, and the comparison with normative data.
Activity monitors	These instruments (e.g., *Actigraph* and *Sensewear Armband*) provide an indication of intensity, frequency and duration of physical activity in free-living conditions.
Heart rate monitor	Heart rate monitoring has been widely used in physical activity research and several instruments are available (e.g, *Casio, Polar, Suunto*).
Pedometers	These cheap, non-invasive devices are easy to administer and can help to promote behavioral changes. The step counters are an objective measure of common activity behavior and are sometimes used as an alternative to activity monitors.
Direct observation	The goal is to measure in a quantitative or qualitative way the behavioral aspects of physical activity. More than in other fields, this technique becomes increasingly more important, not only for research but also as a tool for the coaches. Observation techniques, for example the LOFOPT (Van Coppenolle et al., 1989; Carraro, et al., 2000), are inexpensive and after some training sessions, easy to administer. The disadvantage is that they are time consuming. Observers must be trained.
Indirect calorimetry and doubly labelled water	This technique is a gold standard for estimating the energy expenditure through biological markers that reflect the rate of metabolism in the body. This approach is not applicable in clinical practice.
Measures in motor and health-related fitness	The components of health related fitness are a basis from which to measure general wellbeing. There are five health related components of fitness: *cardiovascular endurance, muscular strength, flexibility, muscular endurance, body composition*. Additional skill-related fitness, as speed, reaction time, agility, balance, coordination, and power can be assessed. An example of a health-related fitness measure is the EUROFIT test battery (Oja & Tuxworth, 1995).

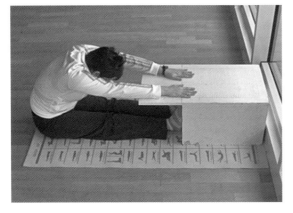

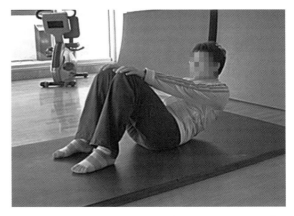

Figure 17.3 - Sit-and-reach. The test aims to evaluate trunk flexibility and hamstring *tightness*.

Figure 17.4 - Dynamic sit-up. The test aims to evaluate trunk muscle strength and endurance.

A plethora of instruments are available today and one of the most prominent problems is the "art" of individualizing the appropriate instrument that fits the research question. We propose three questions as guidelines:

1. *What do I want to assess?* The first crucial and central step is to formulate a clear, detailed, well-founded research question. The quality of your research will depend on your research question.

2. *For what purpose would I measure?* Is the starting point of my research question purely based on research or does it also have a clinical significance? Do you want a reliable statement in regard to influencing and responsible factors of certain behaviors, and in which domain (screening, diagnosis, prognosis of evaluation of an intervention)?

3. *What kind of instrument should I choose?* The choice of the instrument depends on the research question and the goals, or in other words: "what do you want to know" and "about whom?"

The instrument must meet methodological criteria about quality and standardization. To be acceptable, data must be valid, reliable and objective:

- *validity* refers to the appropriateness of the test in measuring what it is designed to measure;
- *reliability* is a measure of the consistency of the data, usually determined by the test-retest method;
- *objectivity* (or inter-rater variability) means that the data are collected without bias by the investigators (Vincent, 2005).

Many tools are freely available, others for a fee. The manageability is very important, several instruments have been developed for research and their length and complexity are not suitable for daily practice. Another decisive argument in the decision of the instrument is the required time investment. Some instruments (e.g., interviews) are time-consuming, others (e.g., questionnaires)

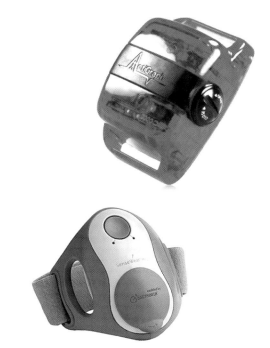

Figure 17.5 - Two examples of portable monitors to record the quantity and intensity of physical activity.

require little time investment.

Check if the instrument is developed and valid for your specific group (children, adults, elderly, athletes, people with intellectual disability, patients, …). Instruments used to evaluate interventions have to be sensitive to small changes.

In Table 17.2 are synthetically described some selected self-report questionnaires related to mental health.

Close to the questionnaires adopted to asses psychological aspects in the treatment of mental health problems, several self-report instruments are used to evaluate different aspects of physical activity participation (e.g., physical habits and attitudes, physical self-perception and description, exertion, anxiety in sport and physical activity, motivation, enjoyment). An overview of some self-report instruments is presented in Table 17.3.

Table 17.2 - A short review of some selected self-report questionnaires related to mental health

The Symptom Check List, SCL-90 (Derogatis, 1977)	SCL-90 is an extensively used self-report questionnaire (90 items) designed to screen for a broad range of psychological problems. It is one of the most widely used measures of psychological problems in clinical practice and research. It is also useful for measuring the progress and outcome of treatments. The subscales are *somatisation, obsessive-compulsivity, interpersonal sensitivity, depression, anxiety, hostility, phobic anxiety, paranoid ideation and psychoticism*. The global severity index is designed to measure the overall psychological distress. Each item is rated on a 5-point Likert scale of distress, ranging from "not at all" (0) to "extremely" (4). The instrument is normed on individuals 13 years and older. Norms are available for adult non patients, adult psychiatric patients, and adolescent non-patients. The questionnaire is accepted worldwide as a reliable and valid instrument.
The Beck Depression Inventory, BDI-II (Beck, Steer, & Brown, 1996)	BDI is an efficient and extensively used 21-item self-reporting questionnaire of the somatic, cognitive, affective, and vegetative symptoms of depression (Beck, Steer, & Brown, 1996). This measure was initially designed by Beck et al. in 1979 to evaluate the overall severity of depression in adults and adolescents aged at least 13 years. The BDI-II has been shown to be a valid and reliable measure of depression severity. Each item is rated on a 4-point Likert scale, ranging from "absent" or "mild" (0) to "severe" (3).The BDI-II is easy to score by counting the responses of the 21 items together. The range of possible total scores is 0-63, with higher scores indicating greater depression. The internal consistency coefficients and test-retest in different groups included patients with psychiatric disorders.
The State and Trait Anxiety Inventory, STAI Y form (Spielberger, 1983)	STAI-Y is a self-report assessment inventory which includes separate measures of state and trait anxiety. It helps distinguish feelings of anxiety and depression. The instrument is the leading measure of anxiety worldwide. It is adapted in more than 40 languages. Psychometric features are good. A version for children is available. *State anxiety inventory* (STATE-A) measures a temporary condition or a transitory emotional state or condition of the human organism that is characterized by subjective, consciously perceived feelings of tension and apprehension and heightened autonomic nervous system activity. State anxiety may fluctuate over time and can vary in intensity. The State Anxiety Inventory is a self-rating scale with 20 items rated on a 4-point intensity scale from not at all (1) to very much so (4). The scores increase in response to physical danger and psychological stress and decrease as a result of relaxation training. *Trait Anxiety inventory* (TRAIT-A) is a 20-item self-rating scale to assess trait anxiety. Trait anxiety refers to a more general and long-standing type of anxiety or to a general tendency to respond with anxiety to perceived threats in the environment. It denotes relatively stable individual differences in anxiety proneness. The items are rated on a 4-point frequency scale (from 1 for "almost never" to 4 for "almost always"). The final scores have a possible range from 20 to 80. Higher scores indicate higher levels of trait anxiety.
The Rosenberg Self-Esteem Scale, RSES (Rosenberg, 1965)	The RSES is a 10-item self-rating scale to evaluate global self-esteem and self-acceptance. The items are scored on a 4-point Likert scale, ranging from 1 (totally disagree) to 4 (totally agree). Higher total scores indicate higher self-esteem. Items 1, 3, 4, 7 and 10 are positively worded; items 2, 5, 6, 8 and 9 negatively. The RSES is regarded as one of the better measurements of global self-esteem.

(continued)

Table 17.2

The Body Attitude Test, BAT (Probst, Vandereycken, & Vanderlinden, 1995)	The BAT is intended to measure the subjective body experience and the attitude towards one's body. The BAT consists of 20 items to be scored on a 6-point scale. With the exception of the negatively keyed items (4 and 9), items are scored as follows: always (5) usually-often-sometimes-rarely and never (0). The maximum score is 100; the higher the score, the more deviating the body experience is. Repeated analysis yielded a stable four factor structure: (1) negative appreciation of body size, (2) lack of familiarity with one's own body, (3) general dissatisfaction, and (4) a rest factor. There are no weightings from factor loadings. The authors developed the scale for female patients suffering from eating disorders but the test can be used for non-clinical males and females, eating disorders and all other mental disorders. The questionnaire is psychometrically robust.
SF-36 Health Survey	The SF-36 is a multipurpose, short-form health survey with 36 questions for measuring health status and outcomes from the individual's point of view. It is a generic measure, as opposed to ones that target specific age, diseases, or treatment groups (Ware, 2004). The survey can be self-administered by people 14 years of age or older or administered by trained interviewers either in person or by telephone. These measures rely upon patient self-reporting and are now widely used by managed care organizations and by Medicare for routine monitoring and assessment of care outcomes in adult people to examine a person's perceived health status. The survey's standardized scoring system yields a profile on 8 health scales and 2 summary measures. *Physical Functioning*, *Role-playing*, *Bodily Pain* and *General Health* scales are included in the *Physical Health* summary measure; *Vitality*, *Social-functioning*, *Role-emotional* and *Mental Health* scales are grouped in the *Mental Health* summary measure.
Visual Analog Scale, VAS	VAS is a measurement instrument for subjective characteristics or attitudes that cannot be directly measured (e.g., perceived fatigue). When responding to a VAS item, respondents specify their level of agreement to a statement by indicating a position along a continuous line between two end-points. At the opposite ends of the line the keywords "very bad" and "very good" are used. This continuous (or *analog*) aspect of the scale differentiates it from discrete scales such as the Likert scale (Grant et al., 1999).
Semantic differential (Osgood, Suci, & Tannenbaum, 1957)	An alternative to the VAS scale is the semantic differential, which asks individuals to respond to bipolar adjectives, that is, pairs of adjectives with opposite meanings. Semantic differentials can be used to describe not only persons, but also the connotative meaning of abstract concepts. Examples of bipolar adjectives are: good/bad, pleasant/unpleasant, relaxed/tense, hot/cold, healthy/unhealthy, nice/awful, delicate/rugged, active/passive, fair/unfair, honest/dishonest, successful/unsuccessful, useful/useless, strong/weak, hard/soft, heavy/light, dominant/submissive, dirty/clean, valuable/worthless, steady/nervous, happy/sad, dynamic/static, stationary/moving, fast/slow.

Table 17.3 - A review of some selected self-report questionnaires related to physical activity

International Physical Activity Questionnaire, IPAQ	IPAQ was developed to measure health-related physical activity in the general population. IPAQ assesses physical activity undertaken across a comprehensive set of domains including: a. leisure time physical activity; b. domestic and gardening (yard) activities; c. work-related physical activity; d. transport-related physical activity. Data collected with IPAQ can be reported as a continuous measure. One measure of the volume of activity can be computed by weighting each type of activity by its energy requirements defined in METs to yield a score in MET/minutes. METs are multiples of the resting metabolic rate and a MET-minute is computed by multiplying the MET score of an activity by the minutes performed. IPAQ consists of a Short Form and Long Form Questionnaire. IPAQ Short Form consists of the 4 topics mentioned above as well as items to provide separate scores on walking, moderate-intensity and vigorous-intensity activity. Computation of the total score for the short form requires summation of the duration (in minutes) and frequency (days) of walking, moderate-intensity, and vigorous-intensity activities. The IPAQ Long Form consists of details about the specific types of activitiesundertaken within each of the four domains mentioned above. The items in the long IPAQ form were structured to provide separate domain. Specific scores for walking, moderate-intensity and vigorous-intensity activity within each of the work, transportation, domestic chores and gardening (yard), and leisure-time domains are all included. Computation of the total scores for the long form requires summation of the duration (in minutes) and frequency (days) for all types of activities in all domains. The development of the IPAQ started by Booth in 1996 and was further developed by an International Consensus Group in 1998 (see http://www.ipaq.ki.se/downloads.htm).
Baecke Questionnaire (Baecke, 1982)	This is a self-administered questionnaire about habitual physical activity developed for the various socioeconomic classes in the general population. It consists of 16 items with different possibilities of answer recorded on a 5-point scale. Three meaningful dimensions can be distinguished within habitual physical activity: 1. occupational physical activity (work index) precoded according to three levels of PA at work; 2. sport during leisure-time (sport index) subdivided into three levels and a sport score calculated from a combination of the intensity of the sport, the amount of time per week, and the proportion of the year during which sport is played regularly; 3. other physical activity during leisure-time (leisure-time index). The total physical activity level is the sum of work, sport and leisure-time indexes. The score for each of the three factors ranges between 1 and 5. A higher score means a higher physical activity level. The test-retest reliability coefficient for work, sport, and leisure time indexes is higher than 0.74.
The Physical Self-Perception Profile, PSPP (Fox & Corbin, 1989)	PSPP is a 30-item questionnaire to measure self-perceptions related to one's physical self based on a hierarchical model. This model has global self-esteem at the apex of the hierarchy, physical self-worth as a domain, and sports competence, physical strength, physical condition, and body attractiveness as subdomains. Furthermore, the PSPP is based on a bottom-up hierarchy, where physical self-perceptions would influence global self-esteem. Each of the five subscales consist of 6 items given in a structured alternative format, with item values ranging from 1 to 4, and roughly half of the items reverse-scored. All item scores in a subscale are summed for a subscale score (ranging from 6 to 24), with high scores indicating high physical self-perceptions and low scores indicating low physical self-perceptions. There are different revised forms of the PSPP. The short with 21 items and the Very Short Form of the Physical Self-Inventory with 12 items (Morin & Maïano, 2010).

(continued)

Table 17.3

The Physical Self-Description Questionnaire, PSDQ (Marsh et al., 1994)	The PSDQ is a multidimensional, physical self-concept instrument designed to measure 11 scales, 9 of which are designed to tap perceptions of the self, related to specific areas of physical fitness and competence: *Strength, Body Fat, Activity, Endurance/Fitness, Sports Competence, Coordination, Health, Appearance, Flexibility.* One subscale (*Global Physical Self-Concept*) measures self-perceptions of global physical competence, and one measures *Global Self-Esteem*. The response format is based on a 6-point true/false Likert-type scale. Higher scores indicate higher physical self-concept. The instrument is appropriate for use with adolescents and adults, and elite and non-elite athletes (Marsh, 1996). Based on the PSDQ normative archive (n = 1,607 Australian adolescents), 40 of 70 items were selected to construct a new short-form (Marsh, Martin, & Jackson, 2010). Both questionnaires are psychometrically robust.
Borg's Rating of Perceived Exertion Scales, RPE (Borg, 1998)	There are a number of RPE scales but the most common are the 15-point scale (6-20) and the 9-point scale (1-10). There is a wide range of indication which speaks for using RPE scale in healthy as well as patients with different pathologies. This is true in clinical work test, rehabilitation, exercise prescription, and also clinical diagnostics of breathlessness and dyspenia, chest pain, angina and muscular-skeletal pain. Moreover, it is extremely applied for athletes.
The Physical Activity and Sport Anxiety Scale, PASAS (Norton, Hope, & Weeks, 2004)	The PASAS is a 16-item self-report questionnaire to measure the social anxiety in physical activities and sports. The items are scored on a 5-point Likert scale, ranging from 1 (absolutely not true for me) to 5 (absolutely true for me). Higher total scores indicate higher experience of social anxiety in physical activities and sports. This brief measure demonstrated in a sample of healthy subjects an excellent internal consistency across a number of samples, an excellent temporal stability, and good convergent and divergent validity.
Motivation for Physical Activities Measure-Revised, MPAM-r (Frederick & Ryan, 1993)	The MPAM-r collects information on the motivation of physical activity. This questionnaire has 30 items divided into 5 categories: interest and enjoyment (7 items), competence (7 items), appearance (6 items), fitness (5 items) and social contact (5 items). The items are scored using a 7-point Likert scale. There are two distinct types of motivation: intrinsic (interest, enjoyment and competence) and extrinsic motivation (appearance and social contact). Fitness includes both intrinsic and extrinsic motivation. The internal consistency determined using the Cronbach's alpha range from 0.78 to 0.92.
The Situational Motivation Scale, SIMS (Guay, Vallerand, & Blanchard, 2000)	The SIMS is designed to assess the constructs of intrinsic motivation, identified regulation, external regulation, and amotivation (Deci & Ryan, 1985). The SIMS is composed of 4 internally consistent factors and represents a brief and versatile self-report measure of situational intrinsic motivation, identified regulation, external regulation and amotivation. Each subscale is composed of 4 items rated on a 7 point Likert scale ranging from 1 (does not correspond at all) to 7 (corresponds exactly).
The Physical Activity Enjoyment Scale, PACES (Motl et al., 2001)	Enjoyment has been implicated as a determinant of physical activity, but advances in understanding have been limited by the use of measures that were not adequately validated (Motl et al., 2001). Assessing motivation for and enjoyment of physical activity is an important step in the promotion of an active lifestyle. The PACES, originally proposed by Kendzierski and De Carlo (1991), is a 16-item scale, with 9 pro and 7 con items. PACES has been validated in different languages (Carraro, Young, & Robazza, 2008). Items are scored on a 5-point Likert scale ranging from 1 (disagree a lot) to 5 (agree a lot). High scores on the pro items and low scores on the con items would indicate a high enjoyment of physical activity. A total enjoyment score can also be obtained by reversing con item scores and adding them to pros item scores. With this procedure, total enjoyment scores can range from 16 to 80 (maximum enjoyment).

Sport activities in leisure time for people with psychiatric disorders 18

Ilaria Ferri & Amber De Herdt

18.1 INTRODUCTION

The role of sport and physical activity (PA) in the prevention and treatment of mental health disorders is extensively discussed in previous chapters of this book. Besides the effects of PA on somatic and mental symptoms (Tordeurs, et al., 2011; Knöchel, et al., 2012), a third component, the social aspect of sport and PA, has to be highlighted in detail.

The aim of the current chapter is 1) to discuss the background of sport as a social integration tool for patients with psychiatric disabilities and 2) to present the principal European Sport organizations (international, national and local sport clubs) for people affected by mental health problems.

18.2 BACKGROUND: SPORT AND DISABILITY

Sports and PA involve humans in a multidimensional perspective. Being physically active not only influences both physical and mental health, it also teaches people how to deal with limits, difficulties, wellbeing and enjoyment. It enhances learning and developmental processes. Sport and PA represent a metaphor of life, with joy and pain: an opportunity to know and test themselves, to acquire self-esteem, to come into contact with other people, to interact and create relationships. In modern society, being physically active represents a human right, but reflection on "ability and disability," accessibility, advantages and inclusion shows that the possibility to do PA and sport is not always self-evident. In 1975 the European Sports Ministers discussed the idea of a "European Sport for All Charter" endowed with a common pro-

gram based on the conviction that the values of sport would contribute to the fulfilment of the ideals of the Council of Europe. On September 24, 1976 the charter was officially adopted and provided the framework for sports policy in Europe. Later, in 1992, in order to provide a common set of principles for all Europe, the Council of Europe prescribed the Code of Sports Ethics (revised in 2001) as a complement to the European Sport Charter (www.coe.int). It is based on the principle that "ethical considerations leading to fair play are integral, and not optional elements, of all sports activity, sports policy and management, and apply to all levels of ability and commitment, including recreational as well as competitive sport." In these documents, governments have committed themselves to providing their citizens with opportunities to practice sport under well-defined conditions. Sport must be:

- accessible to everybody;
- available for children and young people in particular;
- healthy and safe, fair and tolerant, building on high ethical values;
- capable of fostering personal self-fulfilment at all levels;
- respectful of the environment;
- protective of human dignity;
- against any kind of exploitation of those engaged in sport.

Within this frame, at the beginning of the 21st century, the dialogue on accessibility, advantages and inclusion involved a shift in focus from disabilities to abilities and capacities (van Hilvoorde & Landeweerd, 2010). As Van Hilvoorde and Landeweerd suggest: "Disability is not regarded a characteristic (that is present all the time) but a state that may be present in certain environments or results from specific interaction with other people." From this point of view disability is not considered a static definition, a natural state of being, but rather a socio-cultural construction. The environment is thought of as a place of relations and possibilities where everyone can realize their potential for growth. From these ideas generated the modern concept of "adaptation." Doll-Tepper et al., in a multinational perspective, defined Adapted Physical Activity (APA), a more adequate term in the landscape of movement: "APA refers to movement, physical activity and sports in which special emphasis is placed on the interests and capabilities of individuals with limiting conditions, such as the disabled, health impaired or aged" (Doll-Tepper et al., 1990). Later Sherrill and Dunn presented APA as a "cross-disciplinary theory and practice related to lifespan activity of individuals whose function, structure, or appearance requires expertise in assessing and adapting ecosystems and facilitating societal changes necessary for: a) equal access, b) integration/inclusion, c) lifespan wellness, d) movement success, and e) empowerment/self-actualization" (Sherrill & Dunn, 1996).

People affected by mental diseases are often excluded from and stigmatized in common social contexts like school, work and recreational environments. Such situations create social isolation and the perception that you are on your own and misunderstood in these difficult situations. For these reasons, "social support" represents the most important predictive factor for a positive progress in chronic psychiatric illness (WHO, 2003). Sports and PA can be considered a healthy occasion to "come out," to "come between" other people, and to "discover" capabilities and possibilities that people in suffering situations often forget. Lennart Nordenfelt, the philosopher of health, suggests an interesting "ability-centered theory of health" in which he underlines how "the ability of health should be related to the realization of the person's *vital goal*" (van Hilvoorde & Landeweerd, 2010). The challenge of sport and PA is to give individuals opportunities and possibilities to participate in the ways and to the extent they choose to participate (Nordenfelt, 2006). Mental illness in general is very difficult to accept and deal with. Sometimes it seems invisible, silent; sometimes its manifestations are excessive and uncontrollable. Diagnosis can require a lot of time and several consultations, and this fact weighs on a person's families, friends, and colleagues, but first of all it entails suffering for

the ill person; what follows is the complex and difficult way to accept the diagnosis, to find a cure, to live with special requirements consequent with medications and good practice. Lot of personal stories tell of the sensation of inability, describe loss of stimulus and confidence in our selves, and report the absolute lack of a sense of life. The change from illness to cure and from cure to health can be facilitated by social interaction, by people that come into contact with patients either from care or familiar settings. Sport clubs become, in this perspective, meeting places for every kind of athlete, and this is why PA has to be adapted to every kind of limitation. "Sport for all" means that sport gives people an occasion to take part, to be inside a group, to have a role, to establish new contacts with others, and to promote inter-human relationships.

Sport and PA becomes the environment where abilities and capacities find the possibility to be expressed as they are. It is a way to contrast isolation-creating networks. Furthermore, sport is a vehicle for education, an instrument for personal and social training, but first of all it is an important means to promote a healthy lifestyle. Stigma must be fought where rooted: in society. Only when citizens come into contact with disadvantaged people they can meet themselves, start to know and interact with social distress and this part of reality. Sports and leisure PA can enhance social participation and provide a unique basis for the practice of social skills (Dinomais et al., 2010). In extent, the organization of "mixed" activities, where persons with a psychiatric disability can take part in regular sports clubs, provides a starting point for social inclusion and rehabilitation. The reintegration of persons with a psychiatric disability in daily life is an important social theme on a global scale. Many national organizations are occupied with this challenge, and try to provide support for the engagement in work and social activities of these people.

18.3 SPORT FEDERATIONS IN EUROPE FOR PEOPLE WITH A MENTAL DISABILITY

The integration of three policy fields – mental health care, sports, and social administration – resulted in the birth of sport organizations for people with a psychiatric disability. Nevertheless, the frame of many sport clubs shifted throughout the years, depending on changing needs and new

PHYSICAL ACTIVITY AND MENTAL HEALTH – A Practice-Oriented Approach

Table 18.1 - International sport federations for people with a disability

Organization	Members
IFAPA *(International Federation of Adapted Physical Activity)*	International, cross-disciplinary, professional organization of individuals, institutions and agencies supporting, promoting and disseminating information about APA, disability sport and all aspects about sport, movement and exercise science for individuals with all abilities.
International Paralympic Committee (IPC)	International non-profit organization formed and run by 170 National Paralympic Committees (NPCs) from five regions and four disability specific international sport federations (IOSDs).
Special Olympics	International organization that provides year-round sports training and athletic competition in a variety of Olympic-type sports for children and adults with intellectual disabilities, giving them continuing opportunities to develop physical fitness, demonstrate courage, experience joy, and participate in a sharing of gifts, skills and friendship with their families, other Special Olympics athletes, and the community.

legislature. The rise of the biopsychosocial model in psychiatry in the late seventies/early eighties, led to a growing interest in improving rehabilitation of persons affected by a chronic illness. The biopsychosocial model is a general model or approach which posits that biological, psychological (which entails thoughts, emotions, and behaviors), and social factors all play a significant role in human functioning in the context of disease or illness. Today, most sport and recreation organizations in the field of mental health try to support their members by offering a safe sporting place (structured environment), a variation of sport activities, and social support to stimulate social integration and capacities. To achieve individual successes, the following cornerstones are important: offering different kinds of activities, offering different degrees of integration, and the adaptation of activities to the specific capabilities of each individual athlete. Despite the fact that structure, goals, members, and provided activities may differ between several sport federations and sport clubs, all are driven by the same ambition: "to create a forum for sport and social interaction between healthy athletes and athletes affected by a mental illness, and to stimulate sport participation in people with mental health problems." Sport federations in Europe are organized on different levels: international organizations, national organizations, and local sport clubs for different regions in a country. Table 18.1. gives an overview of international sport organizations for people with a disability. Some examples for people with psychiatric illness are reported in Table 18.2. Data

Table 18.2 - Some examples of Sport and Leisure Organizations in Europe

Organization	Dimension	Country
U.I.S.P. Unione Italiana Sport per tutti (www.uisp.it)	National	Italy
A.N.P.I.S. Associazione Nazionale Polisportive per l'Integrazione Sociale (www.anpis.it)	National	Italy
Psylos Psychiatrie, Lichamelijke opvoeding en Sport (www.psylos.be)	National	Belgium
REAKT (www.reakt.nl)	National	The Netherlands
ACTENZ (www.actenz.nl)	National	The Netherlands
Bellaria Solidarietà (www.solidarieta.gsbellaria.it)	Local	Italy
The Activities Development Service, Manzil Resource Centre, Oxford (www.oxfordhealth.nhs.uk)	Local	England
ASBA Association "Sofia" Bratislava	Local	Slovakia
La Maison Bleue (www.alamaisonbleue.org)	Local	France

retrieval in the vast area of the EU underlined very different situations and the lack of a European register of associations. Authors would be grateful for every contribution that will sustain this purpose.

18.4 INTERNATIONAL SPORT ORGANIZATIONS FOR PEOPLE WITH A DISABILITY

The most important international sport federations for people with a disability are the IFAPA (International Federation in Adapted Physical Activity), the International Paralympic Committee (IPC), and the Special Olympics. Currently, no specific international organizations exist for people with mental health problems. Nevertheless, the growing cooperation of several national sport federations has established an international forum where organizations for people with a mental disability can interact.

18.4.1 National sport organizations

Several countries in the EU have national sport clubs and recreation organizations for people affected by mental health problems. Both general goals and activities of such organizations will be highlighted in detail in the next paragraphs.

Goals

Most sport federations for people with mental health problems have two major targets. As patients with a psychiatric disability are often sedentary, the first focal point is to stimulate *participation* in sport activities. To achieve this goal, a qualitative offering of sports activities is organized. To motivate people toward a more active life style, choice of activities is very important: each person, regardless of restrictions, should be able to choose any sport and any accommodation or club. As regular physical activity has been shown to have major benefits for both physical and mental health in patients with mental issues, health care workers have to create the space and environment for those patients to be physically active and play sports.

The second aim is to *achieve social integration* and *improve social skills* of patients with mental health problems. By trying to reach as high an integration as possible of these people into the sport landscape, the social stigma that rests on a psychiatric disorder can be tackled.

Activities

The activities organized by different sport federations for people with disabilities can be situated on a continuum of activities. The Flemish federation for sport and recreation in mental health care (Psylos) defined four factors that have to be taken into account in order to draw up this continuum.

These factors are 1) the type of disability (motor, visual, auditory or mental handicap, mental health issues, multiple disabilities), 2) the branch of sports (individual sports, team sports, adapted sports), 3) kind of sports (recreational, competitive-recreational, professional sports), and 4) degree of integration (exclusive, special branch for people with disabilities, inclusive). The degree of integration was used as the starting point for this continuum. Table 18.2 gives an example for each degree of integration.

Each country presents different opportunities to choose a sport activity for regular use, in line with local sport traditions: football, basketball, volleyball, and swimming are the most famous, but different organizations also organize special activities on weekends or holidays, usually exploiting natural environment or people's motor habits. These are group activities such as bike riding, guided walking, adventure activities, day trips, etc. All members can join these activities. New social contact can be made and new sport interest can be established.

18.4.2 Local sport clubs

National Associations like Psylos (Belgium) and UISP-ANPIS (Italia) are further organized into local sport clubs for different regions in a country.

In Belgium, the Flemish Federation of Sport and Recreation in Mental Health, "Psylos," is an overarching national organization with different local sport clubs for each province. An example of such a local organization is the Psylos sport club of Kortenberg. This local organization provides several sports and special activities for its members.

In Italy UISP and ANPIS are national organizations that promote a wide set of sport activities in different regions. They promote sport and physical activity for a healthier style of life, proposing "sport for all" as a socio-cultural approach and intent.

The example of Bellaria Solidarietà

Bellaria Solidarietà is a local sport club born in 2000 from a "contamination project" between the Adult Mental Health Unit (UFSMA) ASL 5 Pisa and the Sport Club Bellaria Cappuccini, in Pontedera, a village in the region of Tuscany (Italy). Bellaria Solidarietà brings together people with psychiatric illness, health workers, and volunteers that originally met each other just to play football as a recreational activity. This group decided early on to adhere to ANPIS and to participate at the regional championship USIP-ANPIS. In 2006 the meeting with the sport club Bellaria Cappuccini signaled an important step on the way to integration: the sport club in fact enthusiastically received the group in its structures, giv-

ing a home to the whole group's initiative. In these years the project has grown-up, and now Bellaria Solidarità offers the possibility to play football, basketball, volleyball, swimming, archery, sailing, and fencing to anyone who wants to participate, with particular attention to people suffering from psychiatric disorders. The teams have regular weekly trainings, with qualified coaches. For each discipline there is the possibility to participate in regional or national championships managed by the UISP or the ANPIS organizations. Every year the sport club organizes a meeting called "Palla in rete" (Ball in the net) to promote sport and physical activity for these "special teams." Participants come from Italy and other countries. The ideals of the sport club underline how discomfort, as well as a disability, whether social or mental, can limit daily life and relationships. Sport can be an instrument of equality and integration as well as an excellent tool for rehabilitation, through the respect of common rules which deal with themselves and others, to overcome a malaise.

References

Abrantes, A., Strong, D., Cohn, A., Cameron, A., Greenberg, B., Mancebo, M., et al. (2009). Acute changes in obsessions and compulsions following moderate-intensity aerobic exercise among patients with obsessive-compulsive disorder. *Journal of Anxiety Disorders, 23,* 923-927.

Acil, A. A., Dogan, S., & Dogan, O. (2008). The effects of physical exercises to mental state and quality of life in patients with schizophrenia. *Journal of Psychiatric and Mental Health Nursing, 15,* 808-815.

Adkins, E. C., & Keel, P. K. (2005). Does "excessive" or "compulsive" best describe exercise as a symptom of bulimia nervosa? *International Journal of Eating Disorders, 38(1),* 24-9.

Adlard, P., & Cotman, C. (2004). Voluntary exercise protects against stress-induced decreases in brain-derived neurotrophic factor protein expression. *Neuroscience, 124(4),* 985-992.

Ahlström, S., & Österberg, E. (2004/2005). International perspectives on adolescent and young adult drinking. *Alcohol Research & Health, 28(4),* 258-268.

Alberti, K. G., Zimmet, P., & Shaw, J. (2006). Metabolic syndrome-a new world-wide definition. A Consensus Statement from the International Diabetes Federation. *Diabetic Medicine, 23,* 469-480.

Aldana, S. G., Sutton, L. D., & Jacobson, B. H. (1996). Relationship between leisure time physical activity and perceived stress. *Perceptual and Motor Skills, 82,* 315-321.

Alexander, N., Kuepper, Y., Schmitz, A., Osinsky, R., Kozyra, E., & Hennig, J. (2009). Gene-environment interactions predict cortisol responses after acute stress: implications for the etiology of depression. *Psychoneuroendocrinology, 34,* 1294-1303.

Allison, D. B., Fontaine, K. R., Heo, M., Mentore, J. L., Cappelleri, J. C., Chandler, L. P., et al. (1999).The distribution of body mass index among individuals with and without schizophrenia. *Journal of Clinical Psychiatry, 60,* 215-220.

Alpers, G., & Tuschen-Caiffier, B. (2001). Negative feelings and the desire to eat in bulimia nervosa. *Eating Behaviors, 2,* 339-352.

Al-Talib, N. I., & Griffin, C. (1994). Labelling effect on adolescent's self-concept. *International Journal of Offender Therapy and Comparative Criminology, 38,* 47-57.

Altemeier, W., & Horwitz, E. (1997). The role of the school in the management of attention-deficit hyperactivity disorder. *Pediatric Annals, 26(12),* 737-744.

Amaral, J. D. (2004). *Jogos cooperativos.* São Paulo: Phorte.

American Association on Intellectual and Developmental Disabilities (AAIDD) 11th Edition Implementation Committee (2010). Public comments regarding draft definition of intellectual disability.

American Association on Mental Retardation (1992). *Mental retardation definition, classification and systems of supports.* (9th ed.) Washington DC: American Association on Mental Retardation.

American College of Sports Medicine (1982). Position Statement on the Use of Alcohol in Sports. *Medicine & Science in Sports & Exercise, 14(6),* ix-xi.

American College of Sports Medicine (2009). *A.C.S.M.'s guidelines for exercise testing and prescription* (8th ed.). Baltimore: Williams & Wilkins.

American Psychiatric Association (2013). *Diagnostic and statistical manual of mental disorders.* (5th ed.). Washington DC: American Psychiatric Association.

American Psychiatric Association (2000). *Diagnostic and statistical manual of mental disorders* (4th ed.). Washington, DC: American psychiatric Association.

American Psychiatric Association (1994). *Diagnostic and statistical manual of mental disorders* (4th ed.). Washington DC: American Psychiatric Association.

American Psychiatric Association (1990). *Schizophrenia.* Arlington, Virginia: Pamphlet by American Psychiatric Association.

American Psychiatric Association (2013). DSM-5 Development. http://www.dsm5.org/ Pages/Default.aspx.

Anderson, B. J., Rapp, D. N., Baek, D. H., McCloskey, D. P., Coburn-Litvak, P. S., & Robinson, J. K. (2000). Exercise influences spatial learning in the radial arm maze. *Physiology & Behavior, 70,* 425-429.

Anderson, D. J., McGovern, J. P., & Dupont, R. L. (1999). The origins of the Minnesota model of addiction treatment: a first person account. *Journal of Addictive Diseases, 18(1),* 107-114.

Andreasen, N. C, & Black, D.W. (1995). *Introductory textbook of psychiatry.* Washington, DC: American Psychiatric Press.

Andrews, J. P., & Andrews, G. J. (2003). Life in a secure unit: the rehabilitation of young people through the use of sport. *Social Science and Medicine, 56,* 531-550.

Angevaren, M., Aufdemkampe, G., Verhaar, H. J., Aleman, A., & Vanhees, L. (2008). Physical activity and enhanced fitness to improve cognitive function in older people without known cognitive impairment. *Cochrane Database System, 16(2).*

Angold, A., & Costello, E. J. (2001). The epidemiology of disorders of conduct: Nosological issues and comorbidity. In J. Hill, & B. Maughan (Eds.), *Conduct disorders in childhood and adolescence* (pp. 126-168). Cambridge, UK: Cambridge University.

Anstiss, T. (1991). A randomized controlled trial of aerobic exercise in the treatment of the alcohol dependent. *Medicine & Science in Sports & Exercise, 23,* 116-118.

Antonini, P. R., Seiler, R., & Mengisen, W. (2004). Relationship of coping style with type of sport. *Perceptual and Motor Skills, 98,* 479-486.

Antonovsky, A. (1987). *Unraveling the mystery of health. How people manage stress and stay well.* San Francisco: Jossey-Bass.

Antshel, K. M., & Remer, R. (2003). Social skills training in children with attention deficit hyperactivity disorder: A randomized controlled clinical trial. *Journal of Clinical Child and Adolescent Psychology, 32,* 153-165.

Archie, S. M., Goldberg, J. O., Akhtar-Danesh, N., Landeen, J., McColl, L., & McNiven, J. (2007). Psychotic disorders, eating habits, and physical activity: who is ready for lifestyle changes? *Psychiatric Services, 58,* 233-239.

Archie, S. M., Wilson, J. H., Osborne, S., Hobbs, H., & McNiven, J. (2003). Pilot study: access to fitness facility and exercise levels in olanzapine-treated patients. *Canadian Journal of Psychiatry, 48,* 628-632.

Armstrong, L. E., & VanHeest, J. L. (2002). The unknown mechanism of the overtraining syndrome: clues from depression and psychoneuroimmunology. *Sports Medicine, 32(3),* 185-209.

Arns, M., De Ritter, D., Strehl, U., Breteler, M., & Coenen, A. (2009). Efficacy of neurofeedback treatment in ADHD: The effects on inattention, impulsivity and hyperactivity: A meta-analysis. *Clinical EEG and Neuroscience, 40(3),* 180-189.

Aron, A. R., Fletcher, P. C., Bullmore, E. T., Sahakian, B. J., & Robbins, T. W. (2003). Stop signal inhibition disrupted by damage to right inferior frontal gyrus in humans. *Nature Neuroscience, 6,* 115-116.

Ashley, C.D., Smith, J.F., Robinson J.B., Richardson, M.T. (1996). Disordered eating in female collegiate athletes and collegiate females in advanced program of study: a preliminary investigation. *International Journal of Sport and Nutrition, 6,* 391-401.

Åstrand, P.-O. (2004). Physiology related to school physical education from a historic perspective to the 21st century. In M.-K. Chin, L. D. Hensley, P. Cote & S.-H. Chen (Eds.), *Global perspectives in the integration of physical activity, sports, dance, and exercise science in physical education: From theory to practice* (pp. 3-11). Hong Kong: The Hong Kong Institute of Education.

Aubin, G., Stip, E., Gelinas, I., Rainville, C., & Chapparo, C. (2009). Daily activities, cognition and community functioning in persons with schizophrenia. *Schizophrenia Research, 107,* 313-318.

Aucouturier, B. (2005). *La méthode Aucouturier, fantasmes d'action et pratique psychomotrice.* Brusselles: De Boeck Université.

Azrin, N. H., Vinas, V., & Ehle, C. T. (2007). Physical activity as reinforcement for classroom calmness of ADHD children: a preliminary study. *Child & Family Behavior Therapy, 29(2),* 1-8.

Baecke, J., Burema, J., Frijters, E. (1982). A short questionnaire for the measurement of habitual physical activity in epidemiological studies. *American Journal of Clinical Nutrition, 36,* 936-942.

Bahrke, M. S., Morgan, W. P. (1978). Anxiety reduction following exercise and meditation. *Cognitive Therapy and Research, 2(4),* 323-333.

Baigent, M. F. (2005). Understanding alcohol misuse and comorbid psychiatric disorders. *Current Opinion in Psychiatry, 18(3),* 223-228.

Bailey, R. (2005) Evaluating the relationship between physical education, sport and social inclusion. *Educational Review, 57,* 71-90.

Bailey, R. (2006). Physical education and sport in schools: a review of benefits and outcomes. *Journal of School Health, 76,* 397-401.

Baker, C. W. & Brownell, K. D. (2000). Physical activity and maintenance of weight loss: physiological and psychological mechanisms. In C. Bouchard (Ed.), *Physical Activity and Obesity* (pp. 311-328). Champaign, IL: Human Kinetics.

Bandura, A. (1977). Toward a unifying theory of behavioral change. *Psychological Review, 84,* 191-215

Barabasz, A., & Barabasz, M. (2000). Treating ADHD with hypnosis and neurotherapy. *Child Study Journal, 3,* 25-44.

Barbour, K., Edenfield, T., & Blumenthal, J. (2007). Exercise as a treatment for depression and other psychiatric disorders: a review. *Journal of Cardiopulmonary Rehabilitation and Prevention, 27,* 359-367.

Barkley, R. A. (1990). *Attention-deficit hyperactivity disorder.* New York: Guilford Press.

Barkley, R. A. (1997). Behavioral inhibition, sustained attention, and executive functions: constructing a unifying theory of ADHD. *Psychological Bulletin, 121(1),* 65-94.

Barkley, R. A. (2002). Major life activity and health outcomes associated with attention-deficit/hyperactivity disorder. *Journal of Clinical Psychiatry, 63*(Suppl. 12), 10-15.

Barkley, R. A., Fischer, M., Smallish, L., & Fletcher, K. (2006). Young adult outcome of hyperactive children: adaptive functioning in major life activities. *Journal of the American Academy of Child and Adolescent Psychiatry, 45(2),* 192-202.

Barry, C. T., Frick, P. J., & Killian, A. L. (2003). The relation of narcissism and self-esteem to conduct problems in children: A preliminary investigation. *Journal of Clinical and Child Adolescent Psychology, 32,* 139-152.

Barry, R. J., Clarke, A. R., McCarthy, R., Selikowitz, M., MacDonald, B. & Dupuy, F. (2012). Caffeine effects on resting-state electrodermal levels in AD/HD suggest an anomalous arousal mechanism. *Biological Psychology, 89(3),* 606-608.

Bassarath, L. (2001). Conduct disorder: a biopsychosocial review. *Canadian Journal of Psychiatry/Revue Canadienne de Psychiatrie, 46,* 609-616.

Beals, K. (2004). *Disordered eating among athletes. A comprehensive guide for health professionals.* Champaign, IL: Human Kinetics.

Beals, K. A., Brey, R. A. & Gonyou, J.B. (1999). Understanding the female athlete triad : eating disorders, amenorrhea and osteoporosis. *Journal of School Health, 69,* 337-340.

Beals, K., & Manore, M. (1994). The prevalence and consequences of subclinical eating disorders in female athletes. *International Journal of Sport and Nutrition, 4,* 175-195.

Beals, K., & Manore, M. (2000). Behavioral, psychological and physical characteristics of female athletes with subclinical eating disorders. *International Journal of Sport Nutrition and Exercise Metabolism, 10(2),*128-143.

Beck, A.T., Steer, R.A., & Brown, G.K. (1996). *Beck depression inventory -second edition (BDI-II).* San Antonio, TX: The Psychological Corporation.

Beck, A.T., Steer, R.A., & Carbin, M.G. (1988). Psychometric properties of the Beck Depression Inventory: twenty-five years of evaluation. *Clinical Psychology Review, 8(1)*, 77-100

Beebe, L., Tian, L., Morris, N., Goodwin, A., Allen, S., & Kuldau, J. (2005). Effects of exercise on mental and physical health parameters of persons with schizophrenia. *Issues in Mental Health Nursing, 26*, 661-676.

Berchicci, M., & Bertollo, M. (2009). Il contributo psicomotorio nell'intervento multidisciplinare con un bambino con ADHD. *Psicomotricità, 13*, 23-32,

Berger, B. G. (1996). Psychological benefits of an active lifestyle: What we know and what we need to know. *Quest, 48*, 330-353.

Berren, M. R., Hill, K. R., Merikle, E., Gonzalez, E., Santiago, J. (1994). Serious mental illness and mortality rates. *Hospital and Community Psychiatry, 45*, 604-605.

Bertollo, M., & Carraro, A. (2002). Psychophysical activation related to cognitive performance in ADHD children. In D. Milanovic & F. Prot (Eds.), *Kinesiology New Perspectives, Proceedings Book* (pp 738-741). Opatija: Croatia.

Beumont, P. J., Arthur, B., Russell, J. D., & Touyz, S. W. (1994). Excessive physical activity in dieting disorder patients: Proposals for a supervised exercise program. *International Journal of Eating Disorders, 15*, 21-36.

Bianchi, G., Rossi, V., Muscari, D., Magalotti, D., Zoli, M.; Pianoro Study Group (2008). Physical activity is negatively associated with the metabolic syndrome in the elderly. *QJM: An International Journal of Medicine, 101*, 713-721.

Biddle, S. J. H. (1995). Exercise and psychosocial health. *Research Quarterly for Exercise and Sport, 66(4)*, 292-297.

Biddle, S. J. H. (1997). Cognitive theories of motivation and the physical self. In K.R. Fox (Ed.), *The physical self* (pp. 59-82). Champaign, IL: Human Kinetics.

Biddle, S. J. H., Fox, K. R., & Boutcher, S. H. (2000). *Physical Activity and Psychological Well-Being*. London: Routledge.

Biddle, S. J. H., Gorely, T. & Stensel, D. J. (2004) Health-enhancing physical activity and sedentary behaviour in children and adolescents. *Journal of Sports Sciences, 22*, 679-701.

Biddle, S. J. H., Whitehead, S. H., O'Donovan, T. M. & Nevill, M. E. (2005). Correlates of participation in physical activity for adolescent girls: a systematic review of recent literature. *Journal of Physical Activity & Health, 2*, 421-432.

Biddle, S. J. H., & Mutrie, N. (2008). *Psychology of physical activity determinants, well-being & interventions* (2nd ed.). Abingdon, Oxon, UK: Routldge.

Biddle, S. J. H., & Mutrie, N. (2001). *Psychology of physical activity. Determinants, well-being and interventions*. London: Routledge.

Birbaumer, N., & Schmidt, R. F. (2006). *Biologische Psychologie*. Heidelberg: Springer Medizin Verlag.

Birmingham, C. L., & Beumonts, P. J. V. (2004). *Medical management of eating disorders: a practical handbook for healthcare professionals*. Cambridge: University Press.

Bish, C. L., Michels Blanck, H., Maynard, L. M., Serdula, M. K., Thompson, N. J., & Kettel Khan, L. (2006). Health-related quality of life and weight loss among overweight and obese U.S. adults, 2001 to 2002. *Obesity, 14*, 2042-2053.

Black, D., Lawson, J., & Fleishmann, S. (1999). Excessive alcohol use by non-elite sportsmen. *Drug and Alcohol Review, 18(2)*, 201-205.

Blake, H., Mo, P., Malik, S., & Thomas, S. (2009). How effective are physical activity interventions for alleviating depressive symptoms in older people? A systematic review. *Clinical Rehabilitation, 23(10)*, 873-887.

Blanchard, C. M., Rodgers, W.M., Spence, J. C., & Courneya, K. S. (2001). Feeling state responses to acute exercise of high and low intensity. *Journal of Science and Medicine in Sport, 4*, 30-38.

Blanchard, E. B., Greene, B., Scharff, L., & Schwarz-McMorris, S. P. (1993). Relaxation training as a treatment for irritable bowel syndrome. *Biofeedback and Self Regulation, 18(3)*, 125-132.

Bliss, E. L., & Ailion, J. (1991). Relationship of stress and activity to brain dopamine and homovanillic acid. *Life Sciences, 1(10)*, 1161-1169.

Blumenthal, J., Babyak, M., Moore, K., Craighead, W., Herman, S., Khatri, P., et al. (1999). Effects of exercise training in older patients with major depression. *Archives of Internal Medicine, 159*, 2349-2356.

Blumenthal, J. A., Friedrikson, M., Kuhn, C. M., Ulmer, R. L., Walsh-Riddle, M. & Appelbaum, M. (1990). Aerobic exercise reduces levels of cardiovascular and sympathoadrenal responses to mental stress in subjects without prior evidence of myocardial ischemia. *American Journal of Cardiology, 65*, 93-98.

Bonci, C. M., Malina, R. M., Granger, L. R., Johnson, C. L., Milne, L. W., Ryan, R. R., & Vanderbunt, E. M. (2008). National athletic trainer association position statement : preventing detecting and managing disordered eating in athletes. *Journal of Athletic Training, 43*, 80-108.

Bordua, D. (1960). *Sociological theories and their implications for juvenile delinquency*. Washington, DC: Government printing office.

Borg, G. (1998). External, physiological and psychological factors and perceived exertion. In G. Borg (Ed), *Borg's perceived exertion and pain scales* (pp. 68-74). Champaign, IL: Human Kinetics.

Borges, K. (1995). Atividades físicas para pacientes psiquiátricos no instituto raul soares. *IX Congresso Brasileiro de Ciências do Esporte*. Vitória.

Borges, K. (1997). *Futebol: recurso na reabilitação de pacientes com transtornos mentais*. II congresso Brasileiro da Sociedade de Atividade Motora Adaptada. Uberlândia: Sobama – Universidade Federal de Uberlândia.

Borges, K. (1998). *Atividade física para os usuários de saúde mental de belo horizonte*. I Convenção das Escolas de Educação Física de Minas Gerais. Belo Horizonte: Escola de Educação Física da Universidade Federal de Minas Gerais.

Borges, K. (1998). *Lei anti-manicomial e educação física: perspectiva de intervenção da atividade física adaptada junto ao paciente psiquiátrico*. I Congresso Brasileiro de Atividade Motora Adaptada (pp. 71-71). Campinas: Imprensa da Universidade de Campinas.

Borges, K. (1998). *Proposta de registro de planejamento de atividades físicas para usuários do serviço de saúde mental de belo horizonte*. III Simpósio Mineiro de Ciências do Esporte e I Forum Nacional de Administração Esportiva.

Viçosa: Gráfica Universitária Universidade Federal de Viçosa.

Borges, K. (2000). *E viva a diferença*. Belo Horizonte: Governo de Minas Gerais.

Borges, K. (2005). *Influência da atividade física na qualidade de vida de sujeitos com transtornos mentais: estudo realizado nos centros de convivência do município de belo horizonte*. Unpublished doctoral dissertation, Universidade do Porto. Portugal.

Borges, K., Marques, U., & Silva, M. (2003). *Physical activity, leisure, quality of life and psychotic syndrome: description and critical reflection on an assessment methodology*. 14th ISAPA. Seoul: College of Human Movement & Performance.

Borges, K., Marques, U., & Silva, M. (2005). Questionnaire on socio-demographics and leisure: an evaluation process. *Book of Procedures of the 15th International Symposium of Adapted Physical Activity, Verona, 167*.

Borges, K., Marques, U., & Silva, M. (2006). Afastamento social e lazer: avaliação de indivíduos com transtornos mentais. *Revista brasileira de educação física e esporte,* 222-223.

Borges, K., Marques, U., & Silva, M. (2007). Goals in life of participants with severe mental disabilities are associated with leisure skills. *Sobama Journal, 12(1)*, 227-230.

Boutcher, S. H., & Hamer, M. (2006). Psychobiological reactivity, physical activity, and cardiovascular health. In E. O. Acevedo & P. Ekkekakis (Eds.), *Psychobiology of physical activity* (pp. 161-176). Champaign, IL: Human Kinetics.

Boutcher, S. H. (2000) Cognitive performance, fitness and ageing. In: , S., Fox, K. R., Boutcher, & S. J. H., Biddle (Eds.), *Physical activity and psychological well-being: an evidence based approach*. London: Routledge.

Bradshaw, T., Lovell, K., & Harris, N. (2005). Healthy living interventions and schizophrenia: a systematic review. *Journal of Advanced Nursing, 49*, 634-654.

Brand, S., Gerber, M., Pühse, U., & Holsboer-Trachsler, E. (2010). Depression, hypomania and dysfunctional cognitions as mediators between stress and insomnia: The best advice is not always found on the pillow! *International Journal of Stress Management, 17*, 114-134.

Brandl-Bredenbeck, H. P. (2006). Physical activity and risk behavior in young people. In J. Diniz, F. Carreiro da Costa, & M. Onofre. *AIESEP World Congress – Active Lifestyles: The Impact of Education and Sport* (pp 23-40). Lisboa: Edições.

Brazil's Health Ministry. (2009). O SUS de A a Z. [portal. saude.gov.br/portal/arquivos/pdf/sus_3edicao_completo.pdf].

Breier, J. I., Gray, L. C., Klaas, P., Fletcher, J. M., & Foorman, B. (2002). Dissociation of sensitivity and response bias in children with attention-deficit/hyperactivity disorder during central auditory masking. *Neuropsychology, 16(1)*, 28-34.

Brewerton, T. D., Stellefson, E. J., Hibbs, N., Hodges, E. L., & Cochrane, C. E. (1995). Comparison of eating disorder patients with and without compulsive exercising. *International Journal of Eating Disorders, 17(4)*, 413-416.

Briar, S., & Piliavin, I. (1965). Delinquency, situational inducements, and commitment to conformity. *Social Problems, 13*, 35-45.

Broadbent, D. E. (1958). *Perception and communication*. London: Pergamon Press.

Brody, J. E. (1981). Effects of beauty found to run surprisingly deep. *New York Times, 1*, C1-C3.

Bron, M. (1994). Demente ouderen in de psychomotorische therapie: een verslag van een behandeling. *Bewegen en hulpverlening, 11*, 171-180.

Broocks, A., Meyer, T., Bandelow, B., George, A., Bartmann. U., Hillmer-Vogel, U., et al. (1997). Exercise avoidance and impaired endurance capacity in patients with panic disorder. *Neuropsychobiology, 36*, 182-187.

Broocks, A., Bandelow, B., Pekrun, G., George, A., Meyer, T., & Bartmann, U. (1998). Comparison of aerobic exercise, clomipramine, and placebo in the treatment of panic disorder. *American Journal Psychiatry, 155*, 603-609.

Broota, A., & Dhir, R. (1990). Efficacy of two relaxation techniques in depression. *Journal of Personality and Clinical Studies, 6*, 83-90.

Brosse, A., Sheets, E., Lett, H., & Blumenthal, J. (2002). Exercise and the treatment of clinical depression in adults: recent findings and future directions. *Sports Medicine, 32*, 741-760.

Brower, K. J. (1993). Anabolic steroids. *Psychiatric Clinics of North America, 16*, 97-103.

Brown, A., Liu-Ambrose, T., Tate, R., & Lord, S. R. (2009). The effect of group-based exercise on cognitive performance and mood in seniors residing in intermediate care and self-care retirement facilities: a randomised controlled trial. *British Journal of Sports Medicine, 43*, 608-614.

Brown, D. R. (1990). Exercise, fitness, and mental health. In C. Bouchard, R. J. Shepard, T. Stephens, J. R. Sutton, & B. D. McPherson (Eds.), *Exercise, fitness, and health: a consensus of current knowledge* (pp 607-627). Champaign, IL: Human Kinetics.

Brown, J. D. (1991). Staying fit and staying well: Physical fitness as a moderator of life stress, *Journal of Personality and Social Psychology, 60*, 555-561.

Brown, R., Abrantes, A., Read, J., Marcus, B., Jakicic, J., Strong D., et al. (2009). Aerobic exercise for alcohol recovery: rationale, program description, and preliminary findings. *Behavior Modification, 33(2)*, 220-249.

Brown, R., Abrantes, A., Strong, D., Mancebo, M., Menard, J., Rasmussen, S., et al. (2007). A pilot study of moderate-intensity aerobic exercise for obsessive compulsive disorder. *Journal Nervous and Mental Disease, 195*, 514-520.

Brown, S. (1997). Excess mortality of schizophrenia: a meta-analysis. *British Journal of Psychiatry, 171*, 502-508.

Brown, S., Birtwistle, J., Roe, L., & Thompson, C. (1999). The unhealthy lifestyle of people with schizophrenia. *Psychological Medicine, 3*, 697-701.

Bruce, B., Thernlund, G., & Nettelbladt, U. (2006). ADHD and language impairment: A study of the parent questionnaire FTF (Five to Fifteen). *European Child and Adolescent Psychiatry, 15(1)*, 52-60.

Buchman, A. S., Wilson, R. S., Bennett, D. A. (2008) Total daily activity is associated with cognition in older persons. *American Journal of Geriatric Psychiatry, 16*, 697-701.

Budgett, R. (1990). Overtraining syndrome. *British Journal of Sports Medicine,24(4)*, 231-236.

Burijon, B. N. (2007). *Biological bases of clinical anxiety*. New York: Norton & Company.

Bush, G., Valera, E. M., & Seidman, L. J. (2005). Functional neuroimaging of attention deficit/hyperactivity disorder: a review and suggested future directions. *Biological Psychiatry, 57(11)*, 1273-1284.

Byrne, D. G., & Mazanov, J. (2003). Adolescent stress and future smoking behaviour. A prospective investigation. *Journal of Psychosomatic Research, 54*, 313-321.

Byrne, S., & McLean, N. (2001). Eating disorders in athletes: a review of the literature. *Journal of Science and Medicine in Sport, 4*, 145-159.

Cacioppo, J. T., Berntson, G. G., Malarkey, W. B., Kiecolt-Glaser, J. K., Sheridan, J. F., Poehlmann, K. M., et al. (1998). Autonomic, neuroendocrine, and immune responses to psychological stress: The reactivity hypothesis. *Annals of the New York Academy of Science, 840*, 664-673.

Calfas, K. J., & Taylor, W. C. (1994) Effects of physical activity on psychological variables in adolescents. *Pediatric Exercise Science, 6*, 406-423.

Callaghan, P. (2004). Exercise: a neglected intervention in mental health care? *Journal of Psychiatric and Mental Health Nursing, 11*, 476-483.

Cameron, L. D, & Leventhal, H. (2003). *The self-regulation of health and illness behavior.* London: Routledge.

Cannon, W. B. (1929). *Bodily changes in pain, hunger, fear and rage.* New York: Appleton-Century-Crofts.

Capasso, R. M., Lineberry, T. W., Bostwick, J. M., Decker, P. A., & St Sauver, J. (2008). Mortality in schizophrenia and schizoaffective disorder: an Olmsted County, Minnesota cohort: 1950-2005. *Schizophrenia Research, 98*, 287-294.

Cardoso, C. S. (2001). *Adaptação transcultural para o Brasil de uma escala de qualidade de vida para pacientes com esquizofrenia: Escala QLS .* Unpublished Master's thesis, Universidade Federal de Minas Gerais, Belo Horizonte, Brazil.

Carey, G. B., & Sidmore, K. A. (1994). Exercise attenuates the anti-lipolytic effect of adenosine in adipocytes isolated from miniature swine. *International Journal of Obesity and Related Metabolic Disorders, 18(3)*, 155-160.

Carmeli, E., Zinger-Vaknin, T., Morad, M., & Merrick, J. (2005). Can physical training have an effect on well-being in adult with mild intellectual disability? *Mechanisms of Ageing and Development, 126*, 299-304.

Carney, C. P., Jones, L., & Woolson, R. F. (2006). Medical comorbidity in women and men with schizophrenia: a population-based controlled study. *Journal of General, Internal Medicine, 21*, 1133-1137.

Carr, D. B., Bullen, B. A., Skrinar, G. S., Arnold, M. A., Rosenblat, M. Beitins, I. Z., et al. (1981). Physical conditioning facilitates the exercise-induced secretion of beta-endorphin and beta-lipotropin in women. *New England Journal of Medicine; 305*, 560-563.

Carraro, A., Cognolato, S., & Fiorellini, A. (2000). Una griglia di osservazione per l'attività fisica adattata con pazienti psichiatrici. *Giornale Italiano di Psicologia dello Sport, 1(1)*, 13-15.

Carraro, A., Mioni, D., & Pessa, G. (2002). Physical activity and alcohol dependence. In D. Milanovic & F. Prot (Eds.). *Kinesiology New Perspective* (pp. 503-506). Zagreb: University of Zagreb.

Carraro, A., Young, M.C., & Robazza, C. (2008). A contribu-tion to the validation of the Physical Activity Enjoyment Scale in an Italian sample. *Social Behavior and Personality, 36(7)*, 911-918.

Carroll, D., &. Seers, K. (1998). Relaxation for the relief of chronic pain: a systematic review. *Journal of Advanced Nursing, 27(3)*, 476-487.

Carron, A., Hausenblas, H., & Mack, D. (1996). Social influence and exercise: a meta-analysis. *Journal of Sport Exercise and Psychology, 18*, 1-16.

Carter-Morris, P. & Faulkner, G. (2003). A football project for service users: the role of football in reducing social exclusion. *Journal of Mental Health Promotion, 2*, 24-30.

Casey, D. E., Haupt, D. W., Newcomer, J. W., Henderson, D. C., Sernyak, M. J., Davidson, M. et al. (2004). Antipsychotic-induced weight gain and metabolic abnormalities: implications for increased mortality in patients with schizophrenia. *Journal of Clinical Psychiatry, 65*(Suppl. 7), 4-18.

Casper, R. (2006). Review the 'drive for activity' and "restlessness" in anorexia nervosa: potential pathways. *Journal of Affective Disorders, 92(1)*, 99-107.

Caterino, M. C., & Polak, E. D. (1999). Effects of two types of activity on the performance of second-, third-, and fourth-grade students on a test of concentration. *Perceptual and Motor Skills, 89(1)*, 245-248.

Centorrino, F., Wurtman, J. J., Duca, K. A., Fellman, V. H., Fogarty, K. V., Berry, J. M. et al. (2006). Weight loss in overweight patients maintained on atypical antipsychotic agents. *International Journal of Obesity, 30*, 1011-1016.

Centros de Atenção Psicosocial. (2009). Ministério da Saúde - Brasil. [http://www.dgsaude.min-saude.pt/pns/vol2_227.html].

Chaouloff, F. (1989): Physical exercise and brain mono-amines: a review. *Acta Physiologica Scandinavica; 137*, 1-13.

Cherkasova, M. V., & Hechtman, L. (2009). Neuroimaging in attention-deficit hyperactivity disorder: beyond the frontostriatal circuitry. *Canadian Journal of Psychiatry, 54(10)*, 651-664.

Chida, Y., & Steptoe, A. (2010). Greater cardiovascular responses to laboratory mental stress are associated with poor subsequent cardiovascular risk status: a meta-analysis of prospective evidence. *Hypertension, 55*, 1026-1032.

Chodzko-Zajko, W. J., Schuler, P. B., Solomon Henl B., & Ellis, N. (1992) The influence of age and physical fitness on automatic and effortfull cognitive processing. *International journal of aging and human development, 35*, 265-285.

Christiansen, T., Bech, M., Lauridsen, J., & Nielsen, P. (2006). Demographic changes and aggregate health-care expenditure in Europe. In *Social welfare policies* (ENEPRI Policy Briefs No. 32). Brussels: CEPS - The Centre for European Policy Studies.

Clark, D., Lynch, K., Donovan, J., & Block, G. (2001). Health problems in adolescents with alcohol use disorders: self-report, liver injury, and physical examination findings and correlates. *Alcoholism: Clinical and Experimental Research, 25(9)*, 1350-1359.

Claytor, R. P. (1991). Stress reactivity: Hemodynamic adjustments in trained and untrained humans, *Medical Science and Sports Exercise, 23,* 873-881.

Cluphf, D., O'Connor, J., & Vanin, S. (2001). Effects of aerobic dance on the cardiovascular endurance of adults with intellectual disabilities. *Adapted Physical Activity Quarterly, 18,* 60-71.

Cohen, A. K. (1955). *Delinquent boys: the culture of the gang.* New York, NY: Free Press.

Cohen, S., & Edwards, J. R. (1989). Personality characteristics as moderators of the relationship between stress and disorder. In R. W. Neufeld (Ed.), *Advances in the investigation of psychological stress* (pp. 235-283). New York: Wiley.

Cohen, S., & Williamson, G. M. (1988). Perceived stress in a probability sample of the United States. In S. Spacapan & S. Oskamp (Eds.), *The social psychology of health* (pp. 31-67). Newbury Park: Sage.

Cohen, S., Kamarck, T., & Mermelstein, R. (1983). A global measure of perceived stress. *Journal of Health and Social Behavior, 24,* 385-396.

Colcombe, S. J., . Erickson, K. I., Raz, N., Webb, A. G., Cohen, N, J, McAuley, E., et al. (2003). Aerobic fitness reduces brain tissue loss in aging humans. *Journal of Gerontology, 58,* 176-180.

Colcombe, S., & Kramer, A. F. (2003). Fitness effects on the cognitive function of older adults: a meta-analytic study. *Psychological Science, 14,* 125-130.

Coldham, E. L., Addington, J., & Addington, D. (2002). Medication adherence of individuals with a first episode of psychosis. *Acta Psychiatrica Scandinavica, 106,* 286-290.

Connolly, M., & Kelly, C. (2005). The Royal College of Psychiatrists, lifestyle and physical health in schizophrenia. *Advances in Psychiatric Treatment, 11,* 125-132.

Conti, L. (1999). *Repertorio delle scale di valutazione in psichiatria.* Firenze: SEE.

Cook, B., & Hausenblas, H. (2011). Eating disorder-specific health-related quality of life and exercise in college females. *Quality Of Life Research, 20(9),* 1385-1390.

Cooper, C. L. (2003). Stress prevention in the police. *Occupational Medicine, 53,* 244-245.

Corrêa, W. (1995). *I torneio nacional de futebol de salão Franco Basaglia torneio realizado no II encontro nacional da luta antimanicomial.* Unpublished master's thesis, Belo Horizonte: Escola de Educação Física, Fisoterapia e Terapia Ocupacional da Unversidade Federal de Minas Gerais.

Correll, C. U., Frederickson, A. M., Kane, J. M., & Manu, P. (2006). Metabolic syndrome and the risk of coronary heart disease in 367 patients treated with second-generation antipsychotic drugs. *Journal of Clinical Psychiatry, 67,* 575-583.

Côrtes, G. P. (2002). Conhecimento escolar e cultura popular: os caminhos para a Educação do Novo Milênio. *Revista da Comissão Mineira de Foclore,* 57-64.

Costa, C. (2007). *Percepção de liberdade no lazer dos trabalhadores de Saúde Mental dos Centros de Referência em Saúde Mental e Centros de Convivência da Prefeitura Municipal de Belo Horizonte.* Unpublished master's thesis, Porto, Portugal: Faculdade de Ciências do Desporto e de Educação Física da Universidade do Porto.

Cotman, C. W., & Berchtold, N. C. (2007). Physical activity and the maintenance of cognition: Learning from animal models. *Alzheimer's and Dementia, 3,* S30-S37.

Cotman, C., Berchtold, N., Christie, L. (2007). Exercise builds brain health: key roles of growth factor cascades and inflammation. *Trends in Neurosciences, 30,* 464-472.

Craft, L. L., & Landers, D. M. (1998). The effect of exercise on clinical depression and depression resulting from mental illness: a meta-analysis. *Journal of Sport and Exercise Psychology, 20,* 339-357.

Crews, D. J., & Landers, D. M. (1987). A meta-analytic review of aerobic fitness and reactivity to psychosocial stressors. *Medicine & Science in Sports & Exercise, 19,* 114-130.

Crouch, R. B. (1989). *Occupational Therapy in Psychiatry and Mental Health.* Cape Town: CTP Book Printers.

Dalgalarrondo, P. (2000). *Psicopatologia e Semiologia dos Transtornos Mentais.* Porto Alegre: Artes Médicas.

Damen, J., Ouwens, M. (2008) Toegepaste relaxatie: antwoorden vanuit de psychomotorische therapie op storende preoccupaties. *Tijdschrift voor vaktherapie, 4,* 3-7.

Daumit, G. L., Goldberg, R. W., Anthony, C., Dickerson, F., Brown , C. H., Kreynebuhl J., et al. (2005). Physical activity patterns in adults with severe mental illness. *Journal of Nervous and Mental Disease, 193,* 641-646.

Davenport, B. R. & Bourgeois, N. M. (2008). Play, aggression, the preschool child, and the family: A review of the literature to guide empirically informed play therapy with aggressive preschool children. *International Journal of Play Therapy, 17(1),* 2-23.

Davidson, S., Judd, F., Jolley, D., Hocking, B., Thompson, S., & Hyland, B. (2001).Cardiovascular risk factors for people with mental illness. *Australian and New Zealand Journal of Psychiatry, 35,* 196-202.

Davies, D. M., Ashton, C. H., Rao, J. G., Rawlins, M. D., Routledge, P. A., Savage, R. L., et al. (1977). Comprehensive clinical drug information service: first years' experience. *British Medical Journal, 1,* 89-90.

Davis, C. (2000). Exercise abuse. *International Journal of Sport Psychology, 31,* 278-289.

Davis, C., & Cowles, M. A. (1989). Comparison of weight and diet concerns and personality factors among female athletes and non-athletes. *Journal of Psychosomatic Research, 33,* 527–536.

Davis, C., & Fox, J. (1993). Excessive exercise and weight preoccupation in women. *Addictive Behaviors, 18,* 201-211.

Davis, C. & Kaptein, S. (2006). Anorexia Nervosa with excessive exercise: a phenotype with close links to obsessive-compulsive disorder. *Psychiatry Research, 142(2-3),* 209-217.

Davis, C., Kaptein, S., Kaplan, A. S., Olmsted, M. P., & Woodside, D. B. (1998). Obsessionality in Anorexia Nervosa: the moderating influence of exercise. *Psychosomatic Medicine, 60(2),* 192-197.

Davis, C., Katzman, D. K., Kaptein, S., Kirsh, C., Brewer, H., Kalmbach, K., Olmsted, M. P., Woodside, D. B., & Kaplan, A. S. (1997). The prevalence of high-level exercise in the eating disorders: etiological implications. *Comprehensive Psychiatry, 38(6),* 321-326.

Davis, C., Kennedy, S. H, Ralevski, E. & Dionne, M. (1994). The role of physical activity in the development and maintenance of eating disorders. *Psychological Medicine, 24,* 957-967.

Davis, C., Kennedy, S. H., Ralevski, E., Dionne, M., Brewer, H., Neitzert, C., et al. (1995). Obsessive compulsiveness and physical activity in Anorexia Nervosa and high-level exercising. *Journal of Psychosomatic Research, 39(8),* 967-976.

Dawson, P., & Guare, R. (2004). *Executive skills in children and adolescents: A practical guide to assessment and intervention.* New York: Guilford Press.

De Coverley Veale, D. M. W. (1987). Exercise dependence. *British Journal of Addiction, 87,* 735-40.

De Geus, E. J., Lorenz, J. P. & Van Doornen, P. (1993). The effects of fitness training on thè physiological stress response. *Work & Stress, 7,* 141-159.

De Haan, L. (2009). Bewegen. *Tijdschr.Psychiatr, 51,* 275-277.

De Hert, M., Dekker, J., Wood, D., Kahl, K., & Müller, H. (2009). Cardiovascular disease and diabetes in people with severe mental illness: Position statement from the European Psychiatric Association (EPA), supported by the European Association for the Study of Diabetes (EASD) and the European Society of Cardiology. *European Psychiatry, 24(6),* 412-424.

De Hert, M., Schreurs, V., Vancampfort, D., & Van Winkel, V. (2009). Metabolic syndrome in people with schizophrenia: a review. *World Psychiatry, 8,* 15-22.

De Vries, H. A. (1976). Immediate and long-term effects of exercise upon resting muscle action potential, *Journal of Sports Medicine and Physical Fitness, 8,* 1-11.

De Zwaan, M., & Friederich, H. C. (2006). Binge eating disorder. *Therapeutische Umschau, 63,* 529-533.

Deci, E. L., & Ryan, R. M. (1985). *Intrinsic motivation and self-determination in human behavior.* New York: Plenum.

Deci, E. L., & Ryan, R. M. (2000). The 'what' and 'why' of goal pursuits: human needs and the self-determination of behaviour. *Psychological Inquiry, 11,* 227-268.

Deelman, B., Eling, P., de Haan, E., & van Zomeren, E. (2004). *Klinische neuropsychologie.* Boom: Amsterdam.

Deimel, H. (1983). *Sporttherapie bei psychotischen Erkrankungen : Entwicklung, Methodik und Ergebnisse.* Berlin: Marhold.

DeKlyen, M., & Speltz, M. L. (2001). Attachment and conduct disorder. In J. Hill & B. Maughan (Eds.), *Conduct disorders in childhood and adolescence* (pp. 320-345). Cambridge, UK: Cambridge University Press.

Derogatis, L. R. (1977). *SCL-90-R: Administration scoring and procedures manual.* Baltimore, MD: Clinical Psychometric Research.

Detweiler, M. B., Murphy, P. F., Kim, K.Y., Myers, L. C., & Ashai, A. (2009). Scheduled medications and falls in dementia patients utilizing a wander garden. *American Journal of Alzheimer's Disease and Other Dementias, 14,* 322-332.

Devenport, B. R., & Bourgeois, N. M. (2008). Play, aggression, the preschool child, and the family: A review of literature to guide empirically informed play therapy with aggressive preschool children. *International Journal of Play Therapy, 17(11),* 2-23.

Di Michele, V. & Bolino, F. (2004). The natural course of schizophrenia and psychopathological predictors of outcome. A community-based cohort study. *Psychopathology, 37,* 98-104.

Dickerson, S. S., & Kemeny, M. E. (2004). Acute stressors and cortisol responses: A theoretical integration and synthesis of laboratory research. *Psychological Bulletin, 130,* 355-391.

Dickstein, S. G., Bannon, K., Castellanos, F., & Milham, M. P. (2006). The neural correlates of attention-deficit hyperactivity disorder: An ALE meta-analysis. *Journal of Child Psychology and Psychiatry, 47(10),* 1051-1062.

Dilip, V., Jeste, M. D. (2000) Geriatric psychiatry may be the mainstream psychiatry of the future. *American Journal of Psychiatry, 157,* 1912-1914.

Dinas, P. C., Koutedakis, Y., & Flouris, A. D. (2011). Effects of exercise and physical activity on depression. *Irish Journal of Medical Sciences, 180,* 319-325.

Dinomais, M., Gambart, G., Bruneau, A., Bontoux ,L., Deries, X., Tessiot, C., et al. (2010). Social functioning and self-esteem in young people with disabilities participating in adapted competitive sport. *Neuropediatrics, 41(2),* 49-54.

Dishman, R. K., & Buckworth, J. (1996). Increasing physical activity: a quantitative synthesis. *Medicine & Science in Sports & Exercise, 28,* 706-719.

Dishman, R. K. (1997). Brain monoamines, exercise, and behavioral stress: animal models. *Medicine & Science in Sports & Exercise, 29(1),* 63-74.

Dishman, R. K., & Jackson, E. M. (2000). Exercise, fitness, and stress. *International Journal of Sport Psychology, 31,* 175-203.

Dishman, R. K., Berthoud, H. R., Booth, F. W., Cotman, C. W., Edgerton, V. R., Fleshner, M. R. et al. (2006). Neurobiology of exercise. *Obesity, 14,* 345-356.

Dishman, R. K., Washburn, R. A., & Heath, G.W. (2004). *Physical Activity Epidemiology.* Champaign, IL: Human Kinetics.

Doll-Tepper, G., Dahms C., Doll, B., & von Selzman, H. (Eds.). (1990). *Adapted physical activity: An interdisciplinary approach.* Berlin: Springer-Verlag.

Donadia, G. (2007). *Autismo: características e estrátegias no contexto da Educação Física.* Unpublished master's thesis, Belo Horizonte: Escola de Educação Física, Fisoterapia e Terapia Ocupacional da Unversidade Federal de Minas Gerais.

Donaghy, M., Ralston, G., & Mutrie N. (1991). Exercise as a therapeutic adjunct for problem drinkers. *Journal of Sports Sciences, 9(4),* 440.

Donaghy, M., & Ussher, M. (2005). Exercise intervention in drug and alcohol rehabilitation. In G. Faulkner & A. Taylor (Eds), *Exercise, Health and Mental Health* (pp. 48-69). London: Routledge.

Donnelly, J. E., Blair, S. N., Jakicic, J. M, Manore, M. M., Rankin, J. W, & Smith, B. K. (2009). American College of Sports Medicine Position Stand. Appropriate physical activity intervention strategies for weight loss and prevention of weight regain for adults. *Medicine & Science in Sports & Exercice, 41,* 459-471.

Donnelly, P. (1981). Athletics and juvenile delinquency: A comparative analysis of the literature. *Adolesence, 16,* 415-431.

Douglas, V. I. (1988). Cognitive deficits in children with attention deficit disorder with hyperactivity. In L. M. Bloomingdale & J. Sergeant (Eds.), *Attention deficit disorder: Criteria, cognition, intervention* (pp. 65–81) [Book supplement to the *Journal of Child Psychology and Psychiatry, 5*]. New York: Pergamon Press.

Draheim, C. C., McCubbin, J. A., & Williams, D. P., (2002). Differences in cardiovascular disease risk between non-diabetic adults with Down syndrome and mental retardation. *American Journal on Mental Retardation, 107,* 201-211.

Dröes, R. M. (1992). Beweging als middel in de (re)activering en (re)socialisering van demente ouderen: over de ontwikkeling van bewegingsprogramma's. *Bewegen en hulpverlening, 9,* 118-136.

Dröes, R. M. (1994). Psychomotorische therapie in het verpleeghuis voor demente patiënten. *Bewegen en hulpverlening, 11,* 151-170.

Dröes, R.M. (2001). Bewegingsactivering bij demente bejaarden. In H. Van Coppenolle, & J. Simons (Eds.), *Van Observatie naar psychomotorische therapie.* Acco: Leuven.

Dröes, R. M. (2001). Psychomotorische therapie voor ouderen met dementie. In M. Probst, & R. Bosscher (Eds.), *Ontwikkelingen in de psychomotorische therapie.* Zeist: Cure & Care publishers.

Dröes, R.M., Goffin, J., Bos, J., Oudhof, J. (1999). Bijdrage van de psychomotorische therapie in de behandeling van mensen met dementie. *Bewegen en hulpverlening, 16,* 43-63.

Duncan, J., & Owen, A. M. (2000). Common regions of the human frontal lobe recruited by diverse cognitive demands. *Trends in Neurosciences, 23,* 475-483.

Dunn, A., Trivedi, M. H., Kampert, J., Clark, C., & Chambliss, H. (2005). Exercise treatment for depression efficacy and dose response. *American Journal of Preventive Medicine, 28(1),* 1-8.

Dunn, A. L., & Dishman, R. K. (1991). Exercise and the neurobiology of depression. *Exercise and Sport Sciences Reviews, 19,* 41-98.

Duraiswamy, G., Thirthalli, J., Nagendra, H. R., & Gangadhar, B. N. (2007). Yoga therapy as an add-on treatment in the management of patients with schizophrenia-a randomized controlled trial. *Acta Psychiatrica Scandinavica, 116,* 226-232.

Dustman, R. E, Emerson, R., & Shearer, D. (1994). Physical activity, age, and cognitive-neuropsychological function. *Journal of Aging and Physical Activity, 2,* 143-181.

Dykens, E. M., Rosner, B. A. & Butterbaugh, G. (1998). Exercise and sports in children and adolescents with developmental disabilities: Positive physical and psychosocial effects. *Child and Adolescent Psychiatric Clinics of North America, 7,* 757-771.

Edenfield, T. (2007). Exercise and mood: Exploring the role of exercise in regulating stress reactivity in bipolar disorder. Unpublished doctoral dissertation, University of Maine-Orono.

Edginton, C. R., Jordan, D. J., DeGraaf, D. G., & Edginton, S. (1998). *Leisure and Life Satisfaction: Foundation Perspectives.* Boston: Mc Graw-Hill.

Edwards, N., Gardiner, M., Ritchie, D. M., Baldwin, K., Sands, L. (2008). Effect of exercise on negative affect in

residents in special care units with moderate to severe dementia. *Alzheimer Disease and Associated Disorder, 22(4),* 362-368.

Eichner, E. (1989). Chronic fatigue syndrome: searching for the cause and treatment. *The Physician and SportsMedicine, 17(6),* 142-52.

Ekeland, E., Heian, F., & Hagen, K. B. (2005). Can exercise improve self-esteem in children and young people? A systematic review of randomised controlled trials. *British Journal of Sports Medicine, 39,* 792-798.

Ekkekakis, P., & Acevedo, E. O. (2006). Affective responses to acute exercise: Toward a psychobiological dose-response model. In E. O. Acevedo & P. Ekkekakis (Eds.), *Psychobiology of physical activity* (pp. 91-110). Champaign, IL: Human Kinetics.

Ekwall, A., Lindberg, A., & Magnusson, M. (2009). Dizzy-Why not take a walk? Low level physical activity improves quality of life among elderly with dizziness. *Gerontology, 55(6),* 652-659.

Elliot, R. O., Dobbin, A. R., Rose, G. D., & Soper, H. V. (1994). Vigorous, aerobic exercise versus general motor training activities: effects on maladaptive and stereotypic behaviors with both autism and mental retardation. *Journal of Autism and Developmental Disorders, 24,* 565-576.

Ellis, N., Crone, D., Davey, R., & Grogan, S. (2007). Exercise interventions as an adjunct therapy for psychosis: a critical review. *British Journal of Clinical Psychology, 46 (1),* 95-111.

El-Sayed, M. S., Ali, N., & El-Sayed Ali, Z. (2005). Interaction between alcohol and exercise physiological and haematological implications. *Sports Medicine, 35(3),* 257-269.

Emery, C. F. & Blumenthal, J. A. (1988). Effects of exercise training on psychological functioning in healthy type A men. *Health Psychology, 2,* 367-379.

Emery, C. F, Huppert, F., & Schein, R. L. (1995). Relationship among age, exercise, health and cognitive function in a British sample. *The Gerontologist, 35(3),* 378-385.

Engels, H. J., Currie, J. S., Lueck, C. C., & Wirth, J. C. (2002). Bench/step training with and without extremity loading. Effects on muscular fitness, body composition profile, and psychological affect. *Journal of Sports Medicine and Physical Fitness; 42(1),* 71-78.

Enright, P. L. (2003). The six-minute walk test. *Respiratory Care, 48,* 783-785.

Epling, W. F. & Pierce, W. D. (1996). An overview of activity anorexia. In W. F. Epling & W. D. Pierce (Eds.), *Activity Anorexia theory, research and treatment* (pp. 3-12). New Jersey, NJ: Lawrence Erlbaum Associates.

Eppley, K. R., Abrams, A. I., & Shear, J. (1989). Differential effects of relaxation techniques on trait anxiety: a meta-analysis. *Journal of Clinical Psychology, 45(6),* 957-974.

Erickson, K. I., & Kramer, A. (2009). Aerobic exercise effects on cognitive and neural plasticity in older adults. *British Journal of Sports Medicine, 43,* 22-24.

Erickson, K. I., Prakash, R. S., Voss, M. W., Chaddock, L., Hu, L., Morris, K. S., et al. (2009). Aerobic fitness is associated with hippocampal volume in elderly humans. *Hippocampus, 19,* 1030-1039.

Ermalinski, R., Hanson, P., Lubin, B., Thornby, J., & Nahormek, P. (1997). Impact of a body-mind treatment component on alcoholic inpatients. *Journal of Psychosocial*

Nursing and Mental Health Services, 35(7), 39-45.

Etnier, J. L., Nowell, P. M., Landers, D. M., & Sibley, B. A. (2006). A meta-regression to examine the relationship between aerobic fitness and cognitive performance. *Brain Research Reviews, 52*, 119-130.

Etnier, J. L., Salazar, W., Landers, D. M., Petruzzello, S. J., Han, M. & Nowell, P. (1997). The influence of physical fitness and exercise upon cognitive functioning: A meta-analysis, *Journal of Sport and Exercise Psychology, 19*, 249-277.

Ettema, T., de Lange, J., Droes, R.M., Mellenbergh, D., & Ribbe, M. (2005). Handleiding Qualidem: een meetinstrument kwaliteit van leven bij mensen met dementie in verpleeg- en verzorgingstehuizen, Versie 1. [Manual Qualidem: a measuring quality of life in people with dementia in nursing homes, version 1]. VUmc/EMGO-instituut, afdeling Psychiatrie en afdeling Huisarts-, Sociale en Verpleeghuisgeneeskunde.

Evans, R., Levy, L., Sullenberger, T., & Vyas, A. (1991). Self concept and delinquency: The on-going debate. *Journal of Offender Rehabilitation, 16*, 59-74.

Ewing, G., McDermott, S., Thomas-Kroger, M., Whitner, W., & Pierce, K. (2004). Evaluation of a cardiovascular health program for participants with mental retardation and normal learners. *Health Education and Behavior, 31*, 77-87.

Exner, C., Hebebrand, J., Remschmidt, H., Wewetzer, C., Ziegler, A., Herpertz, S., Schweiger, U., Blum, W.F., Preibisch, G., Heldmaier, G., & Klingenspor, M. (2000). Leptin suppresses semi-starvation induced hyperactivity in rats: implications for anorexia nervosa. *Molecular Psychiatry, 5(5)*, 476-481.

Expert panel on detection and evaluation of high blood cholesterol in adults (2001). Executive summary of the third report of the expert panel on detection, evaluation, and treatment of high blood cholesterol in adults (Adult Treatment Panel III). *Journal of the American Medical Association, 285*, 2486-2497.

Ey, H. B. P., & Brisset, C. H. (1978). *Tratado de Psiquiatría*. Barcelona: Toray-Masson.

Fabel, K., & Kempermann, G. (2008). Physical activity and the regulation of neurogenesis in the adult and aging brain. *Neuromolecular Medicine, 10*, 59-66.

Fagiolini, A, Frank, E., Scott, J. A., Turkin, S., & Kupfer, D. J.(2005). Metabolic syndrome in bipolar disorder: findings from the Bipolar Disorder Center for Pennsylvanians. *Bipolar Disorders, 7*, 424-430.

Fagiolini, A., & Chengappa, K. N. R. (2007). Weight gain and metabolic issues of medicines used for bipolar disorder. *Current Psychiatry Reports, 9*, 521-528.

Fairburn, C.G., Cooper, Z., & Shafran, R. (2003). Cognitive behaviour therapy for ED: A "transdiagnostic" theory and treatment. *Behaviour Research and Therapy, 41*, 509-528.

Farmer, M. E., Locke, B. Z., Moscicki, E. K., Dannenberg, A. L., Larson, D. B., & Radloff, L. S. (1988). Physical activity and depressive symptoms: the NHANES I epidemiologic follow-up study. *American Journal of Epidemiology, 128*, 1340-1351.

Faulkner, G. (2005). Exercise as an adjunct treatment for schizophrenia. In G. Faulkner & A. Taylor (Eds.), Exercise, health and mental health: Emerging relationships (pp. 27-45). London: Routledge.

Faulkner, G. & Biddle, S. (1999). Exercise as an adjunct treatment for schizophrenia: a review of the literature. *Journal of Mental Health, 8*, 441-457.

Faulkner, G., & Carless, D. (2006). Physical activity in the process of psychiatric rehabilitation: theoretical and methodological issues. *Psychiatric Rehabilitation Journal, 29(4)*, 258-266.

Faulkner, G., Cohn, T., & Remington, G. (2006). Validation of a physical activity assessment tool for individuals with schizophrenia. *Schizophrenia Research, 82*, 225-231.

Faulkner, G., Cohn, T., Remington, G., & Irving, H. (2007). Body mass index, waist circumference and quality of life in individuals with schizophrenia. *Schizophrenia Research, 90*, 174-178.

Faulkner, G., & Taylor, A. (2005). *Exercise, Health and Mental Health Emerging relationships*. London: Routledge Taylor and Francis Group.

Favaro, A., Caregaro, L., Tenconi, E., Bosello, R., & Santonastaso, P. (2009). Time trends in age of onset of anorexia nervosa and bulimia nervosa. *Journal of Clinical Psychiatry, 70*, 1715-1721.

Favaro, A., Ferrara, S., & Santonastaso, P. (2003). The spectrum of eating disorders in young women: a prevalence study in a general population sample. *Psychosomatic Medicine, 65*, 701-708.

Favaro, A., Ferrara, S., & Santonastaso, P. (2007). Self-injurious behavior in a community sample of young women: relationship with childhood abuse and other types of self-damaging behaviors. *Journal of Clinical Psychiatry, 68*, 122-131.

Favaro, A., & Santonastaso, P. (2008). The value of anorexia nervosa subtypes. *American Journal of Psychiatry, 165*, 772-773.

Fazio, R. H., Effrein, E. A., & Falender, V. J. (1981). Self-perceptions following social interactions. *Journal of Personality and Social Psychology, 41*, 232-242.

Feighner, J. P., Robins, E., Guze, S. B., Woodruff, R. A., Winokur, G., & Munoz, R. (1972). Diagnostic criteria for use in psychiatric research. *Archives of General Psychiatry, 26*, 57-63.

Feist, G. J., Bodner, T. E., Jacobs, J. F., Miles, M., & Tan, V. (1995). Integrating top-down and bottom-up structural models of subjective well-being: A longitudinal investigation. *Journal of Personality and Social Psychology, 68*, 138-150.

Fernhall, B., & Pitetti, K. H. (2001). Limitations to physical work capacity in individuals with mental retardation. *Clinical Exercise Physiology, 3*, 176-185.

Fernandes da Fonseca, A. (1997). *Psiquiatria e Psicopatologia*. Lisboa: Fundação Calouste Gulbenkian.

Fiore, T. A., Becker, E. A., & Nero, R. C. (1993). Educational interventions for students with ADD. *Exceptional Children, 60*, 771-773.

Fleischhacker, W. W., Cetkovich-Bakmas, M., De Hert, M., Hennekens, C. H., Lambert, M., Leucht, S. et al. (2008). Comorbid somatic illnesses in patients with severe mental disorders: clinical, policy, and research challenges. *Journal of Clinical Psychiatry, 69*, 514-519.

Fogarty, M., Happell, B., & Pinikahana, J. (2004). The benefits of an exercise program for people with schizophrenia: a pilot study. *Psychiatric Rehabilitation Journal, 28*, 173-176.

Forcier, K., Stroud, L. R., Papandonatos, G. D., Hitsman, B., Reiches, M., Krishnamoorthy, J., et al. (2006). Links between physical fitness and cardiovascular reactivity and recovery to psychological stressors: A meta-analysis. *Health Psychology, 25,* 723-739.

Fossati, M., Amati, F., Painot, D., Reiner, M., Haenni, C., & Golay, A. (2004). Cognitive-behavioral therapy with simultaneous nutritional and physical activity education in obese patients with binge eating disorder. *Eating Weight Disorders, 9,* 134-138.

Fosson, A., Knibbs, J., Bryant-Waugh, R., & Lask, B. (1987). Early onset anorexia nervosa. *Archives of Disease in Childhood, 62(2),* 114-118.

Fox, D. J., Tharp, D. F., & Fox, L. C. (2005). Neurofeedback: An alternative and efficacious treatment for Attention-Deficit/Hyperactivity Disorder. *Applied Psychophysiology and Biofeedback, 30(4),* 365-373.

Fox, K. R. (1997). *The physical self.* Champaign, IL: Human Kinetics.

Fox, K. R. (1997). The physical self and processes in self-esteem development. In K. R. Fox (Ed), *The Physical self: From motivation to well-being* (pp. 111-139). Champaign, IL: Human Kinetics.

Fox, K. R. (2000). Physical activity and mental health promotion: the natural partnership. *International Journal of Mental Health Promotion, 2,* 4-12.

Fox, K. R. (2000). Self-esteem, self-perceptions and exercise. *International Journal of Sport Psychology, 31,* 228-240.

Fox, K. R., & Corbin, C. B. (1989). The physical self-perception profile: development and preliminary validation. *Journal of Sport and Exercise Psychology, 11,* 408-430.

Fox, K. R., Stathi, A., McKenna, K., & Davis, M. G. (2007). Physical activity and mental well-being in older people participating in the better ageing project. *European Journal of Applied Physiology, 100,* 591-602.

Frederick, C. M. & Ryan, R. M. (1993). Differences in motivation for sport and exercise and their relationship with participation and mental health. *Journal of Sport Behavior, 16,* 125-145.

Frick, P. J. (1998). *Conduct disorders and severe antisocial behaviour.* New York, NY: Plenum.

Frick, P. J. (2001). Effective interventions for children and adolescents with conduct disorder. *Canadian Journal of Psychiatry/Revue Canadienne de Psychiatrie, 46,* 597-608.

Friedman, R., Tappen, R. M. (1991). The effect of planned walking on communication in Alzheimer's disease. *Journal of the American Geriatric Society, 39,* 650-654.

Froelich, J. C. (1997). Opioid peptides. *Alcohol Health and Research World, 21,* 132-135.

Frostig, M. (1975). *Frostig motorio. L'educazione mentale mediante il movimento. Guida per l'insegnante.* Torino: Omega.

Fuchs, R., & Klaperski, S. (2012). Sportliche Aktivität und Stressregulation *[Exercise and stress regulation].* In R. Fuchs & W. Schlicht (Eds.), *Sport und seelische Gesundheit.* Göttingen: Hogrefe.

Fuchs, T., Birbaumer, N., Lutzenberg, W., Gruzelier, J. H., & Kaiser, J. (2003). Neurofeedback treatment for Attention-Deficit/Hyperactivity Disorder: A comparison with methylphenidate. *Applied Psychophysiology and Biofeedback, 28(1),* 1-12.

Gailliot, M. T., & Baumeister, R. F. (2007). The physiology of willpower: Linking blood glucose to self-control. *Personality and Social Psychology Bulletin, 11,* 303-327.

Gaitanis, P., Tooley, G., & Edwards, B. (2005). Physical activity, emotional stress, sleep disturbances, and daily fluctuations in chronic fatigue symptomatology. *Journal of Applied Biobehavioral Research, 10,* 69-82.

Galper, D. I., Trivedi, M. H., Barlow, C. E., Dunn, A. L., & Kampert, J. B. (2006). Inverse association between physical inactivity and mental health in men and women. *Medicine & Sciences in Sports & Exercise, 38,* 173-178.

Gapin, J., & Etnier, J. (2009). Physical activity and cognitive performance in children with attention deficit hyperactivity disorder (ADHD)-Does physical activity participation predict executive function? *Journal of Sport & Exercise Psychology, 31,* S11-S12.

Garriott, J. (2008). *Garriott's medicolegal aspects of alcohol, fifth edition.* Tucson, AZ: Lawyers & Judges Publishing Company.

Gaudiano, B., Weinstock, L., & Miller, I. (2008). Improving treatment adherence in bipolar disorder: a review of current psychosocial treatment efficacy and recommendations for future treatment development. *Behavior Modification, 32,* 267-301.

Gerber, M. (2008). *Sport, stress und gesundheit bei jugendlichen [Exercise, stress and health among adolescents].* Schorndorf: Hofmann.

Gerber, M., Hartmann, T., Lang, C., Lüthy, M., & Brand, S. (2010). *Stressmanagement im Sportunterricht. Ein Trainingsprogramm in 8 Modulen. Broschüre für BerufsschülerInnen [Coping training in physical education. A training program in 8 modules. Students' manual].* Dübendorf: Helsana Versicherungen AG.

Gerber, M., Holsboer-Trachsler, E., Pühse, U., & Brand, S. (2011). Elite sport is not an additional source of distress for adolescents with high stress levels. *Perceptual and Motor Skills, 112,* 581-599.

Gerber, M., Kellmann, M., Hartmann, T., & Pühse, U. (2010). Do exercise and fitness buffer against stress among Swiss police and emergency response service officers? *Psychology in Sport and Exercise, 11,* 286-294.

Gerber, M., & Pühse, U. (2009). Do exercise and fitness protect against stress-induced health complaints? A review of the literature. *Scandinavian Journal of Public Health, 37,* 801-819.

Gevensleben, H., Holl, B., Albrecht, B., Vogel, C., Schlamp, D., Kratz, O., et al. (2009). Is neurofeedback an efficacious tratment for ADHD? A randomized controlled clinical trial. *Journal of Child Psychology and Psychiatry, 50(7),* 780-789.

Giannetti, E. (2002). *Felicidade diálogo sobre o bem-estar na civilização.* São Paulo: Companhia das Letras.

Ginis, K. A., Latimer, A. E., McKechnie, K., Ditor, D. S., McCartney, N., Hicks, A. L., et al. (2003). Using exercise to enhance subjective well-being among people with spinal cord injury: The mediating influences of stress and pain. *Rehabilitation Psychology, 48,* 157-164.

Girardi, N. L., Shaywitz, S. E., Shaywitz , B. A., Marchione, K., Fleischman, S. J., Jones, T. J, et al (1995). Blunted catecholamine responses after glucose ingestion in children with attention deficit disorder. *Pediatric Research, 38,* 539-542.

Glass, R. M. (1999). Treating depression as a recurrent or chronic disease [editorial]. *Journal of American Medical Association, 28(1),* 83-84.

Glenister, D. (1996). Exercise and mental health: a review. *Journal of the Royal Society of Health, 2,* 7-13.

Gold, S. M., Zakowski, S. G., Valdimarsdottir, H. B., & Bovbjerg, D. H. (2003). Stronger endocrine responses after brief psychological stress in women at familial risk of breast cancer. *Psychoneuroendocrinology, 28,* 584-593.

Goodman, E., Whitaker, R. (2002). A prospective study of the role of depression in the development and persistence of adult obesity. *Pediatrics, 110,* 497-504.

Goodwin, R. D (2003). Association between physical activity and mental disorders among adults in the United States. *Preventive Medicine, 36,* 698-703.

Gothelf, D., Falk, B., Singer, P., Kairi, M., Phillip, M., Zigel, L., et al. (2002). Weight gain associated with increased food intake and low habitual activity levels in male adolescent schizophrenic inpatients treated with olanzapine. *American Journal of Psychiatry, 6,* 1055-1057.

Graham, A., & Reid, G., (2000). Physical fitness of adult with intellectual disability: a 13-year follow-up study. *Research Quarterly for Exercise and Sport, 71,* 152-161.

Grant, K. E., Compas, B. E., Thurm, A. E., McMahon, S. D., & Gipson, P. Y. (2004). Stressors and child and adolescent psychopathology: Measurement issues and prospective effects. *Journal of Clinical Child & Adolescent Psychology, 33,* 412-425.

Grant, K. E., Compas, B. E., Thurm, A. E., McMahon, S. D., Gipson, P. Y., Campbell, A. J., et al. (2006). Stressors and child and adolescent psychopathology: Evidence of moderating and mediating effects. *Clinical Psychological Journal, 26,* 257-283.

Grant, S., Aitchison, T., Henderson, E., Christie, J., Zare S., McMurray, J., & Dargie, H. (1999). A comparison of the reproducibility and the sensitivity to change of visual analogue scales, Borg scales, and Likert scales in normal subjects during submaximal exercise. *CHEST,* 116,1208-1217.

Greco, M., & Carvalho, A. (1994). *Centro de Convivência para Pacientes Psiquiátricos do Bairro São Paulo.* Belo Horizonte: Secretaria de Municipal de Saúde.

Green, A. I., Drake, R. E., Brunette, M. F., & Noordsy, D. L. (2007). Schizophrenia and co-occurring substance use disorder. *American Journal of Psychiatry, 164,* 402-408.

Gregg, L., Barrowclough, C., & Haddock, G. (2007). Reasons for increased substance use in psychosis. *Clinical Psychogyl Review, 27,* 494-510.

Griest, J. H., Klein, M. H., Eischens, R. R., Faris, J., Gurman, A.S., & Morgan, W. P. (1979). Running as treatment for depression. *Comprehensive Psychiatry, 20(1),* 41-54.

Grilo, C. M. (2006). Obesity: assessment and treatment. In *Eating and Weight Disorders* (pp. 143-184). New York: Psychology Press.

Grossman, H. J. (1983). *Classification in mental retardation.* Washington, DC: American Association on Mental Deficiency.

Grundy, S. M., Cleeman, J. I., Daniels, S. R., Donato, K. A., Eckel, R. H., Franklin, B. A. et al. (2005). Diagnosis and management of the metabolic syndrome: an American Heart Association/National Heart, Lung, and Blood Institute Scientific Statement. *Circulation, 112,* 2735-2752.

Guay, F, Vallerand, R. J., & Blanchard, C. (2000). On the assessment of situational intrinsic and extrinsic motivation: the Situational Motivation Scale (SIMS). *Motivation and Emotion,* 24, 3, 175-213.

Guérin, F., Marsh, H. W., & Famose, J. P. (2003). Construct salidation of the Self-Description Questionnaire II with a french sample. *European Journal of Psychological Assessment, 19,* 142-150.

Guest, A. M., & McRee, N. (2009). A school-level analysis of adolescent extracurricular activity, delinquency, and depression: The importance of situational context. *Journal of Youth and Adolescence, 38,* 51-62.

Guicciardi, M., Castelli, D. & Lussu, C. (1999). Contributo alla validazione della scala di consapevolezza corporea ed efficienza fisica del CBA-Sport [Contribution to the validation of the scale of body awareness and physical efficiency of the CBA-Sport]. In F. Marini (Ed.), *II fare della psicologia.* Cagliari: CUEC.

Guidetti, L., Franciosi, E., Gallotta, M. C., Emerenziani, G. P., & Baldari, C., (2010). Could sport specialization influence fitness and health of adults with mental retardation? *Research in Developmental Disabilities, 31(5),* 1070-1075.

Gustafsson, G., Lira C. M., Johansson, J., Wisén, A., Wohlfart, B., Ekman, R., et al. (2009). The acute response of plasma brain-derived neurotrophic factor as a result of exercise in major depressive disorder. *Psychiatry Research, 169(3),* 244-248.

Guyatt, G., Gutterman, D., Baumann, M., Addrizzo-Harris, D., Hylek, E., Phillips, B., et al. (2006). Grading strength of recommendations and quality of evidence in clinical guidelines: report from an American college of chest physicians task force. *Chest, 129,* 174-181.

Hall, G.S. (1902). *Youth.* New York, NY: Appleton.

Hallal, P. C. Victora, C. G., Azevedo , M. R. & Wells, J. C. K. (2006). Adolescent physical activity and health: A systematic review. *Sports Medicine, 36(12),* 1019-1030

Hallowell, E. M., & Ratey, J. J. (1992). Adults ADHA:50 tips of management. Retrieved from http://www.addresources. org/?q=print/node/253

Haltom, C. (2004). Eating disorder survival guide for family and friends: exercise. In C. Haltom. (Ed.), *A Stranger at the Table: Dealing with Your Child's Eating Disorder.* Carrollton, TX: Hewell Publishing.

Hamer, M., Taylor, A., & Steptoe, A. (2006). The effect of acute exercise on stress related blood pressure responses: A systematic review and meta-analysis. *Biological Psychology, 71,* 183-190.

Hand, G. A., Phillips, K. D., & Wilson, M. A. (2006). Central regulation of stress reactivity and physical activity. In E. O. Acevedo & P. Ekkekakis (Eds.), *Psychobiology of physical activity* (pp. 189-202). Champaign, IL: Human Kinetics.

Handapp, R. M., & Dykens, E. M., (2003). Mental retardation (intellectual disability). In E. J. Mash & R. A. Barkley (Eds), *Child Psychopathology* (2nd ed., pp. 486-519). New York, NY: The Guilford Press.

Hanin, Y. L. (Ed.). (2000). *Emotions in sport.* Champaign, IL: Human Kinetics.

Hannaford, C. P., Harrell, E. H., Cox, K. (1988). Psycho-physiological effects of a running program on depression and anxiety in a psychiatric population. *Psychological Record, 38 (1),* 37-48.

Hansen, C. J., Stevens, L. C., Coast, J. R. (2001). Exercise duration and mood state: how much is enough to feel better? *Health Psychology, 20(4),* 267-275.

Harter, S. (1993). Vision of self: beyond the me in the mirror. In J. E Jacobs (Ed.), *Developmental Perspectives on Motivation* (pp. 99-144). Lincoln: University of Nebraska Press.

Harter, S., Whitesell, N. R., & Junkin, L. J. (1998). Similarities and differences in domain-specific and global self-evaluations of learning-disabled, behaviorally disordered, and normally achieving adolescents. *American Educational Research Journal, 35,* 653-680.

Harvey, W., & Reid, G. (2005). Attention-Deficit/Hyperactivity disorder: APA research challenges. *Adapted Physical Activity Quarterly, 22,* 1-20.

Harvey, W. J., Reid, G., Bloom, G. A., Staples, K., Grizenko, N., Mbekou, V., et al. (2009). Physical activity experiences of boys with and without ADHD. *Adapted Physical Activity Quarterly, 26,* 131-150.

Haskell, W. L., Lee, I. M., Pate, R. R., Powell, K. E., Blair, S. N., Franklin, B. A. et al. (2007). Physical activity and public health: updated recommendation for adults from the American College of Sports Medicine and the American Heart Association. *Medicine & Science in Sports & Exercise, 39(8),* 1423-1434.

Hasson-Ohayon, I., Kravetz, S., Roe, D., Rozencwaig, S., & Weiser, M. (2006). Qualitative assessment of a verbal and non-verbal psychosocial interventions with persons with severe mental illness. *Journal of Mental Health, 15,* 343-353.

Hausenblas, H. A., & Carron, A. (1999). Eating disorders indices and athletes: an integration. *Journal of Sport and Exercise Psychology, 21,* 230-258.

Hausenblas, H. A., Cook, B., & Chittester, N. (2008). Can exercise treat eating disorders. *Exercise and Sport Sciences Reviews, 36,* 43-47.

Hausenblas, H. A., & Down, D. S. (2002). Exercise dependence: a systematic review. *Psychology of Sport and Exercise, 3,* 89-123.

Hausenblas, H. A., & Fallon, E. (2006). Exercise and body image: a meta-analysis. *Psychology & Health, 21,* 33-47.

Hebebrand, J., Exner, C., Hebebrand, K., Holtkamp, C., Casper, R.C., Remschmidt, H., Herpertz-Dahlmann, B., & Klingenspor, M. (2003). Hyperactivity in patients with anorexia nervosa and in semistarved rats: evidence for a pivotal role of hypoleptinemia. *Physiology and Behavior, 79(1),* 25-37.

Hennekens, C. H., Hennekens, A. R., Hollar, D., & Casey, D. E. (2005). Schizophrenia and increased risks of cardiovascular disease. *American Heart Journal, 150,* 1115-1121.

Herbert, J., & Martinez, M. (2001). Neural Mechanisms underlying aggressive behaviour. In J. Hill & B. Maughan (Eds.), *Conduct disorders in childhood and adolescence* (pp. 67-102). Cambridge, UK: Cambridge University Press.

Heyn, P., Abreu, B. C., Ottenbacher, K. J. (2004). The effects of exercise training on elderly persons with cognitive impairment and dementia: a meta-analysis. *Archives of Physical Medicine and Rehabilitation, 85(10),* 1694-1704.

Hill, J. (2001). Biosocial influences on antisocial behaviours in childhood and adolescence. In J. Hill & B. Maughan (Eds.), *Conduct disorders in childhood and adolescence* (pp. 103-125). Cambridge, UK: Cambridge University Press.

Hill, J. (2002). Biological, psychological and social processes in the conduct disorders. *Journal of Child Psychology and Psychiatry, 43,* 133-164.

Hill, J. W. (1987). Exercise prescription. *Primary Care, 14 (4),* 817-825.

Hill, J. O., & Wyatt, H. R. (2005). Role of physical activity in preventing and treating obesity. *Journal of Applied Physiology, 99,* 765-770.

Hillebrand, J. J., Koeners, M. P., de Rijke, C. E., Kas, M. J., & Adan, R.A. (2005). Leptin treatment in activity-based anorexia. *Biological Psychiatry, 15(58),*165-71.

Hillman, C. H., Castelli, D. & Buck, S. M. (2005). Aerobic fitness and cognitive function in healthy preadolescent children. *Medicine Science of Sport and Exercise, 37,* 1967-1974.

Hillman, C. H., Erickson, K. I. & Kramer, A. F. (2008). Be smart, exercise your heart: exercise effects on brain and cognition. *Nature Reviews Neuroscience, 9,* 58-65.

Hinshaw, S. P. (1992). Academic underachievement, attention deficits, and aggression: Comorbidity and implications for intervention. *Journal of Consulting and Clinical Psychology, 60(6),* 893-903.

Hirschfield, R. M., Keller, M. B., Panico, S., Arons, B. S., Barlow, D., Davidoff, F. et al. (1997). The national depressive and manic-depressive association consensus statement on the undertreatment of depression. *Journal of the American Medicine Association, 277,* 333-340.

Hirschi, T. (1969). *Causes of delinquency.* Berkeley, CA: University of California Press.

Hobfoll, S. E. (1998). *Stress, culture, and community. The psychology and philosophy of stress.* New York: Plenum Press.

Hobson, M. L., & Rejeski, W. J. (1993). Does the dose of acute exercise mediate psychophysiological responses to mental stress. *Journal of Sport & Exercise Psychology, 15,* 77-87.

Hoffman, M. D., & Hoffman, D. R. (2008). Exercisers achieve greateracute exercise-induced mood enhancement than nonexercisers. *Archives of Physical Medicine and Rehabilitation, 89,* 358-363.

Hoffmann, J. P., & Gray Cerbone, F. (1999). Stressful life events and delinquency escalation in early adolescence. *Criminology, 37,* 343-374.

Holanda Ferreira, A. B. (1986). *Novo Dicionário da Língua Portuguesa.* Rio de Janeiro: Editora Fronteira S. A.

Holmberg, S. K. (1997). Evaluation of a clinical intervention for wanderers on a geriatric nursing unit. *Archives of Psychiatric Nursing, 11,* 21-28.

Holmes, T. H., & Rahe, R. H. (1967). The Social Readjustment Scale. *Journal of Psychosomatic Research, 11,* 213-218.

Hölter, G. (2011). *Bewegungstherapie bei psychischen Erkrankungen.* Köln, Germany: Deutscher Ärzte-verlag.

Holtkamp, K., Hebebrand, J., & Herpertz-Dahlmann, B.

(2004). The contribution of anxiety and food restriction on physical activity levels in acute Anorexia Nervosa. *International Journal of Eating Disorders, 36(2)*, 163-171.

Hong, S. (2000). Exercise and psychoneuroimmunology. *International Journal of Sport Psychology, 31*, 204-227.

Hopman-Rock, M., Staats, P. G. M., Tak, E. C. P. M., Dröes, R. M. (1999). The effects of a psychomotor activation programme for use in groups of cognitively impaired people in homes for the elderly. *International Journal of Geriatric Psychiatry, 14(8)*, 633-642.

Hopman-Rock, M., Staats, P. G. M., Tak, E. C. P. M., Dröes, R. M. (2000). Effecten van een bewegingsactiveringsprogramma voor dementerende ouderen in verzorgingstehuizen. *Bewegen en hulpverlening, 17*, 151-163.

Howells, F. M., Russell, V. A., Mabandla, M. V., & Kellaway, L. A. (2005). Stress reduces the neuroprotective effect of exercise in a rat model for Parkinson's disease. *Behavioral Brain Research, 165(2)*, 210-220.

Howley, E. T. & Franks, D. B. (1997). *Health fitness instructor's handbook* (3th. ed.). Champaign, IL: Human Kinetics.

Hu, F. B. (2008). Physical Activity Measurements. In F. B. Hu (Ed.), *Obesity Epidemiology* (pp. 119-145). New York: Oxford University Press.

Hu, F. B. (2008). Physical Activity, Sedentary Behaviors, and Obesity. In F.B. Hu (Ed.), *Obesity Epidemiology* (pp. 301-319). New York: Oxford University Press.

Huang, K., Su, T., Chen, T., Chou, Y., & Bai, Y. (2009). Comorbidity of cardiovascular diseases with mood and anxiety disorder: A population based 4-year study. *Psychiatry and Clinical Neurosciences, 63*, 401-409.

Hui, E., Chui, B. T., Woo, J. (2009). Effects of dance on physical and psychological well-being in older persons. *Archives of gerontology and geriatrics, 49*, 45-50.

Huijsman, R., Wielink, G., de Klerk, M. M. Y. (1996). Lichaamsbeweging bij ouderen: een literatuuroverzicht van effecten. *Bewegen en hulpverlening, 13*, 159-182.

Hurtado, J. (1991). *Dicionário de Psicomotricidade-Guia técnico-científico para o terapeuta em Psicomotricidade e ciências afins*. Porto Alegre: Prodil.

Huxley, P. (1998). Quality of Life. In N. T. T. Mueser (Ed.), *Handbook of Social Functioning in Schizophrenia* (pp. 52- 64). Needham Heights: Allyn and Bacon.

Instituto Brasileiro de Geografia e Estatística. (2007). [http://www.ibge.gov.br].

International Society of Sport Psychology (1992). Physical activity and psychological benefits: a position statement from the International Society of Sport Psychology. *Journal of Applied Sport Psychology, 4*, 94-98.

Jablensky, A. (1995). Schizophrenia: recent epidemiologic issues. *Epidemiologic Reviews, 17*, 10-20.

Jackson, E. M., & Dishman, R. K. (2006). Cardiorespiratory fitness and laboratory stress: A meta-regression analysis. *Psychophysiology, 43*, 57-72.

Jacob, R. G., Chesney, M. A., Williams, D. M. (1991). Relaxation therapy for hypertension: design effects and treatment effects. *Annals Behavioral Medicine, 13(1)*, 5-17.

Jacobs, G. D., Rosenberg, P. A., Friedman, R. (1993). Multifactor behavioral treatment of chronic sleep-onset insomnia using stimulus control and the relaxation response: a preliminary study. *Behavior Modification, 17(4)*, 498-509.

Jakicic, J. M. (2003). Physical activity as a therapeutic modality. In R. E. Andersen (Ed.), *Obesity Etiology Assessment Treatment and Prevention* (pp. 203-215). Champaign, IL: Human Kinetics.

Janicki, M. P., Davidson, P. W., Henderson, C. M., McCallion, P., Taets, J. D., Force, L. T., et al. (2002). Health characteristics and health services utilization in older adults with intellectual disability living in community residences. *Journal of Intellectual Disability Research, 46*, 287-298.

Janis, I.L., Mann, L. (1977). Decision making: a psychological analysis of conflict, choice and commitment. New York, NY: Free Press.

Jeannin, A., Narring, F., Tschumper, A., Inderwildi Bonivento, L., Addor, V., Bütikofer, A., et al. (2005). Self-reported health needs and use of primary health care services by adolescents enrolled in post-mandatory schools or vocational training programmes in Switzerland. *Swiss Medical Weekly, 135*, 11-18.

Johnson, J. H., Rasbury, W. C., Siegel, L. J. (1997). *Approaches to child treatment: Introduction to theory, research, and practice*. Boston: Allyn and Bacon.

Johnston, O., Reilly, J. Kremer, J. (2011). Excessive exercise: from quantitative categorization to a qualitative continuum approach. *European Eating Disorders Review, 19*, 237-248.

Jones, J. M., Jones, K. D. (1997). Promoting physical activity in the senior years. *Journal of Gerontological Nursing, 23(7)*, 41-48.

Jonsdottir, I., Rödjer, L., Hadzibajramovic, E., Börjeson, M., & Ahlborg, G. (2010). A prospective study of leisure-time physical activity and mental health in Swedish health care workers and social insurance officers. *Preventive Medicine, 51*, 373-377.

Juckel, G. & Morosini, P. L. (2008). The new approach: psychosocial functioning as a necessary outcome criterion for therapeutic success in schizophrenia. *Current Opinion in Psychiatry, 21*, 630-639.

Kahn, C., & Pike, K. M. (2001). In search of predictors of dropout from inpatient treatment for anorexia nervosa. *International Journal of Eating Disorders, 30*, 237-244.

Kaplan, B., & Sadock, V. (2001). *Pocket handbook of clinical psychiatry, third edition*. Philadelphia, PA: Lippincott Williams & Williams.

Kavussanu, M., & McAuley, E. (1995). Training and optimism: Are highly active individuals more optimistic? *Journal of Sport & Exercise Psychology, 17*, 246-258.

Kazdin, A. E. (1994). *Behaviour modification in applied settings* (5th ed.). Pacific Grove, CA: Brooks/Cole Pub. Co.

Kendler, K. S, First, M. B. (2010). Alternative futures for the DSM revision process: iteration v. paradigm shift. *British Journal of Psychiatry 197*, 263-265.

Kendzierski, D., & De Carlo, K. L. (1991). Physical activity enjoyment scale: two validation studies. *Journal of Sport & Exercise Psychology*, 13, 50-64.

Kerr, J. H. (1987). Structural phenomenology, arousal and performance. *Journal of Human Movement Studies, 13(5)*, 211-229.

Kerr, K. (2000). Relaxation techniques: a critical review.

Critical Reviews in Physical and Rehabilitation Medicine, 12, 51-89.

Keyes, K. M., Hatzenbuehler, M. L., & Hasin, D. S. (2011). Stressful life experiences, alcohol consumption, and alcohol use disorders: the epidemiologic evidence for four main types of stressors. *Psychopharmacology, 218(1),* 1-17.

Kiesling, S. (1983). Brain games. *American Health, 2(1),* 25.

King, A., Rejeski, W. J., Buchner, D. M. (1998). Physical activity interventions targeting older adults: A critical review and recommendations. *American Journal of Preventative Medicine, 15(4),* 316-333.

King, A. C., Frey-Hewitt, B., Dreon, D. M., Wood, P. D. (1989). Diet vs exercise in weight maintenance. The effects of minimal intervention strategies on long-term outcomes in men. *Archive of Internal Medicine, 149(12),* 2741-2746.

Kiphard, E. J. (1994). *Psychomotorik in Praxis und Theorie.* Dortmund: Flottmann.

Kirkbride, J. B., Fearon, P., Morgan, C., Dazzan, P., Morgan, K., Tarrant, J. et al. (2006). Heterogeneity in incidence rates of schizophrenia and other psychotic syndromes: findings from the 3-center AeSOP study. *Archives of General Psychiatry, 63,* 250-258.

Kirschbaum, C., Pirke, K. M., & Hellhammer, D. H. (1993). The Trier Social Stress Test: A tool for investigating psychobiological stress responses in a laboratory setting. *Neuropsychobiology, 28,* 76-81.

Kjaer, M. (1992). Regulation of hormonal and metabolic responses during exercise in humans. *Exercise and Sport Science Review, 20,* 161-184.

Klaperski, S., & Fuchs, R. (2011). Einfluss der Sportaktivität auf die Stressreaktivität bei Frauen *[Influence of exercise on stress reactivity among women].* In K. Hottenrott, O. Stoll & R. Wollny (Eds.), *Kreativität – Innovation – Leistung. Wissenschaft bewegt SPORT bewegt Wissenschaft* (p. 118). Hamburg: Feldhaus.

Klein, D. C., Fencil-Morse, E., & Seligman, M. E. (1976). Learned helplessness, depression, and the attribution of failure. *Journal of Personality and Social Psychology, 33,* 508-516.

Klein, D. A., Mayer, L. E. S., Schebendach, J. E., & Walsh, B.T. (2007). Physical activity and cortisol in Anorexia Nervosa. *Psychoneuroendocrinology, 32,* 539-547.

Knapen, J., Sommerijns, E., Vancampfort, D., Sienaert, P., Pieters, G., Haake, P., et al. (2009). State anxiety and subjective well-being responses to acute bouts of aerobic exercise in patients with depressive and anxiety disorders. *British Journal of Sports Medicine, 43,* 756-759.

Knapen, J., Van de Vliet, P., Van Coppenolle, H., Peuskens, J., & Pieters, G. (2003). Evaluation of cardio-respiratory fitness and perceived exertion for patients with depressive and anxiety disorders: A study on reliability. *Disability and Rehabilitation, 25,* 1312-1315.

Knapen, J., Van de Vliet, P., Van Coppenolle, H., David, A., Peuskens, J., Pieters, G., et al. (2005). Comparison of changes in physical self-concept, global self-esteem, depression and anxiety following two different psychomotor therapy programs in non-psychotic psychiatric inpatients. *Psychotherapy and Psychosomatics, 74,* 353-361.

Knöchel, C., Oertel-Knöchel, V., O'Dwyer, L., Prvulovic, D., Alves, G., Kollmann, B., Hampel, H. (2012). Cognitive and behavioural effects of physical exercise in psychiatric patients. *Progress in Neurobiology, 96(1),* 46-68.

Knol, M., Twisk, J., Beekman, A., Heine, R., Snoek, F., & Pouwer, F. (2006). Depression as a risk factor for the onset of type 2 diabetes mellitus. A meta-analysis. *Diabetologia, 49,* 837-845.

Kobasa, S. C. (1979). Stressful life events, personality, and health: An inquiry into hardiness. *Journal of Personality and Social Psychology, 37,* 1-11.

Kobasa, S. C., Maddi, S. R., & Puccetti, M. C. (1982). Personality and exercise as buffers in the stress-illness-relationship. *Journal of Behavioral Medicine, 5,* 391-404.

Kong, E., Evans, L. K., Guevara, J. P. (2009). Nonpharmacological intervention for agitation in dementia: A systematic review and meta-analysis. *Aging and mental health, 13(4),* 512-520.

Koszewski, W., Chopak, J. S. & Buxton, B. P. (1997). Risk factors for disordered eating in athletes. *Athletic Therapy Today, 3,* 7-11.

Kouvonen, A., Kivimaki, M., Elovainio, M., Virtanen, M., Linna, A., & Vahtera, J. (2005). Job strain and leisure-time physical activity in female and male public sector employees. *Preventive Medicine, 41,* 532-539.

Kowalski, K. C., Crocker, P. R. E., Kowalski, N. P., Chad, K. E., & Humbert, M. L. (2003). Examining the physical self in adolescent girls over time: Further evidence against the hierarchical model. *Journal of Sport and Exercise Psychology, 25,* 5-18.

Krain, A. L., & Castellanos, F. X. (2006). Brain development and ADHD. *Clinical Psychology Review, 26,* 433-444.

Kron, L., Katz, J. L., Gorzynski, G. I., Weiner, H. (1978). Hyperactivity in anorexia nervosa: A fundamental clinical feature. *Comprehensive Psychiatry, 19,* 443-440.

Kumari, V. & Postma, P. (2005). Nicotine use in schizophrenia: the self medication hypotheses. *Neuroscience and Biobehavioral Reviews, 29,* 1021-1034.

Kutcher, S., Aman, M., Brooks, S. J., Buitelaar, J.,van Daalen, E.,Feger, J., et al. (2004). International consensus statement on attention-deficit/hyperactivity disorder (AD-HD) and disruptive behaviour disorders (DBDs): clinical implications and treatment practice suggestions. *European Neuropsychopharmacology, 14(1),* 11-28.

Lacan, J. (1986). O Seminário, Livro 1: *Os escritos técnicos de Freud.* Rio De Janeiro: Jorge Zahar.

Lambourne, K. (2006). The relationship between working memory capacity and physical activity rates in young adults. *Journal of Sport Science and Medicine, 5,* 149-153.

LaMonte, M. J., & Blair, S. N. (2006). Physical activity, cardiorespiratory fitness, and adiposity: contributions to disease risk. *Current Opinion in Clinical Nutrition & Metabolic Care, 9,* 540-546.

Landers, D., & Arent, S. Physical activity and mental health. (2003). In R. N. Singer, H. A. Hausenblas, & C. M. Janelle (Eds.), *The Handbook of Sport Psychology* (pp. 740-765). New York, NY: John Wiley.

Landi, F., Russo, A., & Bernabei, R. (2004). Physical activity and behaviour in the elderly: a pilot study. *Archives of Gerontology and Geriatrics Suppementl, (9),* 235-241.

Lapierre, A., & Aucouturier, B. (1978). I contrasti e la scoperta delle nozioni fondamentali. Milano: Sperling & Kupfer.

Larun, L., Nordheim, L. V., Ekeland, E., Hagen, K. B., & Heian, F. (2006). Exercise in prevention and treatment of anxiety and depression among children and young people. *Cochrane Database of Systematic Reviews, 3,* doi:10.1002/14651858.CD14004691.pub14651852.

Lauriks, S., Dröes, R. M. (2007). Development of the behaviour observation scale for psychomotor therapy for elderly people with dementia (BPMT-dem). Reliability and concurrent validity. *Tijdschr Gerontol Geriatr, 38(2),* 88-99.

Lautenschlager, N. T., Cox, K. L., Flicker, L., Foster, J. K., van Bockxmeer, F. M., Xiao, J., et al. (2008). Effect of physical activity on cognitive function in older adults at risk for Alzheimer disease: a randomized trial. *Journal of American Medicine Association, 300(9),* 1027-1037.

Lavay, B., & McKenzie, T. L. (1991). Development and evaluation of a systematic walk/run program for men with mental retardation. *Education & Training in Mental Retardation, 26(3),* 333-341.

Lawlor, D. A., Hopker, S. W. (2001). The effectiveness of exercise as an intervention in the management of depression: systematic review and meta-regression analysis of randomised controlled trials. *British Medical Journal, 322,* 763-767.

Lawrence, D. M., Holman, C. D., Jablensky, A.V., & Hobb, M. S. (2003). Death rate from ischaemic heart disease in Western Australian psychiatric patients 1980-1998. *British Journal of Psychiatry, 182,* 31-36.

Lazarus, R. S., & Folkman, S. (1984). *Stress, appraisal, and coping.* New York: Springer.

Le Boulch, J. (1979). *Educare con il movimento.* Roma: Armando Editore.

Lee, Y., Park, K., (2007). Does physical activity moderate the association between depressive symptoms and disability in older adults? *International Journal of Geriatric Psychology, 23(3),* 249-256.

Lehman, A. (1996). Measuares of quality of life among persons with severe and persistent mental disorders. *Social Psychiatry and Psychiatric Epidemiology, 32(2),* 78-88.

Leins, U., Goth, G., Hinterberger, T., Klinger, C., Rumpf, N., & Strehl, U. (2007). Neurofeedback for Children with ADHD: A Comparison of SCP and Theta/Beta Protocols. *Applied Psychophysiology and Biofeedback, 32,* 73-88.

Leka, S., Griffiths, A., & Cox, T. (2003). *Work organisation and stress. Systematic problem approaches for employers, managers and trade union representatives (Protecting Workers' Health Series No. 3).* Geneva: Word Health Organization.

Leloup, D. (2007). Fitness maakt jong. *Bodytalk,* 34-35.

Leppämäki S. (2006). The effect of exercise and light on mood. Publications of the National Public Health Institute KTL A8/2006. Helsinki: National Public Health Institute (NPHI).

Leppämäki, S. J., Partonen, T. T., Hurme, J., Haukka, J. K., & Lonnqvist, J. K. (2002). Randomized trial of the efficacy of bright-light exposure and aerobic exercise on depressive symptoms and serum lipids. *Journal of Clinical Psychiatry, 63(4),* 316-321.

Lett, H., Blumenthal, J., Babyak, M., Sherwood, A., Strauman, T., & Robins, C. (2004). Depression as a risk factor for coronary artery disease: evidence, mechanisms, and treatment. *Psychosomatic Medicine, 66,* 305-315.

Leucht, S., Burkard, T., Henderson, J., Maj, M., & Sartorius, N. (2007). Physical illness and schizophrenia: a review of the literature. *Acta Psychiatrica Scandinavica, 116,* 317-333.

Levy, K. S. C. (1997). The contribution of self-concept in the etiology of adolescent delinquency. *Adolescence, 32,* 671-686.

Li, R. (1981). Activity therapy and leisure counseling for the schizophrenic population. *Therapeutic Recreation Journal, 15(4),* 47-49.

Lieberman, J., Stroup, T., & Perkins, D. (2006). The american psychiatric publishing textbook of schizophrenia (1st ed.). Washington DC: American Psychiatric Publishing.

Ljungqvist, A., Jenoure, P. J., Engebretsen, L., Alonso, J. M., Bahr, R., Clough, A. F., BDS Hons, de Bondt G., Dvorak, J., Maloley, R., Matheson, G., Meeuwisse, W., Meijboom, E.J., Mountjoy, M., Pelliccia, A., Schwellnus, M., Sprumont, D., Schamasch, P., Gauthier, J.B. & Dubi, C. (2009). The international olympic committee (CIO) consensus statement on periodic health evaluation of elite athletes. *Clinical Journal of Sports Medicine, 19,* 347-365.

Lima, D. (1999). *Estudo Comparativo do Tempo de Reação entre usuários do Centro de convivência São Paulo e não Usuários.* Unpublished master's thesis, Unversidade Federal de Minas Gerais, Belo Horizonte, Brazil.

Lindamer, L. A., McKibbin, C., Norman, G. J., Jordan, L., Harrison, K., Abeyesinhe, S. et al. (2008). Assessment of physical activity in middle-aged and older adults with schizophrenia. *Schizophrenia Research, 104,* 294-301.

Littbrand, H., Lundin-Olsson, L., Gustafson, Y., & Rosendahl, E. (2009). The effect of a high-intensity functional exercise program on activities of daily living: a randomized controlled trial in residential care facilities. *Journal of the American Geriatrics Society, 57(10),* 1741-1749.

Liu-Ambrose, T., & Donaldson, M. (2009). Exercise and cognition in older adults: is there a role for resistance training programmes? *British Journal of Sports Medicine, 43,* 25-27.

Loas, G., Fremaux, D., Marchand, M. P. (1995). Factorial structure and internal consistency of the French version of the twenty-item Toronto Alexithymia Scale in a group of 183 healthy probands. *Encephale, 21,* 117-22.

Lobitz, W. C., Brammell, H. L., Stoll, S., & Niccoll, A. (1983). Physical exercise and anxiety management training for cardiac stress management in a nonpatient population. *Journal of Cardiopulmonary Rehabilitation and Prevention, 3,* 683-688.

Lollgen, H., Bockenhoff, A., & Knapp, G. (2009). Physical activity and all-cause mortality: an updated meta-analysis with different intensity categories. *International Journal of Sports Medicine, 30,* 213-224.

Lomeo, R. (2009). *Percepção de liberdade no lazer dos familiares dos usuários dos centros de convivência da prefeitura municipal de belo horizonte.* Unpublished master's thesis, Faculdade de Ciências do Desporto e de Educação Física da Universidade do Porto. Porto, Portugal.

Long, B. C. & Flood, K. R. (1993). Coping with Work stress:

Psychological benefits of exercise. *Work & Stress, 7,* 109-119.

Long, C., Smith, J., Midgley, M., & Cassidy, T. (1993). Over-exercising in anorexic and normal samples: behaviors and attitudes. *Journal of Mental Health, 2,* 321-327.

Loovas, O., Schreibman, L., Koegel, R., & Rehm, R. (1971). Selective responding by autistic. *Journal of Abnormal Psychology, 77,* 211-222.

Lorente, F., Peretti-Watel, P., Griffet, J., & Grélot, L. (2003). Alcohol use and intoxication in sport university students. *Alcohol & Alcoholism, 38(5),* 427-430.

Lotan, M., Merrick, J. & Carmeli, E. (2005). Physical activity in adolescence. A review with clinical suggestions. *International Journal of Adolescent Medicine and Health, 17,* 13-21.

Lubar, J. F. (1991). Discourse on the development of EEG diagnostics and biofeedback for attention-deficit/hyperactivity disorders. *Biofeedback and Self-Regulation, 16,* 202-225.

Lubar, J. F., & Shouse, M. N. (1976). EEG behavioral changes in a hyperactive child concurrent training of the sensorimotor rhythm (SMR). A preliminary report. *Biofeedback and Self Regulation, 9(1),* 1-23.

Luepker, R., Evans, A., McKeigue, P., & Reddy, K. (2004). Cardiovascular survey methods Geneva: World Health Organization.

Luppino, F. S., de Wit, L. M., Bouvy, P. F., Stijnen, T., Cuijpers, P., Penninx, B. W. J. H., et al. (2010). Overweight, obesity, and depression a systematic review and meta-analysis of longitudinal studies. *Archives of General Psychiatry, 63,* 220-229.

Lutz, R., Lochbaum, M., Lanning, B., Stinson, L., & Brewer, R. (2007). Cross-lagged relationships among leisure-time exercise and perceived stress in blue-collar workers. *Journal of Sport and Exercise Psychology, 29,* 687-705.

Lutz, R., Stults-Kolehmainen, M., & Bartholomew, J. (2010). Exercise caution when stressed: Stages of change and the stress-exercise participation relationship. *Psychology of Sport & Exercise, 11,* 560-567.

Lynam, D. R., & Henry, B. (2001). The role of neuropsychological deficits in conduct disorders. In J. Hill & B. Maughan (Eds.), *Conduct disorders in childhood and adolescence* (pp. 235-263). Cambridge, UK: Cambridge University Press.

MacDonncha, C., Watson, A. W. S., McSweeney, T., & O'Donovan, D. J. (1999). Reliability of Eurofit physical fitness items for adolescent males with and without mental retardation. *Adapted Physical Activity Quarterly, 16,* 86-95.

MacGillivray, S., Arroll, B., Hatcher, S., Ogston, S., Ried, I., Sullivan, F., et al.(2003). Efficacy and tolerability of selective serotonin reuptake inhibitors compared with tricyclic antidepressants in depression treated in primary care: Systematic review and metaanalysis. *British Medical Journal, 326,* 1014.

Mackie, S., Shaw, P., Lenroot, R., Pierson. R., Greenstein, D. K., Nugent, T. F., et al. (2007). Cerebellar development and clinical outcome in attention deficit hyperactivity disorder. *American Journal of Psychiatry, 164(4),* 647-655.

MacLeod, C. M. (1991). Half a century of research on the Stroop effect: An integrative review. *Psychological Bulletin, 109,* 163-203.

Maïano, C., Bégarie, J, Morin, AJ, Ninot, G. (2011). Assessment of physical self-concept in adolescents with intellectual disability: content and factor validity of the very Short Form of the Physical Self-Inventory. *Body Image, 8(4)*:404-410.

Maïano, C., Morin A.J.S., Monthuy-Blanc, J., Garbarino, J.-M. & Stephan, Y. (2009). Eating disorders inventory: Assessment of its construct validity in a non clinical French sample of adolescents. *Journal of Psychopathology and Behavioral Assessment, 31,* 387-404.

Maïano, C., Ninot, G., Bilard, J., & Albernhe, T. (2002). Outcome of specialized schooling on self-esteem in adolescents with severe learning disabilities and behavior disorders. *European Review of Applied Psychology, 52,* 103-118.

Majorek, M., Tuchelmann, T., & Heusser, P. (2004). Therapeutic eurythmy-movement therapy for children with attention deficit hyperactivity disorder (ADHD): a pilot study. *Complementary Therapies in Nursing and Midwifery, 10,* 46-53.

Maletzky, B., & Klotter, J. (1974). Smoking and alcoholism. *American Journal of Psychiatry, 131,* 445-447.

Malina, R., Bouchard, C., Bar-Or, O. (2004). *Growth, maturation, and physical activity.* Champaign IL: Human Kinetics.

Mandle, C. L., Jacobs, S. C., Arcari, P. M. (1996). The efficacy of relaxation response interventions with adult patients: a review of the literature. *Journal of Cardiovascular Nursing, 10(3),* 4-26.

Mann, J., Zhou, H., McDermott, S., & Poston, M. (2006). Healthy behavior change of adults with mental retardation: Attendance in a health promotion program. *American Journal on Mental Retardation, 111,* 62-73.

Mannix, E. D., Steinberg, H. O., Faryna, S., Hazard, J., Engel, R. J., Schneider, B. et al. (2005). The role of physical activity, exercise, and nutrition in the treatment of obesity. In D. J. Goldstein (Ed.), *The Management of eating disorders and obesity* (2nd ed., pp. 181-207). Totowa, NJ: Humana Press.

Manson C., Katzmarzyk, P. T. (2009). Variability in waist circumference measurements according to anatomic measurement site. *Obesity, 17(9),* 1789-1795.

Marcotte, A. C., & Stern, C. (1997). Qualitative analysis of graphomotor output in children with attentional disorders. *Child Neuropsychology, 3(2),* 147-153.

Marsh, H. W. (1996). Physical self-description questionnaire: stability and discriminant validity. *Research Quarterly Exercise Sport, 67,* 3, 249-264.

Marsh, H. W. (1997). The measurement of physical self-concept: A construct validation approach. In K. R. Fox (Ed.), *The physical self* (pp. 27-58). Champaign, IL: Human Kinetics.

Marsh, H. W., Martin, A. J., Jackson, S. (2010). Introducing a short version of the physical self- description questionnaire: new strategies, short-form evaluative criteria, and applications of factor analyses. *Journal of Sport Exercise Psychology, 32,* 4, 438-482.

Marsh, H. W., Richards, G. E., Johnson, S., Roche, L., & Tremayne, P. (1994). Physical Self-Description Questionnaire: Psychometric properties and a multitrait-multimethod analysis of relations to existing instruments. *Journal of Sport and Exercise Psychology, 16,* 270-305.

Marsh, H. W., & Yeung, A. S. (1998). Top-down, bottom-up, and horizontal models: The direction of causality in multidimensional, hierarchical self-concept models. *Journal of Personality and Social Psychology, 75*, 509-527.

Marshall, S., & Biddle, S. (2001). The transtheoretical model of behavior change: a meta-analysis of applications to physical activity and exercise. *Annals of Behavioral Medicine, 23*, 229-246.

Martens, M., Dams-O'Connor, K., & Beck, N. (2005). A systematic review of college student-athlete drinking: prevalence rates, sport-related factors, and interventions. *Journal of Substance Abuse Treatment, 31*, 305-316.

Martinsen, E. W. (1990). Benefits of exercise for the treatment of depression. *Sports Medicine, 9 (6)*, 380-389.

Martinsen, E. W. (1994). Physical activity and depression: clinical experience. *Acta Psychiatrica Scandinavica, 89*(Suppl. 377), 23-27.

Martinsen, E., & Biddle, S. J. H. (1995). The effects of exercise on mental health in clinical populations. In S. Biddle (Ed.), *European Perspectives on Exercise and Sport Psychology* (pp. 71-84). Stanningley, UK: Human Kinetics.

Martinsen, E. W., Hoffart, A., & Solberg, O. (1989). Aerobic and non-aerobic forms of exercise in the treatment of anxiety disorders. *Stress Medicine, 5*, 115-120.

Martinsen, E. W., Medhaus, A., Sandvik, L. (1985). Effects of exercise on depression: a controlled study. *British Medical Journal, 291*, 109.

Martinsen, E.W., & Raglin, J. S. (2007). Themed review: anxiety/depression. *American Journal of Lifestyle Medicine, 1(3)*, 159-166.

Martinsen, E. W., & Stanghelle, J. K. (1997). Drug therapy and physical activity. In W. P. Morgan, (Ed.), *Physical activity and mental health* (pp. 81-90). Washington, DC: Taylor and Francis.

Marzolini, S., Jensen, B., & Melville, P. (2009). Feasibility and effects of a group-based resistance and aerobic exercise program for individuals with severe schizophrenia: A multidisciplinary approach. *Mental Health and Physical Activity, 2*, 29-36.

Mason, G., & Wilson, P. (1988). *Sport, recreation and juvenile crime: An assessment of the impact of sport and recreation upon Aboriginal and non-Aboriginal youth.* Canberra, AU: Australian Institute of Criminology.

Mateus, M., Mari, J., Delgado, P., Almeida-Filho, N., Barret, T., Gerolin, J., et al. (2008). The mental health system in Brazil: Policies and future challenges. *International Journal of Mental Health Systems, 2 (12)*, 2-12.

Mathéron, I., Léonard, T., & Bonneval, G. (2002). Entretiens de motivation et groupe de réflexion dans le traitement des patientes anorexiques résistantes. *Journal de Thérapie Comportementale et Cognitive, 12*, 122-130.

Mauerberg-deCastro, E. (2005). *Atividade Física Adaptada.* Ribeirão Preto, São Paulo: Tecmedd.

Maughan, B. (2001). Conduct disorder in context. In J. Hill & B. Maughan (Eds.), *Conduct disorders in childhood and adolescence* (pp. 169-201). Cambridge, UK: Cambridge University Press.

Mauri, M., Castrogiovanni, S., Simoncini, M., Iovieno, N., Miniati, M., Rossi, A., et al. (2006). Effects of an educational intervention on weight gain in patients treated with antipsychotics. *Journal of Clinical Psychopharmacology, 26 (5)*, 462-466.

McArdle, W. D., Katch, F. I., & Katch, V. L. (2007). *Exercise physiology: energy, nutrition, and human performance.* Baltimore, MD: Lippincott Williams & Wilkins.

McAuley, E., & Blissmer, B. (2000). Self-efficacy determinants and consequences of physical activity. *Exercise and Sport Sciences Reviews, 28*, 85-88.

McAuley, E., & Courneya, K. S. (1992). Self-efficacy relationships with affective and exertion responses to exercise. *Journal of Applied Social Psychology, 22*, 312-326.

McDermott, A. Y., Mernitz, H. (2006). Exercise and older patients: prescribing guidelines. *American Family Physician, 74*, 437-444.

McDevitt, J., Wilbur, J. (2006). Exercise and people with serious, persistent mental illness. *American Journal of Nursing, 106(4)*, 50-54.

McDuff, D., & Baron, D. (2005). Substance use in athletics: a sports psychiatry perspective. *Clinics In Sports Medicine, 24*, 885-897.

McPherson, B. D. (1990) *Aging as a social process.* Toronto: Butterworths.

Mechling, H. (2008). Dementia and physical activity. *European Review of Aging and Physical Activity, 5*, 1-3.

Medina, J. A., Netto, T. L. B., Muszkat, M., Medina, A. C., Botter, D., Orbetelli, R., et al. (2010). Exercise impact on sustained attention of ADHD children, methylphenidate effects. *ADHD Attention Deficit Hyperactivity Disorder, 2*, 49-58.

Meehl, P. E. (1992). Factors and taxa, traits and types, differences of degree and differences in kind. *Journal of Personality, 60*, 117-174.

Meeusen, R., & De Meirleir, K. (1995): Exercise and brain neurotransmission. *Sports Medicine, 20*, 160-188.

Meeusen, R., Smolders, I., Sarre, S., De Meirleir, K., Keizer, H., Serneels, M., et al. (1997). Endurance training effects on neurotransmitter release in rat striatum: an in vivo microdialysis study. *Acta Physiologica Scandinavica, 159(4)*, 335-341.

Meleddu, M. & Guicciardi, M. (1998). Self-knowledge and social desirability of personality traits, *European Journal of Personality, 12*, 151-168.

Mellion, M. B. (1985). Exercise therapy for anxiety and depression. *Postgraduate Medical Journal, 77(3)*, 59-66.

Merom, D., Phongsavan, P., Wagner, R., Chey, T., Marnane, C., Steel, Z., et al. (2008). Promoting walking as an adjunct intervention to group cognitive behavioral therapy for anxiety disorders: A pilot group randomized trial. *Journal Anxiety Disorders, 22*, 959-968.

Merton, R. K. (1938). Social structure and anomie. *American Sociological Review, 3*, 672-682.

Meyer, J. M. & Stahl, S. M. (2009). The metabolic syndrome and schizophrenia. *Acta Psychiatrica Scandinavica., 119*, 4-14.

Meyer, T., & Broocks, A. (2000). Therapeutic impact of exercise on psychiatric diseases guidelines for exercise testing and prescription. *Sports Medicine, 30(4)*, 269-279.

Miller, W., & Rollnick, S. (2002). *Motivational interviewing: Preparing people for change.* New York: Guilford Press.

Ministério da Saúde. (2009). [http://www.dgsaude.minsaude.pt/pns/vol2_227.html].

Moghaddam, B. R., Katon, W. J., & Russo, J. (2009). The longitudinal effects of depression on physical activity. *General Hospital Psychiatry, 31*, 306-315.

Mond, J.M., Hay, P., Rodgers, B.& Owen, C. (2006). An update on the definition of excessive exercise in eating disorders research. International *Journal of Eating Disorders, 39*, 147-153.

Monteiro, M. (2008). *Análise de domínios predominantes em atividades de expressão corporal para pessoas com transtornos mentais severos.* Unpublished master's thesis, Escola de Educação Física, Fisoterapia e Terapia Ocupacional da Unversidade Federal de Minas Gerais, Belo Horizonte, Brazil.

Monthuy-Blanc, J., Bonanséa, M., Maïano, C., Therme, P., Lanfranchi, M-C., Pruvost, J., Serra, J-M. (2010). Guide de recommandations : prévention des troubles du comportement alimentaire des sportifs à destination des professionnels et/ou des bénévoles du sport et de la santé. Fédération Française d'Athlétisme : FR.

Monthuy-Blanc, J., Maïano, C., & Therme, P. (2010). Prevalence of eating disorders symptoms in non-elite ballet dancers and basketball players: An exploratory and controlled study among french adolescent girls. *Revue d'Epidémiologie et de Santé Publique, 58*, 415-424.

Monthuy-Blanc, J., Morin, A. J. S., Pauzé, R., & Ninot, G. (2012). Directionality of the relationships between global self-esteem and physical self components in anorexic outpatient girls: An in-depth idiographic analysis. In N. Gotsirize-Columbus (Ed.), *Anorexia: symptoms, treatment and prevention.* New York, NY: Nova Science Publishers.

Monthuy-Blanc, J., Ninot, G., Morin, A. J. S., Pauzé, R., Guillaume, S., Rouvière, N., & Campredon, S. (2008). Utilité d'un carnet de suivi quotidien dans la thérapie de l'anorexie mentale. *Journal de Thérapie Comportementale et Cognitive, 18*, 146-156.

Monthuy-Blanc, J., & Probst, M. (2010). *Self concept and eating disorders: theoretical and practical applications.* Acts of the 18th International Conference of Jubilee Congress on Eating Disorders, Alpbach, Autriche.

Moore, B., & Adams, A. (2008). Exercise as an adjunctive evidence-based treatment. In W. O'Donohue & N. Cummings (Eds.), *Evidence-Based Adjunctive Treatments* (pp. 161-175). Academic Press.

Moore, M. (1982). Endorphins and exercise: a puzzling relationship. *Physician Sports Medicine, 10(2)*, 111-114.

Moore, M., & Weerch, C. (2008). Relationship between vigorous exercise frequency and substance use among first-year drinking college students. *Journal of American College Health, 56(6)*, 686-690.

Moreau, K. L., Degarmo, R., Langley J., McMahon, C., Howley, E. T., Bassett, D. R. Jr., et al. (2001). Increasing daily walking lowers blood pressure in postmenopausal women. *Medicine & Science in Sports & Exercise, 33*, 1825-1831.

Morey, M. C., Sloane, R., Pieper, C. F., Peterson, M. J., Pearson, M. P., Ekelund, C. C., et al. (2008). Effect of physical activity guidelines on pysical function in older adults. *Journal of American Geriatrics Society, 56(10)*, 1873-1878.

Morgan, O. (2005). Approaches to increase physical activity: reviewing the evidence for exercise-referral schemes. *Public Health, 119*, 361-370.

Morgan, W. P. (1997). *Physical activity and mental health.* Bristol, PA: Taylor end Francis.

Morgan, W.P. (1985). Affective beneficence of vigorous physical activity. *Medicine & Science in Sports & Exercise, 17*, 94-100

Morgan, W. P., Brown, D. R., Raglin, J. S., O'Connor, P. J., & Ellickson, K. A. (1987). Psychological monitoring of overtraining and staleness. *British Journal of Sports Medicine, 21(3)*, 107-14.

Morin, A. J, Maïano, C. (2009). Assessment of physical self-concept in adolescents with intellectual disability: content and factor validity of the very short form of the physical self-inventory. *Journal of Autism and Developmental Disorders, 39*, 5, 775-87.

Morin, A. J. S., Maïano, C., Marsh, H. W., & Janosz, M. (2011). The longitudinal interplay of adolescents' global self-esteem and perceived physical appearance: A conditional autoregressive latent trajectory analysis. *Multivariate Behavioral Research, 46(2)*, 157-201.

Morone, N. E., & Greco, C. M. (2007). Mind-body interventions for chronic pain in older adults: a structured review. *Pain Medicine, 8(4)*, 359-375.

Morris, T., & Summers, J. (1995). *Sport Psychology: theory, applications and issues.* Milton, Queensland, Australia: Jacaranda/Wiley LTD.

Morrow, J., Jackson, A., Disch, J., Mood, D. (2010*). Measurement and Evaluation in Human Performance.* Champaign, IL: Human Kinetics.

Morrow, J., Jackson, A., Disch, J., Mood, D. (2011). *Measurement and evaluation in human performance with web study guide.* 4th edition. Champaign, IL: Human Kinetics.

Moses, J., Steptoe, A., Matthews, A., & Edwards, S. (1989). The effects of exercise training on mental well-being in the normal population: a controlled trial. *Journal of Psychosomatic Research, 33(1)*, 47-61.

Motl, Dishman, R.K., Saunders, R., Dowda, M., Felton, G., Pate, R.R. (2001). Measuring enjoyment of physical activity in adolescent girls. *American Journal of Preventive Medicine*, 21, 2, 110-117.

Moura-Lima, F., Borges, K., & Probst, M. (2009). *Life in Movement program in Brazil: assessment strategies.* 17th International Symposium of Adapted Physical Activity. Gavle, Sweden: University of Gavle.

Mudge, A. M., Glebel, A. J., & Cutler, A. J. (2008). Exercise body and mind: an integrated approach to functional independence in hospitalized older people. *Journal of American Geriatrics Society, 56(4)*, 630-635.

Mueser, K. T., Yarnold, P. R., & Bellack, A. S. (1992). Diagnostic and demographic correlates of substance abuse in schizophrenia and major affective disorder. *Acta Psychiatrica Scandinavica, 85*, 48-55.

Müller, C. (1971). Schizophrenia in advanced senescence. *British Journal of Psychiatry,118*, 347-348.

Munsch, S. & Margraf, J. (2003). Prinzipien der verhaltenstherapie der adipositas. In F. Petermann & V. Pudel (Eds.), *Übergewicht und Adipositas* (pp. 223-238). Göttingen: Hogrefe.

Muraven, M., & Baumeister, R. F. (2000). Self-regulation and depletion of limited resources: Does self-control resemble a muscle. *Psychological Bulletin, 126,* 247-259.

Murphy, R., Nutzinger, D. O. & Leplow, B. (2004). Conditional associative learning in eating disorders: a comparison with OCD. *Journal of Clinical and Experimental Neuropsychology, 26,* 190-199.

Murphy, T., Pagano, R., & Marlatt, G. (1986). Lifestyle modification with heavy alcohol drinkers: effects of aerobic exercise and meditation. *Addictive Behaviors, 11,* 175-186.

Musselman, J., & Rutledge, P. (2010). The incongruous alcohol-activity association: physical activity and alcohol consumption in college students. *Psychology of Sport and Exercise, 11,* 609-618.

Mutrie, N., & Fox, K. (2010). *Physical activity and the prevention of mental illness, dysfunction and deterioration.* In BASES' Guidelines on Physical Activity in the Prevention of Chronic Disease: Human Kinetics. The British Association of Sport and Exercise Sciences.

Mutrie, N., & Parfitt, G. (1998). Physical activity and its link with mental, social and moral health in young people. In S. J. H. Biddle, J. Sallis & N. Cavill (Eds.), *Young & Active? Young people and health – enhancing physical activity – evidence and implications* (pp. 49-68). London: Health Education Authority.

Nair, J., Ehimare, U., Beitman, B. D., Nair, S. S., & Lavin, A. (2006). Clinical review: evidence-based diagnosis and treatment of ADHD in children. *Missouri Medicine, 103(6),* 617-621.

Naranjo, C. A., Shear N. H., & Lanctôt K. L. (1992). Advances in the diagnosis of adverse drug reactions. *Journal of Clinical Pharmacology, 32,(10),* 897-904.

Nasrallah, H. A., Meyer, J. M., Goff, D. C., McEvoy, J. P., Davis, S. M., Stroup, T. S. et al. (2006). Low rates of treatment for hypertension, dyslipidemia and diabetes in schizophrenia: data from the CATIE schizophrenia trial sample at baseline. *Schizophrenia Research, 86,* 15-22.

Natvig, G. K., Albrektsen, G., & Qvarnstrøm, U. (2001). School-related stress experience as a risk-factor for bullying behavior. *Journal of Youth and Adolescence, 30,* 561-575.

Newcomer, J. (2005). Second-generation (atypical) antipsychotics and metabolic effects: a comprehensive literature review. *CNS Drugs, 19,* 1-93.

Newcomer, J. W. (2007). Metabolic syndrome and mental illness. *American Journal of Managed Care, 13*(Suppl. 7), 170-177.

Ng, F., Dodd, S., & Berk, M. (2007). The effects of physical activity in the acute treatment of bipolar disorder: a pilot study. *Journal of Affective Disorders, 101,* 259-262.

Nguyen-Michel, S., Unger, J., Hamilton, J., & Spruijt-Metz, D. (2006). Associations between physical activity and perceived stress/hassles in college students. *Stress and Health, 22,* 179-188.

NIH Technology assessment panel on integration of behavioral and relaxation approaches into the treatment of chronic pain and insomnia (1996). Integration of behavioral and relaxation approaches into the treatment of chronic pain and insomnia. *Journal of American Medical Association, 276(4),* 313-318.

Nordenfelt, L. (2006). Replay to the commentaries. *Disability and Rehabilitation, 28,* 1487-1489.

North, T. C, McCullagh, P., & Tran, Z. V. (1990). Effect of exercise on depression. *Exercise and Sports Scientific Reviews, 18,* 379-415.

Norton, P. J., Hope, D. A., Weeks, J. W. (2004). The physical activity and sport anxiety scale (PASAS): scale development and psychometric analysis. *Anxiety, Stress and Coping,* 4, 363-382.

Nylander, L. (1971). The feeling of being fat and dieting in a school population. *Acta Socio-Medica Scandinavia, 1,* 17-26.

O'Brien, C., & Lyons, F. (2000). Alcohol and the athlete. *Sports Medicine, 29,* 295-300.

O'Connor, P. J., Morgan, W. P., & Raglin, J. S. (1991). Psychobiologic effects of 3 d of increased training in female and male swimmers. *Medicine & Science in Sports & Exercise, 23(9),* 1055-1061.

O'Connor, P. J., Raglin, J. S., & Martinsen, E. W. (2000). Physical activity, anxiety and anxiety disorders. *International Journal of Sport Psychology, 31,* 136-155.

O'Kelly, J. G., Piper, W. E., Kerber, R., & Fowler, J. (1998). Exercise groups in an insight-oriented, evening treatment program. *International Journal of Group Psychotherapy, 48,* 85-98.

O'Neal, H. A., Dunn, A. L., & Martinsen, E. W. (2000). Depression and exercise. *International Journal of Sport Psychology, 31,* 110-135.

Oaten, M., & Cheng, K. (2005). Academic examination stress impairs self-control. *Journal of Social and Clinical Psychology, 24,* 254-279.

Oja, P. & Tuxworth, B. (1995). *EUROFIT for adults. Assessment of health related fitness.* Strasbourg: Council of Europe.

Olivardia, R., Harrison, G. Pope, & Hudson, J. I. (2000). Muscle dysmorphia in male weightlifters': A case-control study. *American Journal of Psychiatry, 157(8),* 1291-1296.

Ornelas, G. (1997). *O Ensino do futebol de campo como recurso na reabilitação de pacientes com transtornos mentais.* Unpublished master's thesis,: Escola de Educação Física, Fisoterapia e Terapia Ocupacional da Unversidade Federal de Minas Gerais, Belo Horizonte, Brazil.

Orwin, A. (1984). Treatment of situational phobia. A case for running. *British Journal of Psychiatry, 125,* 95-98.

Osby, U., Correia, N., Brandt, L., Ekbom, A., & Sparen, P. (2000). Mortality and causes of death in schizophrenia in Stockholm county, Sweden. *Schizophrenia Research, 45,* 21-28.

Osei-Tutu, K. E. K., Campagna, P. D. (1998). Psychological benefits of continuous vs. intermittent moderate-intensity exercise. *Medicine & Science & Sports Exercise, 30*(Suppl. 5), 117.

Osgood, C. E., Suci, G., & Tannenbaum, P. (1957). *The measurement of meaning.* Urbana, IL: University of Illinois Press.

Ossip-Klein, D. J., Doyne, E. J., Bowman, E. D., Osborn, K. M., McDougall-Wilson, I. B. & Neimeyer, R. A. (1989). Effects of running or weight lifting on self-concept in clinically depressed women. *Journal of Consulting and Clinical Psychology, 57,* 158-161.

Ost, L. G., & Breitholtz, E. (2000). Applied relaxation vs. cognitive therapy in the treatment of generalized anxiety disorder. *Behaviour Research and Therapy, 38(8),* 777-790.

Otto, M., Church, T., Craft, L., Greer, T., Smits, J., & Trivedi, M. (2007). Exercise for mood and anxiety disorders. *Journal Clinical Psychiatry, 9,* 287-294.

Oudhof, J. (1997). De vergeetachtigen vergeten? Psychomotorische therapie bij demente depressieve ouderen. *Bewegen en hulpverlening, 14,* 52-62.

Pagliari, R., & Peyrin, L. (1995). Norepinephrine release in the rat frontal cortex under treadmill exercise: a study with microdialysis. *Journal of Applied Physiology, 78(6),* 2121-2130.

Palmer, J., Palmer, L. K., Michiels, K., & Thigpen, B. (1995). Effects of type of exercise on depression in recovering substance abusers. *Perceptual and Motor Skills, 80,* 523-530.

Palmer, J., Vacc, N., & Epstein, J. (1988). Adult inpatient alcoholics: Physical exercise as a treatment intervention. *Journal of Studies on Alcohol, 49,* 418-421.

Paluska, S. A., Schwenk, T. L. (2000). Physical activity and mental health: current concepts. *Sports Medicine, 29(3),* 167-80.

Pangrazi, R. P. (2004). *Dynamic physical education for elementary school children* (14th ed.). USA: Pearson education.

Parfitt, G., & Eston, R. (2005). The relationship between children's habitual activity level and psychological well-being. *Acta Paediatrica, 94(12),* 1791-1797.

Park, C. L., Armeli, S., & Tennen, H. (2004). The daily stress and coping process and alcohol use among college students. *Journal of Studies on Alcohol, 65,* 126-135.

Paterson, D. H., Jones, G. R., & Rice, C. L. (2007). Ageing and physical activity: evidence to develop exercise recommendations for older adults. *Canadian Journal of Public Health, 98*(Suppl. 2), 69-108.

Pedersen, B. K. & Saltin, B. (2006). Evidence for prescribing exercise as therapy in chronic disease. *Scandinavian Journal of Medicine and Science in Sports, 16*(Suppl. 1), 3-63.

Peluso, M. A., Assunção, S., Araújo, L. A., & Andrade, L. (2000). Alterações psiquiátricas associadas ao uso de anabolizantes. *Revista de Psiquiatria Clínica, 27(4),* 229-236.

Peluso, M. A., (2003). Alterações de humor associadas a atividade física intensa. Unpublished doctorate thesis, Universidade de São Paulo, São Paulo, Brazil.

Peñas-Lledó, E., Vaz Leal, F. J. & Waller, G. (2002). Excessive exercise in anorexia nervosa and bulimia nervosa: relation to eating characteristics and general psychopathology. *International Journal of Eating Disorders, 31(4),* 370-375.

Penedo, F. J. & Dahn, J. R. (2005). Exercise and well-being: A review of mental and physical health benefits associated with physical activity. *Current Opinion in Psychiatry, 8(2),* 189-193.

Péronnet, F., & Szabo, A. (1993). Sympathetic response to acute psychosocial stressors in humans: Linkage to physical exercise and training. In P. Seraganian (Ed.), *Exercise psychology: The influence of physical exercise on psychological processes* (pp. 172-217). New York: Wiley.

Perri, M. G., Anton, S. D., Durning, P. E., Ketterson, T. U., Sydeman, S. J., Berlant, N. E., et al. (2002). Adherence to exercise prescriptions: Effects of prescribing moderate versus higher levels of intensity and frequency. *Health Psychology, 21(5),* 452-458.

Petrie, T.A. (1996). Difference between male and female college lean sport athletes, nonlean sport athletes and nonathletes on behavioral and psychological indices of eating disorders. *Journal of Applied Sport Psychology, 8,* 218-230.

Petruzzello, S. J., Landers, D. M., Hatfield, B. D., Kubitz, K. A., & Salazar, W. (1991). A meta-analysis of the anxiety-reducing effects of acute and chronic exercise. Outcomes and mechanisms. *Sports Medicine, 11(3),* 143-82.

Physical Activity Guidelines Advisory Committee (2008). *Physical Activity Guidelines Advisory Committee Report, 2008.* Washington, DC: Department of Health and Human Services.

Picchioni, M., & Murray, R. (2007). Schizophrenia. *British Medical Journal, 335,* 91-95.

Piette, J., Richardson, C., & Valenstein, M. (2004). Addressing the needs of patients with multiple chronic illnesses: the case of diabetes and depression. *American Journal of Managed Care, 10,* 41-51.

Pliszka, S. R. (2007). Pharmacologic treatment of Attention-Deficit/Hyperactivity Disorder: Efficacy, safety, and mechanisms of action. *Neuropsychological Review, 17,* 61-72.

Pommering, T. L., Brose, J. A., Randolph, E., Murray, T. F., Purdy, R. W., Cadamagnani, P. E., et al. (1994). Effects of an aerobic exercise program on community-based adults with mental retardation. *Mental Retardation, 32(3),* 218-226.

Pope, H. G., Gruber, A. J., & Choi, P. (1997). Muscle dysmorphia. An under-recognized form of body dysmorphic disorder. *Psychosomatics, 38,* 548-557.

Powell, R. R. (1974). Psychological effects of exercise therapy upon institutionalized geriatric mental patients. *Journal of Gerontology, 29,* 157-161.

Powers, P. (2000). Athletes and eating disorders: protective and risk factors. *Healthy Weight Journal, 14(4),* 59-61.

Prefeitura de Belo Horizonte. (2009). Coordenação de Saúde Mental. Relatório do Coordenador do Centro de Convivência Carlos Prates. Belo Horizonte.[Manuscript].

Probst, M. (2005). The Body Experience in Eating Disorders: Research &Therapy. *European Bulletin of Adapted Physical Activity, 4(1).*

Probst, M., Monthuy-Blanc, J., Postma, M. A., de Greef, M., De Herdt, A., Vansteelandt, K., et al., (2011). *Objective and subjective physical activity levels and psychopathology in persons with anorexia nervosa and bulimia nervosa.* Manuscript submitted for publication.

Probst, M., Pieters, G., Vanderlinden, J. (2008). Body experience assessment in non-clinical male and female subjects. *Eating and Weight Disorders, 14,1,* e16-21.

Probst, M., Pieters, G., Vanderlinden, J. (2008). Evaluation of body experience questionnaire in eating disorders and non-clinical subjects. *International Journal of Eating Disorders, 41,* 657-665.

Probst, M., Simons, J. (2008). Psychomotorische therapie in Vlaanderen: voorstel tot beroepsprofiel en functieomschrijving. In J. Simons (Ed.), *Actuele Themata uit de psychomotorische therapie, Jaarboek 2008* (pp. 11-46). Leuven:Voorburg, Acco.

Probst, M., Vandereycken, W., Van Coppenolle, H., & Vanderlinden, J. (1995). Body Attitude Test for patients with an eating disorder: psychometric characteristics of a new questionnaire. *Eating Disorders, 3,* 133-145.

Probst, M., Vandereycken, W., Vanderlinden, J. (1995). The body attitude test for patients with an eating disorder: psychometric characteristics of a new questionnaire. *Eating Disorder: the Journal of Treatment and Prevention,* 3, 133-145.

Probst, M., Vanderlinden, J. Vandereycken, W., & Van Coppenolle, H. (1999). Over bewegingsdrang en psychomotorische therapie bij anorexia nervosa-patiënten. *Tijdschrift voor Directieve Therapie, 19,* 260-275.

Prochaska, J. O., Velicer, W. F., Rossi, J. S., Goldstein, M. G., Marcus, B.H., Rakowski, W. et al. (1994). Stages of change and decisional balance for 12 problem behaviours. *Health Psychology, 13,* 39-46.

Prochaska, J. O., & Velicer, W. (1997). The transtheoretical model of health behavior change. *American Journal of Health Promotion, 12,* 38-48.

Purdy, D. A., & Richard, S. F. (1983). Sport and juvenile delinquency: An examination and assessment of four major theories. *Journal of Sport Behavior, 6,* 79-83.

Purper-Ouakil, D., Michel, G., Baup, N. & Mouren-Siméoni, M. C. (2002). Aspects psychopathologiques de l'exercice physique intensif chez l'enfant et l'adolescent : mise au point à partir d'une situation clinique. *Annales médico-psychologiques, 160,* 543-549.

Putukian, M. (1998). The female athlete triad. *Clinical Sports and Medicine, 17,* 675-696.

Raglin, J. S. (1990). Exercise and mental health: beneficial and detrimental effects. *Sports Medicine, 9(6),* 323-329.

Raglin, J. S. (1993). Overtraining and staleness: Psychometric monitoring of endurance athletes. In R. B Singer, M. Murphey, & L. K. Tennart (Eds.), *Handbook of Research on Sport Psychology* (pp. 840-850). New York: MacMillan.

Ramaciotti, D., & Perriard, J. (2001). *Les coûts du stress en Suisse [Stress-related costs in Switzerland].* Bern: Staatssekretariat für Wirtschaft (Seco).

Rankin, E. J., Gilner, F. H., Gfeller, J. D. (1993). Efficacy of progressive muscle relaxation for reducing state anxiety among elderly adults on memory tasks. *Perceptual and Motor Skills, 77,* 1395-1402.

Ransford, C. P. (1982). A role for amines in the antidepressant effect of exercise: a review. *Medicine & Science in Sports & Exercise, 4(1),* 1-10.

Rawlins, M. D., Thompson J. W. (1977). Pathogenesis of adverse drug reactions. In D. M. Davies (Ed.), *Textbook of adverse drug reactions* (pp. 10-31). Oxford: Oxford University Press.

Read, J., & Brown, R. (2003). The role of physical exercise in alcoholism treatment and recovery. *Professional Psychology: Research and Practice, 34(1),* 49-56.

Reid, G., O'Connor, J., & Lloyd, M. (2003). *The autism spectrum disorders: physical activity instruction.* Retrived from http://www.thefreelibrary.com/The autism spectrum disorders: physical activity instruction-part… -a0102905083

Rethorst, C., Wipfli, B., & Landers, D. (2009). The antidepressive effects of exercise: A meta-analysis of randomized trials. *Sports Medicine, 39,* 491-511.

Rhea, D.J. (1996). Prevalence of eatingdisbiders in an ethnically diverse urban high school female population. *Journal of Applied Sport Psychology, 8,* S82.

Richardson, C. R., Avripas, S. A., Neal, D. L., & Marcus, S. M. (2005). Increasing lifestyle physical activity in patients with depression or other serious mental illness. *Journal of Psychiatric Practice, 11,* 379-388.

Richardson, C. R., Faulkner, G., McDevitt, J., Skrinar, G. S., Hutchinson, D. S., & Piette, J. D. (2005). Integrating physical activity into mental health services for persons with serious mental illness. *Psychiatric Services, 56,* 324-331.

Rief, W., Hermanutz, M. (1996). Responses to activation and rest in patients with panic disorder and major depression. *British Journal of Clinical Psychology, 35,* 605-616.

Rimmer, J. H., Braddock, D., & Fujiura, G. (1993). Prevalence of obesity in adults with mental retardation: Implication for health promotion and disease prevention. *Mental Retardation, 31,* 105-110.

Rimmer, J. H., Braddock, D., & Marks, B., (1995). Health characteristics and behaviors of adults with mental retardation residing in three living arrangements. *Research in Developmental Disabilities, 16,* 489-499.

Rimmer, J. H., Braddock, D., & Pitetti, K. H. (1996). Research on physical activity and disability: An emerging national priority. *Medicine & Science in Sports & Exercise,28,* 1366-1372.

Rimmer, J. H., Chen, D. M., McCubbin, J. A., Drum, C., & Peterson, J. (2010). Exercise intervention research on persons with disabilities. *American Journal of Physical Medicine & Rehabilitation, 89,* 249-263.

Rimmer, J. H., & Braddock, D. (2002). Health promotion for people with physical, cognitive, and sensory disabilities: An emerging national priority. *American Journal of Health Promotion, 16,* 220-224.

Rimmele, U., Costa Zellweger, B., Marti, B., Seiler, R., Mohiyeddini, C., Ehlert, U., et al. (2007). Trained men show lower cortisol, heart rate and psychological responses to psychological stress compared with untrained men. *Psychoneuroendocrinology, 32,* 627-635.

Rimmele, U., Seiler, R., Marti, B., Wirtz, P. H., Ehlert, U., & Heinrichs, M. (2009). The level of physical activity affects adrenal and cardiovascular reactivity to psychosocial stress. *Psychoneuroendocrinology, 34,* 190-198.

Rintala, P., Pienimaki, K., Ahonen, T., Cantell, M., & Kooistra, L. (1998). The effects of a psychomotor training programme on motor skill development in children with developmental language disorders. *Human Movement Science, 17(4-5),* 721-737.

Rocha, G. (2001). *Verificação da condição cardiorespiratória, do grupo portador de transtornos mentais, participantes do projeto Escola de Futebol.* Unpublished master's thesis, Escola de Educação Física, Fisoterapia e Terapia Ocupacional da Unversidade Federal de Minas Gerais, Belo Horizonte, Brazil.

Roick, C., Fritz-Wieacker, A., Matschinger, Heider, D., Schindler, J., Riedel-Heller, S., et al. (2007). Health habits of patients with schizophrenia. *Social Psychiatry and Psychiatry Epidemiology, 42,* 268-276.

Rolland, Y., Pillard, F., Klapouszczak, A., Reynish, E., Thomas, D., Andrieu, S., et al. (2007). Exercise program for nursing home residents with Alzheimer's disease: a

1-year randomized, controlled trial. *Journal of American Geriatrics Society, 55(2),* 158-165.

Rosenberg, M. (1965). *Society and the adolescence self-image.* Princeton, NJ: Princeton University press.

Rosenbloom, M. J., Rohlfing, T., O'Reilly, A. W., Sassoon, S. A., Pfefferbaum, A., & Sullivan, E. V. (2007). Improvement in memory and static balance with abstinence in alcoholic men and women: selective relations with change in brain structure. *Psychiatry Research: Neuroimaging, 155,* 91-102.

Ross, S. S. (2010). Physical Activity for weight loss. In C. Bouchard, & P. T. Katzmarzyk (Eds.), *Physical Activity and Obesity* (2nd ed., pp. 219-222). Champaign, IL: Human Kinetics.

Rossler, W., Salize, H., van Os, J., & Riecher-Rossler, A. (2005). Size of burden of schizophrenia and psychotic disorders. *European Neuropsychopharmacology, 15,* 399-409.

Rostad, F. G., & Long, B. C. (1996). Exercise as a coping strategy for stress: A review. *International Journal of Sport Psychology, 27,* 197-222.

Rot, M. A., Collins, K. A., Fitterling, H. L. (2009). Physical exercise and depression. *Mount Sinai Journal Of Medicine, 76,* 204-214.

Rowland, A. S., Lesesne, C. A., & Abramowitz, A. J. (2002). The epidemiology of attention-deficit/hyperactivity disorder (ADHD): A public health view. *Mental Retardation and Developmental Disabilities Research Review, 8(3),* 162-170.

Rugulies, R. (2002). Depression as a predictor for coronary heart disease. A review and meta-analysis. *American Journal of Preventive Medicine, 23,* 51-61.

Rumball, J. S., & Lebrun, C. M. (2004). Selected issues for female athlete. *Clinical Journal of Sport Medicine, 14,* 153-160.

Sadock, B., Sadock, V., & Ruiz, P. (2009). *Kaplan and Sadock's Comprehensive Textbook of Psychiatry.* Philadelphia, US: Lippincott Williams & Wilkins.

Sagiv, M. (2009). Safety of resistance traning in the elderly. *European Review of Aging and Physical Activity, 6(1),* 1-2.

Saha, S., Chant, D., & McGrath, J. (2007). A systematic review of mortality in schizophrenia: is the differential mortality gap worsening over time? *Archives of General Psychiatry, 64,* 1123-1131.

Sales, S. M. (1971). Need for stimulation as a factor in social behaviour. *Journal of Personality and Social Psychology, 19,* 124-134.

Sallis, J. F., & Owen, N. (1999). *Physical activity and behavioral medicine.* Thousand Oaks: Sage.

Salmon, P. (2001). Effects of physical exercise on anxiety, depression, and sensitivity to to stress: A unifying theory. *Clinical Psychology Review, 21,* 33-61.

Saporetti, G. (2008). *Análise de atividades recreativas para indivíduos com transtornos mentais severos.* Unpublished master's thesis. Escola de Educação Física, Fisoterapia e Terapia Ocupacional da Unversidade Federal de Minas Gerais, Belo Horizonte, Brazil.

Sarwer, D. B. & Thompson, J. K. (2004). Obesity and body image disturbance. In T. A. Wadden & A. J. Stunkard (Eds.), *Handbook of Obesity Treatment* (pp. 447-464). New York: Guilford Press.

Scheen, A. J., & De Hert, M. (2005). Drug induced diabetes mellitus: the example of atypical antipsychotics. *Revue Medicale de Liege, 60,* 455-460.

Scheen, A. J., & De Hert, M. (2007). Abnormal glucose metabolism in patients treated with antipsychotics. *Diabetes Metabolism, 33,* 169-175.

Schneider, G. M., Jacobs, D. W., Gevirtz, R. N., & O'Connor, D. T. (2003). Cardiovascular haemodynamic response to repeated mental stress in normotensive subjects at genetic risk of hypertension: Evidence of enhanced reactivity, blunted adaptation, and delayed recovery. *Journal of Human Hypertension, 17,* 829-840.

Schnohr, P., Kristensen, T. S., Prescott, E., & Scharling, H. (2005). Stress and life dissatisfaction are inversely associated with jogging and other types of physical activity in leisure time – The Copenhagen City Heart Study. *Scandinavian Journal of Medicine and Science in Sports, 15,* 107-112.

Schoemaker, M. M., Smits-Engelsman, B. C. M. (2005). Neuromotor task training: a new approach to treat children with DCD. In D. Sugden, & M. Chambers (Eds.). *Children with developmental coordination disorder.* London: Whurr.

Schomer, H. H., & Drake, B. (2001). Physical activity and mental health. *International Sport Med Journal, 2(3),* 1-9.

Schomer, H. H, Dunne, T. T. (1994). Emotional transmissions of novice runners during a 7-month marathon training program. *International Journal of Sport Psychology, 25,* 176-186.

Schommer, N. C., Hellhammer, D. H., & Kirschbaum, C. (2003). Dissociation between reactivity of the hypothalamus-pituitary-adrenal axis and the sympathetic-adrenal-medullary system to repeated psychosocial stress. *Psychosomatic Medicine, 65,* 450-460.

Schuler, J. L., & O'Brien, W. H. (1997). Cardiovascular recovery from stress and hypertension risk factors: A meta-analytic review. *Psychophysiology, 34,* 649-659.

Schunk, D. H., & Zimmerman, B. J. (2003). Self-regulation and learning,. In Reynolds, W. M., & Miller, G. E. (Eds.) *Handbook of psychology* (vol. 7) (pp. 59-78). Hoboken NJ: John Wiley & Sons.

Schwartz, A. R., Gerin, W., Davidson, K. W., Pickering, T. G., Brosschot, J. F., Thayer, J. F., et al. (2003). Toward a causal model of cardiovascular responses to stress and the development of cardiovascular disease. *Psychosomatic Medicine, 65,* 22-35.

Schwarzer, R. (2000). *Stress, Angst und Handlungsregulation [Stress, anxiety and action regulation].* Stuttgart: Kohlhammer.

Seagraves, F., Horvat, M., Franklin, C., & Jones, K. (2004). Effects of a school-based program on physical function and work productivity in individuals with mental retardation. *Clinical Kinesiology, 58,* 18-29.

Seers, K., & Carroll, D. (1998) Relaxation techniques for acute pain management: a systematic review. *Journal of Advanced Nursing, 27(3),* 466-475.

Segar, M., Hanlon, J., Jayaratne, T., & Richardson, C. R. (2002). Fitting fitness into women's lives: effects of a gender-tailored physical activity intervention. *Women's Health Issues, 12,* 338-347.

Segrave, J. O. (1983). Sport and juvenile delinquency. *Exercise and Sport Sciences Reviews, 11,* 181-209.

Segrave, J. O., & Hastad, D. H. (1984). Future directions in sport and juvenile delinquency research. *Quest, 36,* 37-47.

Seidell, J. C., & Tijhuis, M. A. R. (2002). Obesity and Quality of life. In C. G. Fairburn & K. D. Brownell (Eds.), *Eating Disorders and Obesity A Comprehensive Handbook* (2nd ed., pp. 388-392). New York: Guilford Press.

Seidenfeld, M. E., Sosin, E., & Rickert, V. I. (2004). Nutrition and eating disorders in adolescents. *Mount Sinai Journal of Medicine, 71(3),* 155-161.

Seligman, M. (1975). *Helplessness: On depression, development, and death.* New York: Freeman.

Selye, H. (1946). The general adaptation syndrome and the diseases of adaptation. *Journal of Endocrinology, 6,* 117-230.

Sernyak, M. J., Leslie, D. L., Alarcon, L. D., Losonczy, M. F., & Rosenheck, R. (2003) Association of diabetes mellitus with use of atypical neuroleptics in the treatment of schizophrenia. *American Journal of Psychiatry, 159,* 561-566.

Sexton, H., Sogaard, A. J., & Olstad, R. (2001). How are mood and exercise related? Results from the Finnmark study. *Social Psychiatry and Psychiatric Epidemiology, 36(7),* 348-35.

Sharpe, J. K., Stedman, T. J., & Byrne, N. M. (2006). Accelerometry is a valid measure of physical inactivity but not of energy expended on physical activity in people with schizophrenia. *Schizophrenia Research, 85,* 300-301.

Sharpe, J. K., Stedman, T. J., Byrne, N. M., Wishart, C., & Hills, A. P. (2006). Energy expenditure and physical activity in clozapine use: implications for weight management. *Australian and New Zealand Journal of Psychiatry, 40,* 810-814.

Shavelson, R. J., Hubner, J. J. & Stanton, G. C. (1976). Self-concept: validation of construct interpretations, *Review of Educational Research, 46,* 407-411.

Sherborne, V. (1990). *Developmental Movement for Children: Mainstream, Special Needs, and Pre-school.* Cambridge: Cambridge University Press.

Sherrill, C., & Dunn, J. M. (1996). Movement and its implication for individuals with disabilities. *Quest, 48,* 378-391.

Shroff, H., Reba, L., Thornton, L. M., Tozzi, F., Klump, K. L., Berettini, W. H., et al. (2006). Features associated with excessive exercise in women with ED. *International Journal of Eating Disorders, 39,* 454-461.

Sibley, B. A., & Etnier, J. L. (2003). The relationship between physical activity and cognition in children: A meta-analysis. *Pediatric Exercise Science, 15,* 243-256.

Siedentop, D., & Tannehill, D. (2000). *Developing teaching skills in physical education.* California: Mayfield Publishing.

Silva, A., & Bastos, S. (2005). Intervenções em Saúde Mental na Proposta da Extensão Universitária. *Proceedings of the VIII Encontro de Extensão da UFMG,* Belo Horizonte, Brazil.

Simão, F., Monteiro, M., Saporetti, G., & Borges, K. (2007). *O ensino da dança folclórica para indivíduos com transtornos mentais severos.* VI Simpósio Nacional de Dança Contemporânea, Belo Horizonte, Brazil.

Sime, W. E. (1987). Exercise in the prevention and treatment of depression. In W. P. Morgan & S. E. Goldston (Eds.), *Exercise and mental health* (pp. 145-52). Washington, DC: Hemisphere.

Sime, W. E. (1997). Guidelines for clinical applications of exercise therapy for mental health. In J. L. Van Raalte & B. W. Brewer (Eds), *Exploring sport and exercise psychology* (pp. 159-187). Washington, DC: American Psychological Association.

Simonoff, E. (2001). Genetic influences on conduct disorders. In J. Hill & B. Maughan (Eds.), *Conduct disorders in childhood and adolescence* (pp. 202-234). Cambridge, UK: Cambridge University Press.

Simpson, M. M., & Goetz, R. R. (2001). Weight gain and antipsychotic medication: differences between antipsychotic-free and treatment periods. *Journal of Clinical Psychiatry, 62,* 694-700.

Singer, R. N. (1988). Strategies and metastrategies in learning and performing self-paced athletic skills. *The Sport Psychologist, 2,* 49-68.

Singh, N. A, Stavrinos, T. M., Scarbek, Y., Galambos, G., Liber, C., & Fiatarone Singh, M. A. (2005). A randomized controlled trial of high versus low intensity weight training versus general practitioner care for clinical depression in older adults. *Journal of Gerontology. Series A. Biological Sciences and Medical Sciences, 60,* 768-776.

Singh, A., Petrides , J. S., Gold, Chrousos, G. P., & Deuster, P. A. (1999). Differential hypothalamic-pituitary-adrenal axis reactivity to psychological and physical stress. *Journal of Clinical Endocrinology and Metabolism, 84,* 1944-1948.

Sinyor, D., Brown, T., Rostant, L., & Seraganian, P. (1982). The role of a physical fitness program in the treatment of alcoholism. *Journal of Studies on Alcohol, 43,* 380-386.

Sinyor, D., Péronnet, F., Brisson, G., & Seraganian, P. (1988). Failure to alter sympathoadrenal response to psychological stress following aerobic training. *Physiology & Behavior, 42,* 293-296.

Siuciak, J. A. Clark, M. S., Rind, H. B., Whittemore, S. R. ,& Russo, A. F. (1998). BDNF induction of tryptophan hydroxylase mRNA levels in the rat brain. *Journal of Neuroscience Research, 52,* 149-158.

Sjöström, M., Hagströmer, M. &, Ruiz, J. R. (2008). *Working paper on physical activity and health.* Retrieved from EU Platform on Diet, Physical Activity and Health [http://ec.europa.eu/health/ph_determinants/life_style/nutrition/platform/docs/ev_20080917_wp_en.pdf].

Sjöström, M., Oja, P., Hagströmer, M., Smith, B. J., & Bauman, A. (2006). Health-enhancing physical activity across European Union countries: the Eurobarometer study. *Journal of Public Health, 14,* 291-300.

Skrinar, G., Huxley, N., Hutchinson, D., Menninger, E., & Glew, P. (2005). The role of a fitness intervention on people with serious psychiatric disabilities. *Psychiatric Rehabilitation Journal, 29(2),* 122-127.

Smolak, L., Murnen, S., & Ruble, A. (2000). Female athletes and eating problems: a meta-analysis. *International Journal of Eating Disorders, 27,* 371-380.

Smolak, L., Murnen, S., & Ruble, A. (2000). Female athletes and eating problems: a meta-analysis. *International Journal of Eating Disorders, 27,* 371-380.

Sniehotta, F. F., Schwarzer, R., Scholz, U., & Schüz, B. (2005). Action planning and coping planning for long-term lifestyle change: Theory and assessment. *European Journal of Social Psychology, 35,* 565-576.

Solenberger, S. E. (2001). Exercise and eating disorders: a 3-year inpatient hospital record analysis. *Eating Behaviors, 2(2),* 151-168.

Somers, J., Goldner, E., Waraich, P., & Hsu, L. (2006). Prevalence and incidence studies of anxiety disorders: A systematic review of the literature. *Canadian Journal of Psychiatry, 51,* 100-103.

Sonnentag, S., & Jelden, S. (2009). Job stressors and the pursuit of sport activities: A day-level perspective. *Journal of Occupational Health Psychology, 14,* 165-181.

Sonstroem, R. J. (1997). The psychological benefits of exercise. *Medicine and Health, Rhode Island, 80(9),* 295-296.

Sonstroem, R., & Morgan, W. (1989). Exercise and self-esteem: Rationale and model. *Medicine & Science in Sports & Exercise, 21,* 329-337.

Sonstroem, R. J. (1982). Exercise and self-esteem: Recommendations for expository research. *Quest, 33,* 124-139.

Sorensen, M. (2006). Motivation for physical activity of psychiatric patients when physical activity was offered as part of treatment. *Scandinavian Journal of Medicine and Sciences in Sports, 16,* 391-398.

Sothmann, M. S. (2006). The cross-stressor adaptation hypothesis and exercise training. In E. O. Acevedo & P. Ekkekakis (Eds.), *Psychobiology of physical activity* (pp. 149-160). Champaign, IL: Human Kinetics.

Sothmann, M. S., Buckworth, J., Claytor, R. P., Cox, R. H., White-Welkley, J. E., & Dishman, R. K. (1996). Exercise training and the cross-stressor adaptation hypothesis. *Exercise and Sport Science Review, 24,* 267-287.

Souza, A., Teixeira-Salmela, L., & Magalhães, L. (2005). Análise das propriedades psicométricas da versão brasileira do Human activity profile. *Revista de Fisioterapia da Universidade de São Paulo, 12,* 165-165.

Sowell, E. R., Peterson, B. S., Thompson, P. M., Welcome, S. E., Henkenius, A. L., & Toga, A. W. (2003). Mapping cortical change across the human life span. *Nature Neuroscience, 6,* 309-315.

Spencer, H. (1873). *Principles of Psychology.* New York, NY: Appleton.

Spieker, M. R. (1996). Exercise dependence in a pregnant runner. *Journal of American Board of Family Practice, 9(2),* 118-121.

Spielberger, C. D. (1983). *Manual for the State-Trait Anxiety Inventory (Form Y).* Palo Alto, CA: Consulting Psychologist Press.

Sprott, J. B., & Doob, A. N. (2000). Bad, sad, and rejected: The lives of aggressive children. *Canadian Journal of Criminology/Revue Canadienne de Criminologie, 42,* 123-133.

Stanish, H. I., & Draheim, C. C. (2004). Comparison of walking habits of men and women with intellectual disabilities. *Research Quarterly for Exercise and Sport, 75,* 112-113.

Stanish, H. I., & Frey, G. C. (2008). Promotion of physical activity in individuals with intellectual disability. *Salud Publica de Mexico, 50*(Suppl. 2), 178-184.

Stefanatos, G. A., & Baron, I. S. (2007). Attention-Deficit/Hyperactivity Disorder: A neuropsychological perspective towards DSM-V. *Neuropsychological Review, 17,* 5-38.

Stein, P. N., Motta, R. W. (1992) Effects of aerobic and non-aerobic exercise on depression and self-concept. *Perceptual and Motor Skills, 74,* 79-89.

Steinacker, J. M., Lormes, W., Kellmann, M., Liu, Y., Reissnecker, S., Opitz-Gress, A., et al. (2000). Training of junior rowers before world championships. Effects on performance, mood state and selected hormonal and metabolic responses. *Journal of Sports Medicine and Physical Fitness; 40(4),* 327-35.

Steiner, B. D., & Gest, K. L. (1996). Do adolescents want to hear preventive counseling messages in outpatient settings? *Journal of Family Practice, 43,* 375-381.

Steptoe, A., & Ayers, S. (2004). Stress, health and illness. In S. Sutton, A. Baum & M. Johnston (Eds.), *The Sage handbook of health psychology* (pp. 169-196). London: Sage.

Steptoe, A., & Butler, N. (1996). Sports participation and emotional wellbeing in adolescents. *Lancet, 347,* 1789-1792.

Steptoe, A., Wardle, J., Pollard, T. M., Canaan, L., & Davies, G. J. (1996). Stress, social support and health-related behavior: A study of smoking, alcohol consumption and physical exercise. *Journal of Psychosomatic Research, 41,* 171-180.

Stetson, B. A., Rahn, J. A., Dubbert, P. M., Wilner, B. I., & Mercury, M. G. (1997). Prospective evaluation of the effects of stress on exercise adherence in community-residing women. *Health Psychology, 16,* 515-520.

Stevens, V. (2004) Effectieve methoden voor meer fysieke activiteit bij 55-plussers. *Vlaams instituut voor Gezondheidspromotie VIG.*

Stice, E. (2002). Risk and maintenance factors for eating pathology: a meta-analytic review. *Psychological Bullettin, 128,* 825-848.

Stice. E., & Shaw, H. (2004). Eating disorder prevention programs: a meta-analytic review *Psychological Bulletin, 130,* 206-227.

Stranahan, A. M, Lee, K., & Mattson, M. P. (2008). Central mechanisms of HPA axis regulation by voluntary exercise. *Neuromolecular Medicine, 10,* 118-127.

Strath, S. J., Swartz, A. M., Bassett, D. R. Jr, O'Brien, W. L., King, G. A., & Ainsworth, B. E. (2000). Evaluation of heart rate as a method for assessing moderate intensity physical activity. *Medicine & Science in Sports & Exercise, 32*(Suppl. 9), 465-470.

Ströhle, A., Graetz, B., Scheel, M., Wittmann, A., Feller, C., Heinz, A., et al. (2009). The acute antipanic and anxiolytic activity of aerobic exercise in patients with panic disorder and healthy control subjects. *Journal of Psychiatric Research, 43,* 1013-1017.

Strømme, P., & Magnus, P. (2000). Correlations between socioeconomic status, IQ and aetiology in mental retardation: a population-based study of Norwegian children. *Social Psychiatry and Psychiatric Epidemiology, 35(1),* 12-18.

Sudi, K., Ottl, K., Payerl, D., Baumgartl, P., Tauschmann, K., & Müller, W. (2004). Anorexia athletica. *Nutrition, 20(7-8),* 657-661.

Sundgot-Borgen, J. (1993). Prevalence of eating disorders in elite female athletes. *International Journal of Sport & Nutrition, 3,* 29-40.

Sundgot-Borgen, J. (1994). Eating disorders in female athletes. *Sports Medicine, 17,* 176-188.

Sundgot-Borgen, J., & Corbin, C. (1987). Eating disorders among female athletes. *The Physician & SportsMedicine, 15,* 88-90.

Sundgot-Borgen, J., & Torstveit, M. K. (2004). Prevalence of eating disorders in elite athletes is higher than in the general population. *Clinical Journal of Sport Medicine, 14,* 25-32.

Sutherland, E. H., & Cressey, D. R. (1966). *Principles of Criminology.* Chicago, IL: Lippincott.

Sutherland, G., Couch, M. A., & Iacono, T., (2002). Health issues for adults with developmental disability. *Research in Developmental Disabilities, 23,* 422-445.

Sutton, J. R., Young, J. D., Lazarus L, et al. (1989). The hormonal response to physical exercise. *Australasian Annual of Medicine, 18,* 84-90.

Swarbrick, M. (2006). A wellness approach. *Psychiatric Rehabilitation Journal, 29(4),* 311-314.

Sweitzer, E. (2005). The relationship between social interest and self-concept in conduct disordered adolescents. *Journal of Individual Psychology, 61,* 55-79.

Tantillo, M., Kesick, C. M., Hynd, G. W., & Dishman R. K. (2002). The effects of exercise on children with attention-deficit hyperactivity disorder. *Medicine & Science in Sports & Exercise, 34(2),* 203-212.

Taylor, C. B., Sallis, J. F., & Needle, R. (1985). The relation of physical activity and exercise to mental health. *Public Health Report, 100(2),* 195-202.

Taylor, A. C. (2000). Physical activity, anxiety, and stress. In S. J. H. Biddle, K. R. Fox & S. H. Boutcher (Eds.), *Physical activity and psychological well-being* (pp. 10-45). London, UK: Routledge.

Teichner, G., & Golden, C. J. (2000). The relationship of neuropsychological impairment to conduct disorder in adolescence: A conceptual review. *Aggression and Violent Behavior, 5,* 509-528.

Temple, V. A., Frey, G. C., & Stanish, H. I., (2006). Physical activity of adults with mental retardation. Review and research needs. *American Journal of Health Promotion, 21,* 2-12.

Teri, L., Gibbons, L. E., McCurry, S. M., Logsdon, R. G., Buchner, D. M., Barlow, et al. (2003). Exercise plus behavioral management in patients with Alzheimer disease: a randomized controlled trial. *Journal of American Medical Association, 290(15),* 2015-2022.

Teychenne, M., Ball, K., Salmon, J. (2008): Physical activity and likelihood of depression in adults: a review. *Preventive Medicine, 46,* 397-411.

Thakker-Varia, S., Alder, J. (2009). Neuropeptides in depression: role of VGF. *Behavioural Brain Research, 11;197(2),* 262-278.

Thiem V, Thomas A, Markin D, Birmingham CL. (2000). Pilot study of a graded exercise program for the treatment of anorexia nervosa. *International Journal of Eating Disorders, 28,* 101-106.

Thirthalli, J., & Jain, S. (2009). Better outcome of schizophrenia in India: a natural selection against severe forms? *Schizophrenia Bulletin, 35(3),* 655-657.

Thomas, J. R., Landers, D. M., Salazar, W., & Etnier, J. (1994). Exercise and cognitive function. In C. Bouchard, R. Shepard & T. Stephens (Eds.). *Physical activity, fitness and health: International proceedings and consensus Statement* (pp. 521-528). Champaign, IL: Human Kinetics.

Thompson, J. K. & Sherman, R. T. (1993). *Helping athletes with eating disorders.* Champaign, IL: Human Kinetics.

Thoren, P., Floras, J. S., Hoffmann, P, & Seals, D. R. (1990). Endorphins and exercise: physiological mechanisms and clinical implications. *Medicine & Science in Sports & Exercise, 22(4),* 417-428.

Tietjens, M. (2001). *Sportliches Engagement und sozialer Rückhalt im Jugendalter. Eine repräsentative Surveystudie in Brandenburg und Nordrhein-Westfalen [Exercise and social support in adolescence. A representative survey study in Brandenburg and North Rhine Westphalia].* Lengerich: Pabst.

Tokumura, M., Yoshiba, S., Tanaka, T., Nanri, S., Watanabe, H. (2003). Prescribed exercise training improves exercise capacity of convalescent children and adolescents with anorexia nervosa. *European Journal of Pediatrics, 162,* 430-1

Tomporowski, P. D. (2003). Effects of acute bouts of exercise on cognition. *Acta Psychologica, 112,* 297-324.

Tordeurs, D., Janne, P., Appart, A., Zdanowicz, N., Reynaert, C. (2011). Effectiveness of physical exercise in psychiatry: A therapeutic approach? *Encephale, 37(5),* 345-532.

Torstveit, M.K., Sundgot-Borgen, J., (2005). The female athlete triad exists in both elite athletes and controls. *Medicine & Science in Sport & Exercise,* 1449-1459.

Torstveit, M. K., & Sungot-Borden, J. (2005). The female athlete triad: are elite athletes at increased risk? *Medicine & Science in Sports & Exercise, 37,* 184-193.

Treasure, J., & Szmukler, G. (1995). Medical complications of chronic anorexia nervosa. In G. Szmukler, C. Dare, & J. Treasure (Eds.), *Handbook of Eating Disorder. Theory, Treatment & Research* (pp. 197-210). New York: John Wiley.

Triplett, N. (1898). The dynamogenic factors in pacemaking and competition. *American Journal of Psychology, 9,* 507-533.

Trivedi, M. H., Greer, T. L., Grannemann, B. D, Chambliss, H. O., & Jordan, A. N. (2006). Exercise as an augmentation strategy for treatment of major depression. *Journal of Psychiatric Practice, 12,* 205-213.

Trost, S. G., Owen, N., Bauman, A. E., Sallis, J. F., & Brown, W. (2002). Correlates of adults' participation in physical activity: review and update. *Medicine & Science in Sports & Exercise, 34,* 1996-2001.

Tsigos, C., & Chrousos, G. P. (2002). Hypothalamic-pituitary-adrenal axis, neuroendocrine factors and stress. *Journal of Psychosomatic Research, 53,* 865-871.

Tsukue, I., & Shohoji, T. (1981). Movement therapy for alcoholic patients. *Journal of Studies on Alcohol, 42,* 144-149.

Tubino, M., Garrido, F. C., & Tubino, F. M. (2007). *Dicionário Enciclopédico Tubino do Esporte.* São Paulo: SENAC.

Twisk, J. W. (2001). Physical activity guidelines for children and adolescents: a critical review *Sports Medicine, 31,* 617-627.

Uchino, B. N., Smith, T. W., Holt-Lunstad, J., Campo, R., & Reblin, M. (2007). Stress and illness. In J. T. Cacioppo, G. Tassinary & G. G. Berntson (Eds.), *Handbook of psychophysiology* (pp. 608-632). Cambridge: Cambridge University Press.

Ussher, M., McCusker, M., Morrow, V., & Donaghy, M. (2000). A physical activity intervention in a community alcohol service. *The British Journal of Occupational Therapy, 63(12)*, 598-604.

Ussher, M., Sampuran, A., Doshi, R., West, R., & Drummond, D. (2004). Acute effect of a brief bout of exercise on alcohol urges. *Addiction, 99*, 1542-1547.

Vaidya, V. A., Marek, G. J., Aghajanian, G. K, & Duma, R. S. (1997). 5-HT2A receptor-mediated regulation of brain-derived neurotrophic factor mRNA in the hippocampus and the neocortex. *Journal of Neuroscience, 17*, 2785-2795.

Valera, E. M., Faraone, S. V., Murray, K. E., & Siedman, L. J. (2007). Meta-analysis of structural imaging findings in attention-deficit hyperactivity disorder. *Biological Psychiatry, 61*, 1361-1369.

Van Coppenolle, H., Simons, J. (1985). Algemene technieken van psychomotorische therapie. Leuven: Acco.

Van Coppenolle, H., Simons, J., Pierloot, R., Probst, M., & Knapen, J. (1989). The Louvain observation scales for objectives in psychomotor therapy. *Adapted Physical Activity Quarterly, 6*, 145-153.

Van Coppenolle, H., Simons, J., Pierloot, R., Vertommen, H., Probst, M., Knapen, J. (1984). Leuvense observatieschalen voor doelstellingen in de psychomotorische therapie. *Vlaams Tijdschrift voor psychomotorische therapie, 11(4)*, 87-91.

Van der Bij, A. K., Laurant, M. G. H., Wensing, M. (2002). Effectiveness of physical activity interventions for older adults: A review. *American Journal of Preventative Medicine, 22(2)*, 120-133.

Van Hilvoorde, I., Landeweerd, L. (2010). Enhancing disabilities: Transhumanism under the veil of inclusion? *Disability and Rehabilitation, 32*, 2222-2227.

Van Praag, H. (2008). Neurogenesis and exercise: Past and future directions. *Neuromolecular Medicine, 10*, 128-140.

Van Wonterghem, G. (1987). Bewegingsactivering bij bejaarden: Vlaamse volkssporten en-spelen. *Vlaams tijdschrift Psychomotorische Therapie, 3*, 58-66.

Vancampfort, D., De Hert, M., Knapen, J., Deckx, S., Demunter, H., Probst, M. (2009) Yoga: een nieuwe evidence-based uitdaging voor de psychomotorische therapie bij mensen met schizofrenie. *Actuele themata uit de psychomotorische therapie*, 53-72.

Vancampfort, D., De Hert, M., Knapen, J., Demunter, H., Deckx, S., Peuskens, J. et al. (2010). State anxiety, psychological distress and positive well-being responses to yoga versus aerobic exercise in people with schizophrenia. *Disability and Rehabilitation, 33(8)*, 684-689.

Vancampfort, D., De Hert, M., Knapen, J., Maurissen, K., Sweers,K., Heip, T., et al. (2011). Test-hertest betrouwbaarheid van de Eurofit testbatterij voor patiënten met schizofrenie [Test-retest reliability of the Eurofit test battery for patients with schizophrenia]. In J. Simons (Ed.). *Actuele themata uit de psychomotorische therapie* (pp. 105-115). Leuven: Acco.

Vancampfort, D., Knapen, J., De Hert, M., Deckx, S., Simons, J., Van Eyck, D. et al. (2009). Physical activity interventions for people with schizophrenia: A critical review. Unpublished work.

Vancampfort, D., Sweers, K., De Hert, M., Probst, M.,

Knapen, J., van Winkel, R.,et al. (2004). Psychiatrie: van diagnose tot behandeling. *Bohn Stafleu Van Loghum*, Houten.

Vandereycken, W., Depreitere, L., & Probst, M (1987). Body-oriented therapy for anorexia nervosa patients. *American Journal of Psychotherapy, 41*, 252-259.

Vandereycken, W., Probst, M., & Van Bellinghen, M. (1992). Treating the distorted body experience of anorexia nervosa patients. *Journal of Adolescent Health, 13*, 403-405.

Vansteelandt, K., Rijmen, F., Pieters, G., Probst, M., & Vanderlinden, J. (2007). Drive for thinness, affect regulation and physical activity in eating disorders: A daily life study. *Behaviour Research and Therapy, 45*, 1717-1734.

Vayer, P. (1982). *Educazione psicomotoria nell'età scolastica.* Roma: Armando Editore.

Vaughan, J.L., King, K.A. & Cottrell, R.R., (2004). Collegiate athletic trainers's confidence in helping female athletes with eating disorders. *Journal of Athletic Training, 39(1)*, 71-76.

Vedamurthachar, A., Janakiramaiah, N., Hegde, J., Shetty, T., Subbakrishna, D., Sureshbabu, S., et al. (2006). Antidepressant efficacy and hormonal effects of Sudarshana Kriya Yoga (SKY) in alcohol dependent individuals. *Journal of Affective Disorders, 94*, 249-253.

Vermeer, A., Bosscher, R. J., & Broadhead, G. D. (Eds.) (1997). *Movement therapy across the life-span.* Amsterdam: VU University Press.

Verret, C., Guay, M. C., Berthiaume, C., Gardiner, P., & Béliveau, L. (2010). A physical activity program improves behaviour and cognitive functions in children with ADHD: An Exploratory Study. *Journal of Attentional Disorders, 16(1)*, 71-80.

Vincent, W. (2005). *Statistics in Kinesiology.* Champaign IL: Human Kinetics.

Vinci, D. M. (1999). The female athlete triad: Body image and disordered eating. *Athletic Therapy Today, 4*, 16-17.

Vitaro, F., Tremblay, R. E., & Bukowski, W. M. (2001). Friends, friendships and conduct disorders. In J. Hill & B. Maughan (Eds.), *Conduct disorders in childhood and adolescence* (pp. 346-378). Cambridge, UK: Cambridge University Press.

Vogel, T., Brechat, P.H., Leprêtre, P.M., Kaltenbach, G., Berthel, M., & Lonsdorfer, J. (2009). Health benefits of physical activity in older patients: A review. *International Journal of Clinical Practice, 63(2)*, 303-320.

Vögele, C. (2003). Sport und Bewegung als Behandlungsansatz. In F. Petermann & V. Pudel (Eds.), *Übergewicht und Adipositas* (pp. 283-302). Göttingen: Hogrefe.

Vogelzangs, N., Kritchevsky, S. B., Beekman, A. T. F., Newman, A. B., Satterfield, S., Simonsick, E. M., Yaffe, K., Harris, T. B., Penninx, B. W. J. H. (2008). Depressive symptoms and change in abdominal obesity in older persons. *Archives of General Psychiatry, 65(12)*, 1386-1393.

Volicer, L., Simard, J., Pupa, J. H., Medrek, R., Riordan, M. E. (2006). Effects of continuous activity programming on behavioral symptoms of dementia. *Journal of American Medical Directors Association, 7*, 426-431.

Von Hausswolff-Juhlin, Y., Bjartveit, M., Lindstrom, E., & Jones, P. (2009). Schizophrenia and physical health problems. *Acta Psychiatrica Scandinavica. Supplementum, 438*, 15-21.

Waddell, C., Lipman, E., & Offord, D. (1999). Conduct disorder: Practice parameters for assessment, treatment, and prevention. *Canadian Journal of Psychiatry/Revue Canadienne de Psychiatrie, 44*(Suppl. 2), 35-42.

Wadden, T. A., Womble, L. G., Stunkard A. J. & Anderson, D. A. (2004). Psychological consequences of obesity and weight loss. In T. A. Wadden & A. J. Stunkard (Eds.), *Handbook of Obesity Treatment* (pp. 144-169). New York: Guilford Press.

Warren, B. J., Stanton, A.L., Blessing, D. L. (1990). Disordered eating patterns in competitive female athletes. *International Journal of Eating Disorders, 9,* 565-569.

Ware, J. E. (2004). SF-36 health survey update. In M. E. Maruish (Ed), *The use of psychological testing for treatment planning and outcomes assessments (*pp. 693-717), Mahwah, NJ: Lawrence Erlbaum Associates Inc. Publisher.

Wei, M., Kampert, J. B., Barlow, C. E., Nichman, N. Z., Gibbson, L. W., Paffenbarger, N. S. et al. (1999). Relationship between low cardiorespiratory fitness and mortality in normal-weight, overweight, and obese men. *Journal of American Medical Association, 282(16),* 1547-1553.

Weinstock, J., Barry, D., & Petry, N. (2008). Exercise-related activities are associated with positive outcome in contingency management treatment for substance use disorders. *Addictive Behaviors, 33,* 1072-1075.

Weiss, G., & Hechtman, L. (1993). *Hyperactive children grown up.* New York: Guilford Press.

Weissman, M. M., Bland, C.R., Canino, G. J., Faravelli, C., Greenwald, S., Hwu, H.-G., et al. (1996). Cross-national epidemiology of major depression and bipolar disorder. *Journal of American Medical Association, 276,* 293-299.

Welden, S., Yesavage, J. A. (1982) Behavioral improvement with relaxation training in senile dementia. *Clinical Gerontologist, 1,* 45-49.

Welk, G. (2002). *Physical activity assessments for health-related research.* Champaign IL: Human Kinetics.

Wemme, K. M., & Rosvall, M. (2005). Work related and non-work related stress in relation to low leisure time physical activity in a Swedish population. *Journal of Epidemiology and Community Health, 59,* 377-379.

Werneck, C. (2000). Lazer, Trabalho e Educação – Relações históricas, questões contempoâneas. Belo Horizonte, MG: Ed. UFMG.

WHO (2003). *Investing in mental health.* Department of Mental Health and Substance Dependence. WHO Library Cataloguing-in-Publication Data.

WHO (2009). *Alcohol and injuries emergency department studies in an international perspective.* Geneve: World Health Organization

WHO (2010). *European Status Report on Alcohol and Health 2010.* Geneve: World Health Organization Regional Office for Europe.

Whorton, J. E., Morgan, R. L., & Nisbet, S., (1994). A comparison of leisure and recreational activities for adults with and without mental retardation. In D. Montgomery (Ed.), *Rural partnerships: Working together Proceeding of the Annual National Conference of the American Council on Rural Special Education* (pp. 174-185). Austin, TX.

Wigal, S., Nemet, D., Swanson, J. M., Regino, R.,Trampush, J., Ziegler, M. G.,et al (2003). Catecholamine response to exercise in children with attention deficit hyperactivity. *Pediatric Research, 53(5),* 756-761.

Willcutt, E. G., & Pennington, B. F. (2000). Comorbidity of reading disability and attention-deficit/hyperactivity disorder: Differences by gender and subtype. *Journal of Learning Disabilities, 33(2),* 179-191.

Williams, M. H. (1996). *Lifetime fitness and wellness* (4th ed.). Madison, WI: Brown & Benchmark.

Williams, M., & Davids, K. (1995). Declarative knowledge in sport: A by-product of experience or a characteristic of expertise. *Journal of Sport & Exercise Psychology, 17,* 259-275.

Williams, M. E., Pulliam C. C., Hunter R., Johnson T. M., Owens J. E., Kincaid J., et al. (2004). The short-term effect of interdisciplinary medication review on function and cost in ambulatory elderly people. *Journal of the American Geriatrics Society, 52(1),* 93-98.

Wilson, P. W., D'Agostino, R. B., Levy, D., Belanger, A. M., Silbershatz, H., & Kannel, W. B. (1998). Prediction of coronary heart disease using risk factor categories. *Circulation, 97,* 1837-1847.

Wing, R. R., & Phelan, S. (2005). Long-term weight loss maintenance. *American Journal of Clinical Nutrition, 82*(Suppl.)*,* 222-225.

Winter, B., Breitenstein, C., Mooren, F. C., Voelker, K., Fobker, M., Lechtermann, A., et al. (2007). High impact running improves learning. *Neurobiology of Learning and Memory, 87,* 597-609.

Wipfli, B., Rethorst, C., & Landers, D. (2008). Anxiolytic effects of exercise: A meta-analysis of randomized trials and dose–response analysis. *Journal of Sport & Exercise Psychology, 30,* 392-410.

Wirth, A. (2003). *Adipositas- Fibel* (2nd ed.). Berlin: Springer.

Wober, C., Wober-Bingol, C., Karwautz, A., Nimmerrichter, A., Deecke, L., & Lesch, O. M. (1999). Postural control and lifetime alcohol consumption in alcohol-dependent patients. *Acta Neurologica Scandinavica, 99,* 48-53.

World Bank. (2008). *Brazil at a glance.* The World Bank Group Press.

World Health Organization (2008). The global burden of disease: 2004 update. Geneva.

World Health Organization, Regional Office for Europe. (2007). The challenge of obesity in the WHO European Region and the strategies for response. Retrieved from http://www.euro.who.int/_data/assets/pdf_file/0010/74746/E90711.pdf

World Health Organization. (1992). *The ICD-10 Classification of Mental and Behavioral Disorders: Clinical Descriptions and Diagnostic Guidelines*, 10th revision. Geneva: World Health Organisation.

World Health Organization. (1998). Obesity: preventing and managing the global epidemic: report of a WHO Consultation on Obesity, Geneva, 3-5 June 1997. Retrieved from http://whqlibdoc.who.int/hq/1998/WHO_NUT_NCD_98.1_%28p1-158%29.pdf

World Health Organization. (2004). Prevention of mental disorders: Effective interventions and policy option: Summary report. Geneva: World Health Organization.

World Health Organization. (2009). [http://www.who.int/mental_health/en/].

World Health Organization. (2010). Global recommendations on physical activity for health. Retrieved from http://whqlibdoc.who.int/publications/2010/9789241599979_eng.pdf

World Health Organization.(2009).[http://www.who.int/mental_health/management/schizophrenia/en/].

Wu, M. K., Wang, C. K., Bai, Y. M., Huang, C. Y., & Lee, S. D. (2007). Outcomes of obese, clozapine-treated inpatients with schizophrenia placed on a six-month diet and physical activity program. *Psychiatric Services, 58,* 544-550.

Yates, A., Leehey, K., & Shisslak, C. M. (1982). Running: An analogue of anorexia? *New England Journal of Medicine, 308,* 251-525.

Yeung, R. R. (1996). The acute effects of exercise on mood state. *Journal of Psychosomatic Research, 2,* 123-141.

Yu, F., Kolanowski, A. M., Strumpf, N. E., Eslinger, P. J. (2006). Improving cognition and function through exercise intervention in Alzheimer's disease. *Journal of Nursing Scholarship, 38(4),* 358-365.

Zhao, G., Zhang, X., Xu, X., Ochoa, M., & Hintze, T. H. (1997). Short-term exercise training enhances reflex cholinergic nitric oxide-dependent coronary vasodilation in conscious dogs. *Circulation Research, 80(6),* 868-876.

Zimetbaum, P., Josephson, M. E. (1998). Evaluation of patients with palpitations. *The New England Journal of Medicine, 338 (19),* 1369-73.

Zimmerman, M., Coryell, W., Corenthal, C., & Wilson, S. (1986). Dysfunctional attitudes and attribution style in healthy controls and patients with schizophrenia, psychotic depression, and nonpsychotic depression. *Journal of Abnormal Psychology, 95,* 403-405.

Zoeller, R. (2007). Physical activity: depression, anxiety, physical activity, and cardiovascular disease: What's the connection? *American Journal of Lifestyle Medicine, 1,* 175-180.

Zuzanek, J., Robinson, J. P., & Iwasaki, Y. (1998). The relationships between stress, health, and physically active leisure as a function of life-cycle. *Leisure Sciences, 20,* 253-275.

Websites

http://www.acsm.org/access-public-information/newsletters/fit-society-page

http://www.acsm-msse.org/pt/re/msse/positionstandards.htm

http://www.actenz.nl/

http://www.cdc.gov/nccdphp/dnpa/physical/index.htm

http://www.coe.int

http://www.icaa.cc/FacilityLocator/Doctors/physiciantools.htm

http://www.ifapa.biz

http://www.oxfordhealth.nhs.uk/?directory=coasters-the-activities-development-service

http://www.paralympic.org

http://www.psylos.be

http://www.reakt.nl/

http://www.shapeup.org/

http://www.solidarieta.gsbellaria.it

http://www.specialolympics.org/

Subjects index